Monoclonal Antibodies: Important Role in Medical Diagnosis and Therapies

Monoclonal Antibodies: Important Role in Medical Diagnosis and Therapies

Editor: Logan Watts

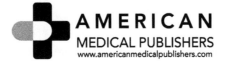
AMERICAN
MEDICAL PUBLISHERS
www.americanmedicalpublishers.com

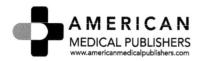

Cataloging-in-Publication Data

Monoclonal antibodies : important role in medical diagnosis and therapies / edited by Logan Watts.
    p. cm.
Includes bibliographical references and index.
ISBN 978-1-63927-735-3
1. Monoclonal antibodies. 2. Monoclonal antibodies--Diagnostic use. 3. Monoclonal antibodies--Therapeutic use.
4. Immunoglobulins. 5. Molecular cloning. 6. Immunology. I. Watts, Logan.
QR186.85 .M663 2023
616.079 3--dc23

American Medical Publishers,
41 Flatbush Avenue,
1st Floor, New York,
NY 11217, USA

ISBN 978-1-63927-735-3 (Hardback)

Contents

Preface

A monoclonal antibody refers to an antibody formed through cloning a distinctive white blood cell. Antibodies are glycoproteins produced through differentiated B lymphocytes known as plasma cells in response to exposure to antigens. The range of antibody responses to different target antigens occurs due to gene recombination process in the hyper-variable areas of antibodies. Monoclonal antibodies (mAbs) are formed through similar clones of B lymphocytes in response to a specific antigen. There are numerous properties of mAbs including antigen-binding site region, identical downstream functional effects, protein sequence and binding affinity for their targets. These antibodies are often given through the subcutaneous route. They are helpful in diagnosing various diseases such as cancer and hormonal disorders. These antibodies are also useful in treating various other conditions like asthma and AIDS. This book elucidates the prospective developments with respect to monoclonal antibodies. It presents researches and studies performed by experts across the globe. Scientists and students actively engaged in the therapeutic applications of antibodies will find this book full of crucial and unexplored concepts.

All of the data presented henceforth, was collaborated in the wake of recent advancements in the field. The aim of this book is to present the diversified developments from across the globe in a comprehensible manner. The opinions expressed in each chapter belong solely to the contributing authors. Their interpretations of the topics are the integral part of this book, which I have carefully compiled for a better understanding of the readers.

At the end, I would like to thank all those who dedicated their time and efforts for the successful completion of this book. I also wish to convey my gratitude towards my friends and family who supported me at every step.

Editor

Monoclonal Antibodies: Leading Actors in the Relapsed/Refractory Multiple Myeloma Treatment

Sonia Morè [1], Maria Teresa Petrucci [2], Laura Corvatta [3], Francesca Fazio [2], Massimo Offidani [1],* and Attilio Olivieri [1]

1   Clinica di Ematologia, Azienda Ospedaliero-Universitaria Ospedali Riuniti di Ancona, 60126 Ancona, Italy; sonia.more@live.it (S.M.); a.olivieri@univpm.it (A.O.)
2   Sezione di Ematologia, Dipartimento di Medicina Traslazionale e di Precisione, Azienda Ospedaliera Policlinico Umberto I, Università "Sapienza" di Roma, 00161 Roma, Italy; petrucci@bce.uniroma.it (M.T.P.); fazio@bce.uniroma1.it (F.F.)
3   UOC Medicina, Ospedale Profili Fabriano, 60044 Fabriano, Italy; laura.corvatta@sanita.marche.it
*   Correspondence: massimo.offidani@ospedaliriuniti.marche.it

Abstract: Multiple myeloma is a complex hematologic malignancy, and despite a survival improvement related to the growing number of available therapeutic options since 2000s, it remains an incurable disease with most patients experiencing relapse. However, therapeutic options for this disease are constantly evolving and immunotherapy is becoming the mainstay of the therapeutic armamentarium of Multiple Myeloma (MM), starting with monoclonal antibodies (MoAbs) as elotuzumab, daratumumab and isatuximab. Elotuzumab, the first in class targeting SLAMF7, in combination with lenalidomide and dexamethasone and daratumumab, directed against CD38, in combination with Rd and with bortezomib and dexamethasone (Vd), have been approved for the treatment of relapsed/refractory MM (RRMM) after they demonstrated excellent efficacy. More recently, another anti-CD38 MoAb named isatuximab was approved by FDA in combination with pomalidomide-dexamethasone (Pd) in the same setting. Many phase II and III trials with regimens containing these MoAbs are ongoing, and when available, preliminary data are very encouraging. In this review we will describe the results of major clinical studies that have been conducted with elotuzumab, daratumumab and isatuximab in RRMM, focusing on phase III trials. Moreover, we will summarized the emerging MoAbs-based combinations in the RRMM landscape.

Keywords: relapsed multiple myeloma; elotuzumab; daratumumab; isatuximab

1. Introduction

The introduction of high-dose therapy in the 1990s and the development of novel classes of drug since the 2000s, led to a significant improved outcome of MM patients [1–3] and recent studies report a 10-year survival until 60% in younger MM patients [4] and a four-year survival of 56% in elderly [5]. However, despite a possible long-lasting remission in some patients, MM remains an incurable disease, and until recently, patients who became non-responsive to immunomodulatory agents (IMiDs) and proteasome inhibitors (PIs) showed an overall survival (OS) of 13 months [6]. These results are consistent with the most recent knowledge on genomic and molecular characterization of MM by next generation sequencing (NGS), showing a lack of universal driver mutation, presence of coexistent subclones and oligoclonality in MM, leading to different type of evolution of the disease over time and drug resistance [7]. Beside biological disease complexity, in patients with relapsed/refractory MM (RRMM) treatment, decisions must take into account two key points. Firstly, the duration of response, progression-free survival (PFS) and OS decrease with successive lines of therapy [8,9], and secondly, the percentage of patients who receive a second-line treatment is 61% as reported by a retrospective European review [10].

Managing RRMM patients can be compared, at present, in order to unravel a skein if we consider all patient-related and disease-related factors to evaluate the choice of therapy in this population. The start of therapy is recommended in patients with clinical relapse as IMWG criteria [11], but it has to also be considered in patients with biochemical relapse, particularly in the presence of a rapid increase in M protein, and specifically when the level of M protein is doubled over two months, having reached at least 1 g/dL in the serum and 0.5 g/24 h in the urine [12,13]. Besides patient factors as age, performance status, frailty, comorbidities, but also patient preference and logistics of drug administration, treatment of relapsed MM should be selected on the basis of disease-related factors. This is because the presence of high-risk features (renal failure, extramedullary MM, high-risk cytogenetic) and therapeutic history, in terms of number of prior lines of therapy, quality and duration of response and toxicity with prior, drugs in order to identify the best approach. Monoclonal antibodies (mAbs) are widely used and represent a breakthrough in the management of hematologic malignancies. Rituximab (mAb against the CD20 antigen) [14], and brentuximab (mAb against CD30 molecules) [15], have significantly improved the outcome of patients with B cell lymphomas and Hodgkin lymphoma. Until now, elotuzumab, mAb targeting SLAM7 in the plasma cells, and daratumumab, mAb binding CD38 molecule, have been approved for the treatment of RRMM. Whereas, several studies evaluated and are assessing another mAb targeting CD38, isatuximab. In this review, we summarized the results of trials conducted so far with these mAbs in RRMM.

2. Elotuzumab

2.1. Elotuzumab Plus Immunomodulatory Drugs (IMiDs)

Elotuzumab is a humanized immunoglobulin G1 kappa (IgG1), specific for human SLAMF7 and it does not show cross-reactivity with non-human homologues or other signaling lymphocyte activation molecule (SLAM) family members [16]. Elotuzumab is actually approved by Food and Drugs Administration (FDA) for the treatment of RRMM patients, in association with lenalidomide-dexamethasone (Elo-Rd) or pomalidomide-dexamethasone (Elo-Pd).

After a phase I study [17] showed no response in patients with advanced MM receiving elotuzumab as single agent, it was evaluated in combination with IMids, starting with thalidomide. Low efficacy was reported with the combination elotuzumab, thalidomide and low-dose dexamethasone (ETd) in a multicenter phase II study [18] with the primary endpoint of evaluating grade 3–4 non-hematological toxicity. Fifty-one patients with a median of 3 prior lines of therapy received elotuzumab 10 mg/kg weekly for the first two cycles and every two weeks thereafter, thalidomide at escalating doses from 50 mg to 200 mg daily and dexamethasone 40 mg weekly. Grade ≥3 non hematological adverse events occurred in 63% of patients mostly fatigue (35%) and peripheral oedema (25%) whereas 15% of patients had an infusion reaction (IRRs). At least a partial response (PR) was achieved by 38% of patients and median PFS was 3.9 months.

Triplet including elotuzumab, lenalidomide and dexamethasone (Elo-Rd) has been assessed in phase I dose escalation study [19], whose primary objective was to identify the maximum tolerated dose (MTD) of elotuzumab, administered at escalating dose from 5 to 20 mg/kg weekly for the first 2 cycles and every two weeks thereafter, combined with lenalidomide (25 mg days 1–21) and dexamethasone (40 mg/weekly). Twenty-eight patients with a median of 3 prior therapies were enrolled. The MTD was not reached up the dose of 20 mg/kg and the most common grade 3–4 adverse events were neutropenia (36%), thrombocytopenia (21%), diarrhoea (11%). Eighty-nine percent of patients developed infusion reaction (consisting on pyrexia, nausea, chills, flushing, rash, chest discomfort) during the first infusion of elotuzumab, mainly of grade 1–2 and resolving within 24 h. As regard response to triplet combination

Elo-Rd, 82% of patients achieved at least a PR, 32% at least very good partial response (VGPR) and 4% a complete response (CR) and the response was not affected by the number of previous therapies received. In the phase II expansion cohort of the same study [20], patients who had received one to three previous lines of therapy (except for lenalidomide, allowed in the phase I study) were assigned to receive either elotuzumab 10 mg/kg or 20 mg/kg combined with lenalidomide and dexamethasone at the same schedules of phase I study. Among 73 patients enrolled, 44% and 11% had received 2, and 3 previous lines of treatment, respectively. Overall, response rates, the main endpoint of the study, were as follows: 84% at least a PR, 56% at least VGPR and 14% at least CR. After a median follow-up of 21.2 months, median PFS was 28.6 months for all patients (32.4 months for the 10 mg/kg group and 25.0 months for the 20 mg/kg group). IRRs occurred in only 8 patients (11%) and were grade 3 only in one patient. As well as the phase I study, the main grade 3–4 adverse events were neutropenia (19%), thrombocytopenia (18%) and diarrhoea (10%).

Based on these results, the phase 3 trials ELOQUENT-2 [21], compared Elo-Rd versus Rd in 646 RRMM patients with a median age of 66 years and a median of 2 lines of prior therapies (range 1–4). Overall, 70% of patients had received bortezomib, 48% thalidomide, 6% lenalidomide and 35% were refractory to their last line of therapy. Elo-Rd group received elotuzumab 10 mg/kg on days 1, 8, 15, and 22 during the first two cycles and every two weeks thereafter, lenalidomide 25 mg days 1–21 and oral dexamethasone 40 weekly whereas the control group received Rd. After a 4-year follow-up [22], ERd significantly improved PFS versus Rd (median 19.4 months versus 14.9 months; HR = 0.71; $p = 0.0004$). The greatest PFS benefit among the subgroups was observed in patients at the median time or further from diagnosis (≥3.5 years) with 1 prior line of therapy, who had a 44% reduction in the risk of progression/death, and in patients with a high-risk MM, who had a 36% reduction in favor of Elo-Rd. The overall response rate (ORR) was 79% with Elo-Rd versus 66% with Rd and at least VGPR was obtained by 35% of Elo-Rd patients versus 29% of Rd group. Elotuzumab did not add hematological or nonhematological toxicity to Rd besides IRRs occurring in 10% of patients, mainly grade 1–2. After a median follow-up of 70.6 months [23], final analysis the study showed a significant OS benefit in patients receiving Elo-Rd versus Rd since median OS was 48.3 versus 39.6 months in the Rd arm (hazard ratio, HR = 0.82; $p = 0.04$) so ELOQUENT-2 represents the first trial to demonstrate a significant OS advantage with an antibody-based triplet regimen in RRMM. Remarkably, OS benefit was maintained across relevant subgroups of patients as well as ≥75 years old (median 48.5 months versus 27.4 months; HR = 0.69), those with 2–3 prior lines of therapy (median 51 months versus 33.6 months; HR = 0.71) and patients with high-risk cytogenetics (median 29.8 months versus 24.8 months; HR = 0.69) [23]. Recently, Gentile et al. [24] reported data of an Italian real-life experience on Elo-Rd administered to 300 RRMM, 41% of whom aged ≥75 years. The results of this retrospective analysis were consistent with ELOQUENT-2 trial since ORR was 77% and median PFS 17.6 months.

Elotuzumab was tested in combination with pomalidomide in the randomized phase II ELOQUENT-3 trial [25], demonstrating that the addiction of elotuzumab to the backbone pomalidomide-dexamethasone (Pd) induces a 46% reduction in progression or death. Sixty patients received Elo-Pd (elotuzumab 10 mg/kg on days 1, 8, 15, 22 for 2 cycles, and 20 mg/kg on day 1 for the next 28-day cycles; pomalidomide 4 mg per day on days 1 to 21 of 28-day cycles; dexamethasone 40 mg weekly) and 57 patients received Pd alone. Patients had a median of 3 (range 2–8) previous therapies and, in Elo-Pd group 68% of patients (versus 72% in PD group) were refractory to both bortezomib and lenalidomide. After a median follow-up of 9.1 months, median PFS was 10.3 versus 4.7 months in Elo-Pd versus Pd groups, respectively (HR 0.54, $p = 0.008$). This advantage was preserved in all the subgroups, also in patients with HR cytogenetic and in lenalidomide-refractory ones. The ORR was 53% in elotuzumab group and 26% in Pd group. As regard safety profile, triplet combination demonstrated to provide a substantial clinical benefit without added clinically relevant toxicities. Main adverse events are pictured in Table 1. In 2018 the combination Elo-Pd had the FDA approval for RRMM who had received at least two previous lines of therapy.

Table 1. Grade 3–4 adverse events (%) reported in randomized phase II and phase III trials with elotuzumab, daratumumab and isatuximab.

Treatment	Neutropenia	Thrombocytopenia	Infections	Pneumonia	Cardiac Disorders	Vascular Events	Neuropathy
ELOQUENT-2 [22] Elo-Rd versus Rd	36 versus 45	21 versus 21	33 versus 26	14 versus 10	5 versus 8	10 versus 8	0
ELOQUENT-3 [25] Elo-Pd versus Pd	13 versus 27	8 versus 5	13 versus 22	5 versus 9	7 versus 4	3 versus 0	0
Jakubowiak [26] Elo-VD versus VD	0	9 versus 17	21 versus 13	8 versus 4	0 versus 1	0	9 versus 12
POLLUX [27] DRd versus Rd	52 versus 37	12.7 versus 13.5	28.3 versus 22.8	7.8 versus 8.2	0	0	0
CASTOR [28] DVd versus Vd	12.8 versus 4.2	45.3 versus 32.9	21.4 versus 19	8.2 versus 9.7	0	6.6 versus 0.8 *	4.5 versus 6.8
CANDOR [29] DKd versus Kd	9 versus 6	24 versus 16	29 versus 16	13 versus 9	7 versus 12	18 versus 13 *	1 versus 1
ICARIA [30] Isa-Pd versus Pd	85 versus 70	31 versus 25	6 versus 1	16 versus 14	0	0	0
IKEMA [31] Isa-Kd versus Kd	19.2 versus 23.8	30 versus 23.8	6 versus 2	16.4 versus 12.3	4 versus 4	20.3 versus 19.7 *	0

Elo-Rd: elotuzumab, lenalidomide, dexamethasone; Elo-Pd: elotuzumab, pomalidomide, dexamethasone; Elo-VD: elotuzumab, bortezomib, dexamethasone; DRd: daratumumab, lenalidomide, dexamethasone; DVd: daratumumab, bortezomib, dexamethasone; DKd: daratumumab, carfilzomib, dexamethasone; Isa-Pd: isatuximab, pomalidomide, dexamethasone; Isa-Kd: isatuximab, carfilzomib, dexamethasone. *: Hypertension.

2.2. Elotuzumab Plus Proteasome Inhibitors (PIs)

The combination of elotuzumab with a PI was tested in a multicenter randomized phase II study [26] comparing elotuzumab, bortezomib and dexamethasone (Elo-VD), with bortezomib-dexamethasone (VD) in 152 RRMM patients, treated with no more than 3 prior lines of therapy who had not to be bortezomib refractory. Overall, 66% and 34% of patients had received one and 2/3 prior lines of therapy, respectively. In Elo-VD group treatment consisted in elotuzumab (10 mg/kg/weekly for cycles 1 and

2, days 1 and 11 for cycles 3–8 and days 1–15 thereafter), bortezomib (1.3 mg/m on days 1, 4, 8, 11) and dexamethasone (20 mg on non-elotuzumab dosing days). Whereas, the control arm received VD. The study met the primary endpoint, since PFS was significantly longer with Elo-VD than VD (median 9.7 months versus 6.9 months; HR = 0.72; p = 0.09, exceeding the prespecified significance level of 2-sided $p \leq 0.3$).

Moreover, patients Elo-VD-treated homozygous for the high-affinity FcγRIIIa V allele had a better trend towards longer PFS compared with those VD-treated with the same characteristic (median 22.3 versus 8.2 months) being FcγRIIIa receptor expressed in NK cells and required to bind Fc part of elotuzumab to induce ADCC. No differences were reported between Elo-Vd and VD in terms of ORR (66% versus 63%) and 2-years OS (73% versus 66%; HR 0.75). The rate of patients went off-treatment because of toxicity was similar in the two arms (13%, versus 19%, respectively). More frequent grade 3–4 adverse events was pneumonia, thrombocytopenia, diarrhoea and anemia which were quite similar in the two arms (Table 1). Elotuzumab infusion reaction occurred in 5% of patients, mainly of grade 1–2.

Nordic Myeloma Study Group [32] assessed elotuzumab in combination with carfilzomib, instead of bortezomib, and dexamethasone (EKd) after 1–3 prior treatment lines and preliminary data showed and ORR of 91% using weekly carfilzomib 70 mg/m^2. Notably, the best responding patients displayed mutation to RAS genes.

Quadruplet elotuzumab-bortezomib-pomalidomide-dexamethasone (Elo-PVd) was studied in a phase 2 trial (NCT02718833) [33] including 48 patients with a median of 3 prior regimens (range 1–9). All patients had received prior lenalidomide, 96% bortezomib, 29% carfilzomib, 33% pomalidomide, 25% daratumumab and were refractory to their last line of therapy. This quadruplet induced an ORR of 61% and a median PFS of 9.8 months. In patients with one prior line of therapy, ORR was 74% and median PFS was not reached. Most frequent grade ≥ 3 haematological adverse event was neutropenia (29%) whereas grade 3–4 pneumonia occurred in 27% of patiens and were the most common non-hematologic toxicities. Patients who received prior pomalidomide, carfilzomib, and/or anti-CD38 monoclonal antibody also benefited.

2.3. Ongoing Clinical Trials with Elotuzumab in RRMM Patients

An ongoing clinical trial (NCT03030261) is evaluating Elo-Pd as induction and consolidation/ maintenace after second ASCT in patients with RRMM. Elo-Pd combination has been compared with elotuzumab in association with PD-1 inhibitor nivolumab (EN) in a phase 2 multiple cohort study (NCT02612779), where enrolling patients relapsed o refractory to prior therapy with lenalidomide. The results are not available yet.

Other quadruplets including elotuzumab are under investigation in the setting of RRMM. A phase II study (NCT03361306) is assessing the efficacy, in term of VGPR, of the combination elotuzumab, carfilzomib, lenalidomide, dexamethasone (Elo-KRd) in patients with no more than one prior line of therapy. Among the different combination therapies that STOMP study (NCT02343042) is evaluating, arm 9 includes patients receiving selinexor, dexamethasone, pomalidomide and elotuzumab (SPEd).

In conclusion, taking into consideration that in the near future a lot of MM patients will be treated with upfront daratumumab-based regimens, elotuzumab would be considered for RRMM setting, having a different mechanism of action. However, studies are needed to confirm the efficacy and safety of elotuzumab in these peculiar group of patients.

3. Daratumumab

3.1. Daratumumab Monotherapy

Daratumumab, the first fully human anti-CD-38 mAb evaluated for the treatment of MM, showed single-agent antitumor activity in the phase 1/2 GEN501 [34] and in the phase II SIRIUS [35] studies. After different doses of daratumumab were explored in the part 1 of GEN501 study [34] without identification of a maximum tolerated dose, the cohort treated with daratumumab at dose of 16 mg/kg in the part 2 of the study achieved an ORR of 36%. In the SIRIUS study [35], 106 patients with RRMM and a median of 5 previous lines of therapy (range 2–14) received daratumumab 16 mg/kg per week for 8 weeks, then every 2 weeks for 16 weeks and every 4 weeks thereafter. The ORR was 29% and after a median follow-up of 9.3 months, median PFS was 3.7 months. A pooled updated analysis of these studies [36] confirmed the significant activity of monotherapy with daratumumab in 148 heavily pretreated and highly refractory MM patients. The ORR for the combined data set was 31% (at least VGPR = 14%) and, after a longer follow-up of 20.7 months, median PFS and OS were 4 months, and 20 months, respectively. Notably, the median PFS was better in patients obtaining at least a PR compared to those with a lower response rate (15 months versus 3 months). Infusion-related reactions (IRRs), mainly consisting of nasal congestion, cough, allergic rhinitis, throat irritation and dyspnea, were documented in 48% of patients but they were of grade ≥3 only in 2.7% of them. Moreover, 96% of these events occurred during the first infusion whereas 7% developed during the second one. Final safety and efficacy results of the combined analysis of GEN501 and SIRIUS [37] have been recently published and show, after a median follow-up of 36.6 months a median OS of 20.5 months with a 3-year OS of 36.5%. The most frequent grade 3–4 side effects reported during treatment were anemia (18%), thrombocytopenia (14%), neutropenia (10%) and infections (9%). Safety profile of daratumumab monotherapy was evaluated in two multicenter early access treatment protocols (EAP) conducted in patients with ≥3 prior lines of therapy. In the first US study by Chari et al. [38], 348 RRMM patients received a median of 8 daratumumab infusions achieving an ORR of 23%. Grade 3–4 IRRs occurred in 8% of patients, mainly during the first infusion. In the Spanish study by Alegre et al. [39], 73 patients after a median of 12 daratumumab infusions achieved an ORR of 24.7% with PFS of 4 months. Only 2.7% of patients developed a grade 3–4 IRR. In a real-world setting [40]. However, daratumumab monotherapy showed little efficacy as reported by a retrospective analysis of 41 patients with a median age of 68 years who had received a median of 4 prior therapies. Despite an ORR of 23% similar to those reported in the GEN501 and SIRIUS studies, median PFS and OS were 1.9, and 6.5 months, respectively.

3.2. Daratumumab Plus IMiDs

Rationale for the combining daratumumab with lenalidomide was based on the in vitro synergistic activity between this mAb and IMiDs, starting from lenalidomide [41]. The phase I/II GEN503 study [42] assessed safety and activity of this triplet (DRd) in 32 patients with a median of 2 prior therapies (range 1–3) who received daratumumab 16 mg/kg (with the scheduleof SIRIUS study) plus lenalidomide (25 mg days 1–21) and dexamethasone (40 mg per week). The final results of this study have been recently published [43], and after a median follow-up of 32.5 months, ORR rate was 81% with 69% of patients achieving at least a VGPR and 44% a CR or better. Median PFS and OS were not reached and 2-year PFS and OS rates were 69%, and 78%, respectively. In relation to toxicities, most common ≥ grade 3 adverse events were neutropenia (84%) and thrombocytopenia (15.6%).

The phase III POLLUX trial [39], with primary endpoint PFS, compared DRd versus Rd alone in 569 patients with RRMM who had previously received ≥1 prior line of therapy. Patients were randomized to Rd (lenalidomide 25 mg days 1–21 of each cycle plus dexamethasone 40 mg weekly) or DRd (Rd plus daratumumab 16 mg/kg every week in cycles 1, 2; every two weeks in cycles 3–6; every 4 weeks thereafter) and 28 days cycles were continued until progression or unacceptable toxicity. Approximately 85% and 18% of patients had been prior exposed to PI and lenalidomide, respectively, but patients refractory to lenalidomide were excluded. Patients who were enrolled in this study were not heavily pre-treated since they had received a median of one prior line of therapy. Updated efficacy data [44], after a median follow-up of 54.8 months, showed a significantly longer PFS for DRd group versus Rd group with a 56% reduction in the risk of progression or death (median 45 months versus 17.5 months; HR = 0.44; $p < 0.0001$). In patients with one prior line of therapy the PFS benefit was even greater with median PFS resulted to be 53.3 in DRd versus 19.6 months in Rd arm (HR = 0.42; $p < 0.0001$). Moreover remarkable efficacy was reported in bortezomib refractory patients treated with DRd (median PFS 34.3 months versus 11.3 months; HR = 0.42; $p = 0.0008$) and in those with high-risk cytogenetics (median PFS 26.8 months versus 8.3 months; HR = 0.37; $p = 0.0056$). Regarding response, significantly higher ORR was seen with DRd versus Rd (93% versus 76%) including ≥ VGPR (81% versus 49%) and ≥ CR (58% versus 24%; all $p < 0.0001$). A sustained Minimal Residual Disease (MRD) negativity at level of 10^{-5} ≥ 6 months and ≥12 months were documented in 20% and 16 patients receiving Drd, respectively (versus 2% and 1% in Rd group). Toxicity profile was similar across the two groups and major adverse events occurred in patients receiving DRd are reported in Table 1. Importantly, considering the median age of MM patients, we found that the results obtained in patients ≥75 years old were consistent with those reported in the overall population, and similar with the rate of grade 3–4 adverse events [45].

The ongoing phase III CONFIRM trial (NCT03836014), whose primary endpoint is OS at 4 years after randomization, is evaluating DRd administered continuously until progression disease versus a fixed duration of 24 months.

The combination daratumumab, pomalidomide and dexamethasone (DPd) has been evaluated in the phase 1b EQUULEUS (MMY1001) study [46], assessing daratumumab in different regimens. One hundred and three patients with a median of 4 (range 1–13) prior therapies, 71% of whom refractory to PIs and IMiDs and 25% at high-risk cytogenetics received daratumumab (at the same dose and schedule of POLLUX trial), pomalidomide (4 mg on days 1–21) and dexamethasone (40 mg weekly). ORR was 60% with 42% of patients obtaining a VGPR or better and 17% a response ≥ CR. The responses were similar across patient subgroups including those with more than 3 lines of prior therapies and those refractory to PIs and IMiDs. After a median follow-up of 13 months, median PFS and OS were was 8.8 and 17.5 months, respectively. In the update of EQUULEUS study [47] after a follow-up of 24.7 months, ORR was 66%, median PFS 9.9 months and median OS 25 months, encouraging results considering the heavily pretreated study population. The most common grade 3–4 side effects, reported with this triplet, were neutropenia (77%), thrombocytopenia (19%), pneumonia (10%) [46]. DPd led to even better results in a less pretreated population enrolled in the arm B of the phase II MM-014 [48], including 112 patients with a median of one line of prior therapies (62.5% at first relapse). All patients have been treated with lenalidomide in the immediate prior line of therapy and 75% of them were lenalidomide refractory. Seventy eight percent of patients achieved ORR, 51% at least VGPR and 24% CR. After a median follow-up of 17.2 months, median PFS was not reached being 75% at 1 years. Notably, in patients lenalidomide, the refractory median PFS was 21.8 months and 1-year PFS 72%. These results showed the benefit of continuing immunomodulation with pomalidomide immediately after lenalidomide, even in case of failure of lenalidomide. Recently, Pierceall et al. [49], analyzing immunophenotipic changes in peripheral blood of patients receiving DPd from MM-14 study, demonstrated enhanced activation/differentiation of B, T and NK cells that is exhibited also in lenalidomide refractory patients. These data could explain the efficacy of DPd in patients heavily pre-treated who are refractory to both, daratumumab and pomalidomide as individual lines of therapy, reported by Emory group [50]. The ongoing phase III APOLLO trial (NCT03180736) comparing DPd versus Pd will address the effects of the addition of daratumumab to Pd in patients with RRMM who have received at least one treatment regimen.

3.3. Daratumumab Plus PIs

Daratumumab was assessed in combination with bortezomib and dexamethasone (DVd) in the phase III CASTOR trial [28] in which Vd (bortezomib 1.3 mg/m^2 on days 1, 4, 8, 11; dexamethasone 20 mg on days 1, 2, 4, 5, 8, 9, 11, 12) given for 8 cycles was compared against DVd (daratumumab 16 mg/kg days 1, 8 and 15 during cycles 1 to 3, once every 3 weeks during cycles 4 to 8 and once every 4 weeks thereafter until progression). The study included 498 patients with RRMM who had previously received a median of two therapies and approximately one-half of patients had been exposed to PIs and IMIDs. IN relation to renal function, the enrolment of patients with a creatinine clearance >20 mL/min was allowed. At the last update [51], after a median follow-up of 50.2 months, median PFS was significantly longer in DVd group versus Vd (16.7 months versus 7.1 months; HR = 0.31; $p < 0.0001$) and this benefit was particularly relevant in patients treated with DVd at first relapse since median PFS resulted 27 months versus 7.9 months (HR = 0.21; $p < 0.0001$). In patients refractory to lenalidomide (any prior line) median PFS was 7.8 versus 4.9 months (HR = 0.44; $p = 0.0002$).

The ORR also improved (85% versus 63%), as did the rate of VGPR or better (63% versus 29%) and CR or better (30% versus 10%) (all $p < 0.0001$). Moreover, patients achieving a sustained MRD-negativity at level of 10^{-5} was significantly higher in the DVd arm since in 10% of patents it lasted at least 6 months (versus 1% in Vd group) and in 7% lasted at least 12 months (versus 0 in Vd group). The most common grade 3 or 4 adverse events are summarized in Table 1. As seen in POLLUX trial most IRRs occurred during the first infusion and were grade 1 or 2.

Phase 1b EQUULEUS study (MMY1001) [52], besides DPd, evaluated the combination daratumumab (16 mg/kg weekly during cycles 1, 2, every two weeks cycles 3–6 and every 4 weeks thereafter), carfilzomib (20 mg/m^2 initial dose escalated to 70 mg/sm weekly) and dexamethasone (40 mg weekly) (DKd) in 85 patients with RRMM. Median number of prior therapies was 2 (range 1–4) and 60% of patients were refractory to lenalidomide. After a median follow-up of 16.6 months, ORR was 84% with 71% of patients achieving at least VGPR. The median PFS was not reached in the all-treated population, but it was 25.7 months in patients refractory to lenalidomide. As regard safety profile, the most frequent grade 3–4 hematologic adverse events were thrombocytopenia (31%) and neutropenia (21%). Grade 3–4 infections occurred in 19% of patients and consisted in pneumonia in 5% of cases. Of note, 10 patients (12%) developed grade 3–4 cardiac events, mainly cardiac failure, that resolved in 8 of them. The efficacy of this triplet has been confirmed in the phase III CANDOR [29,53] in which 466 RRMM patients were randomized to receive Kd (carfilzomib on days 1, 2, 8, 9, 15, 16 at dose of 20 mg/m^2 on days 1 and 2 of cycle 1 and 56 mg/m^2 thereafter; dexamethasone 40 mg weekly) or DKd (Kd plus daratumumab 16 mg/kg with the same schedule of MMY1001 study). Patients had received a median of 2 prior therapies (range 1–2) and 33% were lenalidomide refractory. After a median follow-up of 16.9 months, median PFS, primary endpoint of the study, was not reached in the DKd group and 15.8 in the Kd group (HR = 0.63; $p = 0.0027$). The benefit was observed in all subgroups of patients including those refractory to lenalidomide (HR = 0.47), whereas PFS HR was lower in the bortezomib-refractory group (HR = 0.84). The response rate was significantly higher in patients treated with DKd in terms of ORR (84% versus 75%; $p = 0.0080$) and at least VGPR (69% versus 49%). Moreover 18% of patients in DKd group achieved a MRD rate at 12 months of 18% versus 4% in the Kd group. The most common grade 3–4 toxicities are pictured in Table 1.

In the ongoing phase II DARIA study [54], conducted by the Greek Myeloma Study Group, daratumumab was evaluated, in combination with ixazomib and dexamethasone (IDd), in patients who have received one prior treatment with a lenalidomide-based regimen. Very preliminary results presented at the last EHA Congress showed promising response rates. Another phase II multicenter study is testing IDd (NCT03439293), whereas another one by MD Anderson Cancer Center is evaluating IDd after 3 cycles of DVd in RRMM (NCT03763162).

Phase II studies with quadruplets containing daratumumab plus pomalidomide, carfilzomib and dexamethasone are ongoing (NCT01665794, NCT04176718), whereas preliminary safety data of daratumumab combined with pomalidomide, ixazomib and dexamethasone showed good tolerability and activity [55].

3.4. Daratumumab Plus Venetoclax

An interesting combination under evaluation including daratumumab is that with venetoclax, a selective and potent oral BCL-2 inhibitor that induces apoptosis in MM cell lines and primary samples, particularly those with t(11;14), a cytogenetic abnormality documented in near 20% of MM patients. Moreover, clinical studies demonstrated efficacy of venetoclax in combination with bortezomib and dexamethasone in RRMM [56]. An ongoing phase I/II study [57] is assessing safety and efficacy of venetoclax, daratumumab, dexamethasone with or without bortezomib in RRMM. Twenty-four Patients with t(11;14) and at least one prior line of therapy were treated with venetoclax, daratumumab and dexamethasone (VenDd) in part 1 of study whereas part 2 included 24 patients irrespective of cytogenetics, with 1–3 prior lines of therapy, who received venetoclax, daratumumab, bortezomib and dexamethasone (VenDVd). ORR was 96% with triplet and 92% with quadruplet combination, being ≥ CR rates 54% and 42%, respectively. Remarkably, 21% of patients with t(11;14) who received VenDd obtained MRD negativity at level of 10^{-5}. The most important grade 3–4 adverse events were infections occurring in 21% of patients in the VenDd group and 17% in the VenDVd one. At 12 months, no patients treated with venetoclax at dose of 800 mg daily had progressive disease.

3.5. Daratumumab Plus Selinexor

Promising results in RRMM (≥3 prior lines of therapy) have been obtained, combining daratumumab with selinexor, the first-in-class oral Selective Inhibitor of Nuclear Export (SINE) to be approved with dexamethasone for advanced disease [58]. In a phase Ib/2 study [59] selinexor, in combination with daratumumab and dexamethasone (SDd), was tested at dose of 100 mg weekly or 60 mg twice-weekly; maximum tolerated dose and recommended phase II dose of SDd was found to be selinexor 100 mg, daratumumab 16 mg/kg and dexamethasone 40 mg, administered weekly. Overall, 34 patients with a median of 3 prior therapies were enrolled. Most common grade 3–4 adverse events were thorombocytopenia (32%), neutropenia (26%), fatigue (18%) and nausea (95). ORR was 73% and median PFS 12.5 months. An ongoing phase II study by PETHEMA (SELIBORDARA, NCT03589222) is assessing the quadruplet selinexor, bortezomib, daratumumab and dexamethasone in patients who have received at least 3 prior lines of therapy.

3.6. Intravenous Versus Subcutaneous Daratumumab

Despite the good safety profile, daratumumab, is administered as an intravenous formulation (IV) needing a long infusion time, being 7.0 h for the first infusion, 4.3 h for the second infusion and 3.5 h for subsequent administrations. However, a shorter duration of infusion could result in a reduction of nursing time for each patient, as well as in optimizing the requested time for patients care. For these reasons, daratumumab has been tested as subcutaneous formulation (SC) in 3 clinical trials. The first one was phase 1b dose-escalation PAVO study [60], evaluating safety and PK profile of daratumumab administered sc in combination with the recombinant human hyaluronidase PH20 enzyme (rHuPH20) at dose of 1200 (8 patients) or 1800 mg (45 patients). IRRs occurred mainly during the first infusion in 12.5% and 24.4% of patients receiving 1200 mg, and 1800 mg, respectively, and were generally of grade 1–2. In relation to grade 3–4 adverse events, neutropenia, thrombocytopenia, upper respiratory infections and pneumonia developed in 12.5% each in 1200 mg group patients versus 6.7, 6.7%, 0, and 4.4%, respectively, in 1800 mg group. The 1800 mg dose was comparable in term of PK profile with daratumumab 16 mg/kg IV dose. ORR rates were 42.2%, including 8.9% sCR, in patients receiving 1800 mg versus 25% in those 1200 mg. Parte 2 of PAVO study [61] evaluated a concentrated, pre-mixed co-formulation of daratumumab 1800 mg plus rHuPH20 (DARA SC) administered to 25 patients with a median of 3 (range 2–9) prior lines of therapy. DARA SC was given weekly during cycles 1 and 2, every two weeks during cycles 3–6 and every 4 weeks thereafter. Daratumumab serum concentration following DARA SC was consistent with IV daratumumab as well similar was safety profile. After a median follow-up of 14.2 months, ORR with DARA SC was 52% with 28% of patients achieving VGPG. Moreover median PFS was 12 months for all patients and 11.7 months for those refractory to both PIs and IMiDs. Based on these results, the phase III COLUMBA trial [62] tested the non-inferiority for ORR of daratumumab sc versus daratumumab iv. A total of 522 patients with ≥3 prior lines of therapy were randomized to receive daratumumab sc 1800 mg plus rHuPH20 2000 U/mL or conventional daratumumab iv with the same schedule of PAVO study. After a median follow-up of 7.5 months, primary end-point was met since ORR was 41% in the sc group versus 37% in the iv group. The rates of at least VGPR (19% versus 17%, respectively) and median PFS (5.6 versus 6.1 months, respectively) were similar.

This trial demonstrated that a subcutaneous formulation of daratumumb, needing five minutes for delivery, maintains the same efficacy and safety of original formulation. The ongoing phase II PLEIADES study [63] is assessing daratumumab sc, in combination with standard care in 3 cohorts of both newly diagnosed and RRMM patients. In RRMM cohort, 65 patients received daratumumab sc wth Rd (D-Rd) obtaining an ORR of 90.8% and at least VGPR of 64.6% with less than 5% of patients with toxicities requiring treatment discontinuation. An ongoing randomized phase II study (NCT03871829; LYNX) will evaluate the efficacy and safety of retreatment with daratumumab sc in patients with RRMM previously exposed to daratumumab iv.

In Table 2 we summarized the ongoing clinical studies with daratumumab in RRMM.

Table 2. Ongoing clinical trial with daratumumab in RRMM.

Study	Phase	Treatment	NCT Identifier
Study of ciforadenant in combination with daratumumab in patients with relapsed or refractory multiple myeloma	I	Ciforadenant 100 mg orally twice daily plus daratumumab 16 mg/kg mg iv weekly cycles 1 and 2, every two weeks cycles 3–6 and every 4 weeks thereafter	04280328
Study of melphalan flufenamide (Melflufen) + dex with bortezomib or daratumumab in patients with RRMM (ANCHOR)	I/II	Melflufen 30 mg and 40 mg or 20 mg in day 1 plus daratumumab 16 mg/kg weekly for 8 doses, every other weeks for 8 doses and then every 4 weeks plus dexamethasone or melfuflen (same schedule) plus bortezomib 1.3 mg/sm sc days 1, 4, 8, 11 and dexamethasone	03481556
INCB001158 combined with subcutaneous (SC) daratumumab, compared to daratumumab sc, in relapsed or refractory multiple myeloma	I/II	INCB001158 orally twice daily with dose escalation, plus daratumumab sc 1800 mg weekly cycles 1 and 2, every two weeks cycles 3–6 and every 4 weeks thereafter versus daratumumab sc	03837509
Daratumumab, azacitidine, and dexamethasone for treatment of patients with recurrent or refractory multiple myeloma previously treated with daratumumab	II	Azacitidine iv for 5 days plus daratumumab 16 mg/kg iv weekly for 2 cycles, every 2 weeks for 4 cycles and every 4 weeks thereafter plus dexamethasone	04407442
A study to determine the efficacy of the combination of daratumumab plus durvalumab (D2) in subjects with relapsed and refractory multiple myeloma (FUSION-MM-005)	II	Durvalumab iv 1500 mg on day 2 cycle 1 and on day 1 thereafter plus daratumunimab 16 mg/kg iv weekly cycles 1 and 2, every two weeks cycles 3–6 and every 4 weeks thereafter versus daratumumab sc	03000452

Table 2. *Cont.*

Study	Phase	Treatment	NCT Identifier
A study of JNJ-63723283, an anti-programmed death-1 monoclonal antibody administered in combination with daratumumab, compared with daratumumab alone in partecipants with relapsed or refractory multiple myeloma	II/III	Daratumunìmab 16 mg/kg iv weekly cycles 1 and 2, every two weeks cycles 3–6 and every 4 weeks thereafter plus JNJ-63723283 240 mg iv week 1 on cycle 1 day 2, cycle 1 day 15 then every 2 weeks thereafter versus daratumumab iv	03357952
Evaluation of efficacy and safety of belantamab mafodotin, bortezomib and dexamethasone versus daratumumab, bortezomib and dexamethasone in partecipants with relapsed/refractory multiple myeloma (DREAMM 7)	III	Belantamab mafodotin plus bortezomib and dexamethasone versus daratumumab, bortezomib and dexamethasone (DVd)	04246047
A study comparing JNJ-68284528, a CAR-T therapy directed against B-cell Maturationa Antigen (BCMA), versus pomalidomide, bortezomib and dexametahsone (PVd) or daratumumab, pomalidomide and dexamethasone (DPd) in partecipants with relapsed and lenalidomide-refractory multiple myeloma (CARTIDUDE-4)	III	Pomalidomide 4 mg days 1–14 plus bortezomib 1.3 mg/m^2 days 1, 4, 8, 11 (cycles 1–8) and days 1 and 8 thereafter plus dexamethasone (PVd) or daratumumab 1800 mg sc weekly cycles 1 and 2, every two weeks cycles 3–6 and every 4 weeks thereafter plus pomalidomide 4 mg days 1–21 plus dexamethasone (DPd) versus JNJ-68284528 CAR-T therapy	04181827
Efficacy and safety study of bb2121 versus standard regimens in subjects with relapsed and refractory multiple myeloma (RRMM) (KarMMa-3)	III	Daratumumab, pomalidomide, dexamethasone (DPd) or daratumumab, bortezomib, dexamethasone (DVd) or ixazomib, lenaliodmide, dexametasome (IxaRd) or carfilzomib, dexamethasone (Kd) or elotuzumab, pomalidomide, dexamethasone (EPd) versus bb2121	03651128

4. Isatuximab

4.1. Isatuximab Monotherapy

Isatuximab, an IgG1k chimeric monoclonal antibody directed to CD38, appears to be a strong blocker of the multiple enzymatic functions of the target molecule [64]. It binds to a specific epitope on the human cell surface antigen CD38, which is widely and uniformely expressed on myeloma cells, and it leads to apoptosis of MM cells without crosslinking of the Fc receptors of the antibody [65]. Several clinical trials demonstrated the efficacy of isatuximab in RRMM both in monotherapy and in association with other drugs.

A phase I multicenter dose-escalation study [66] evaluated safety and toxicity of isatuximab monotherapy given at dose ranging from 0.0001 mg/kg to 20 mg/kg in RRMM patients. Overall, 84 patients with a median of 5 (range 1–13) prior lines of therapy were enrolled and 62% of them had received prior carfilzomib or pomalidomide. Maximum tolerated dose (MTD) was not reached and IRRs developed in 47.6% of patients during the first cycle, being of grade 1 and 2 in 94% of cases. As regard efficacy, in patients treated with isatuximab at dose 10–20 mg/kg ORR was 24% and median PFS 3.7 months, consistent with that reported with daratumumab monotherapy. These results have been confirmed in a phase II multicenter randomized study [67] in which patients who had received three or more prior lines of therapy were allocated to receive 4 different doses and schedules of isatuximab as follows: 3 mg/kg every 2 weeks, 10 mg/kg every two weeks, 10 mg/kg every two weeks for 2 cycles and every 4 weeks thereafter, 20 mg/kg weekly during the first cycle and every two weeks thereafter. Overall, 97 patients with a median of 5 (range 2–14) prior lines of therapy were enrolled and among them 83% and 64% were refractory to lenalidomide and pomalidomide, respectively, as well as 74% and 61% were refractory to bortezomib and carfilzomib, respectively. At dose ≥10 mg/kg ORR was 24.3% with 15% of patients achieving a VGPR, median PFS was 4.6 months and median OS was 18.7 months. The part 2 of the same study has been recently published [68]. Patients treated with ≥3 prior lines were randomized to receive isatuximab 20 mg/kg weekly for 4 infusions followed by 20 mg/kg every 2 weeks either as monotherapy (Isa: 109 patients) or in combination with dexamethasone (Isa-dex: 55 patients) 40 mg weekly. The median number of prior lines of therapy was 4 (range 2–10) in both arms. ORR was 23.9% and 43.6% in Isa and Isa-dex arm, respectively ($p = 0.008$). As regard outcome measures, median PFS and OS were 4.9 and 18.9 months for Isa group and 10.2 and 17.3 for Isa-dex group. IRRs occurred in 40% of both groups of patients, mainly of grade 1–2, whereas grade 3–4 neutropenia and infections were the most common toxicities.

4.2. Isatuximab Plus IMiDs

As well as for elotuzumab and daratumumab, also isatuximab was tested in combination with lenalidomide and dexamethasone in a phase 1b dose escalation study [69]. Patients were treated with different doses and schedules of isatuximab with the aim of determining the maximum tolerated dose of isatuximab combined with lenalidomide (25 mg days 1–21) and dexamethasone (40 mg weekly) (Isa-Rd). A total of 57 patients were enrolled; they had received a median of 5 (range 1–12) previous lines therapies, 88% were refractory to any IMiDs-based therapies, 65% to bortezomib and 92% to carfilzomib. The MTD was no reached and the selected dose of isatuximab for further studies evaluating this triplet was 10 mg/kg weekly during cycle 1 and then every two weeks. After a median follow-up of 9 months, ORR for the all population was 51% with a median PFS of 8.5 months. ORR was 52% in lenalidomide-refractory patients and 48% in those who had received ≥3 previous treatment lines. IRRs occurred in 56% of patients, but they were grade 1–2 in 84%. Moreover, the most common grade 3–4 adverse events were neutropenia (60%), thrombocytopenia (38%) and pneumonia (9%). Mikhael et al. [30] found an ORR of 62%, with median PFS of 17.6 months, in a phase Ib dose-escalation study of isatuximab, in association with pomalidomide (4 mg days 1–21) and dexamethasone (40 mg weekly). Also in this study MTD was not reached. Among 45 patients enrolled with a median of 5 prior lines of therapy (range 3–12), 82% were lenalidomide-refractory and the ORR was 56.8%. The incidence of IRRs was similar to that reported with Isa-Rd but the incidence of grade ≥3 neutropenia was higher (84%), as well as that of pneumonia (18%). Based on the promising data from this combination in a very heavily pretreated RRMM population, phase III ICARIA trial [70] compared Isa-Pd versus Pd in 307 RRMM who had previously received ≥2 lines of therapy (median 3, range 2–4). Overall, all patients were previously treated with lenalidomide and proteasome inhibitors, being 93% refractory to lenalidomide and 76% to at least one PI. Treatment consisted of pomalidomide 4 mg days 1–21 and dexametahsone 40 mg weekly in the Pd group with the addition of isatuximab 10 mg/kg weekly in the first cycle and every two weeks thereafter in the Isa-Pd one. After a median follow up of 11.6 months, a 41% reduction of the risk of disease progression or death was reported in Isa-Pd versus Pd group, with a median PFS of 11.5 versus 6.5 months, respectively (HR = 0.59; $p = 0.001$). This benefit was conserved in all subgroups, in particular in lenalidomide-refractory patients (HR = 0.59), high-risk cytogenetic MM (HR = 0.66) and patients with impairment of renal function (HR = 0.50). ORR and ≥ VGPR were 63% and 32% versus 32% and 9% in Isa-Pd and Pd group, respectively. As for safety profile, IRRs were the most relevant adverse events occurring in 38% of patients in Isa-Pd group, 2% of which was grade 3–4. Other grade 3–4 toxicities are reported in Table 1.

The benefits in terms of PFS and ORR was observed in patients ≥75 years old, as shown in a pre-specified subgroup analysis of ICARIA trial [71] comparing Isa-Pd versus Pd, in three age groups as follows: <65 years old, 65–74 and ≥75 years old. The median PFS was significantly longer with

Isa-Pd and similar between three groups (11.5 versus 11.5, versus 11.4, respectively). However, older patients showed a higher rates of serious treatment-emergent adverse events with discontinuation of therapy either in Isa-Pd and in Pd arm.

Another subgroup analysis of ICARIA trial [72] analysed outcome of patients with renal impairment (RI) defined as estimated glomerular filtration rate (eGFR) <60 mL/min/1.73 m^2). Median PFS was 9.5 versus 3.7 months in patients with RI receiving Isa-Pd, and Pd, respectively (HR= 0.50) whereas in patients without RI median PFS was 12.7 versus 7.9 months, respectively (HR = 0.58). Moreover, compared with Pd the addition of isatuximab improved the complete renal response (71.9% versus 38.1%) with a median time to renal response of 3.4 weeks in Isa-Pd versus 7.3 weeks in Pd group.

There were no differences in the IRRs rate between patients with, and without, RI, and the most frequent grade 3–4 non-hematologic adverse events in patients receiving Isa-Pd were infections and pneumonia. In conclusion, Isa-Pd represents a valuable treatment option for patients with RRMM presenting with renal dysfunction, considering that it is not necessary a dose adjustment, differently from lenalidomide.

Finally, benefit of Isa-Pd over Pd was documented also in patients with isolated gain (1q21) as showed in a retrospective analysis from patients enrolled in ICARIA and phase Ib study [73].

4.3. Isatuximab Plus PIs

After a phase 1b study [31] established the feasibility and safety of isatuximab, combined with carfilzomib, the phase III IKEMA trial [74] compared isatuximab, carfilzomib, dexamethasone (Isa-Kd) with carfilzomib, dexamethasone (Kd) in RRMM patients who had received 1–3 previous lines of therapy. At last EHA Congress, Moreau presented results of an interim analysis. Three hundred two patients were randomized to receive Kd (carfilzomib 20 mg/m^2 days 1 and 2 of cycle 1, 56 mg/m^2 days 8, 9, 15, 16 of cycle 1 and subsequent cycles plus dexamethasone 20 mg days 1, 2, 8, 9, 15 and 16) or Kd plus isatuximab (10 mg/kg weekly during cycle 1 and every two weeks thereafter). Patients had received a median of 2 prior lines of therapy (range 1–4), 45% were refractory to IMidDs and 33% to bortezomib. After a median follow-up of 20.7 months median PFS not reached in the Isa-Kd group versus 19.15 months in the Kd one (HR = 0.53; $p<$ 0.0007). This benefit was confirmed among all the subgroups of analysis, in particular HR was 0.59 in lenalidomide-refractory patients, 0.56 in patients previously receiving bortezomib and 0.72 in high-risk cytogenetic subgroup. As for data about OS it is necessary a longer follow-up. No significant difference was found between two arms as regard ORR (86.6% versus 82.9 in Isa-Kd and Kd group, respectively) whereas high quality responses were more frequent in Isa-Kd patients (VGPR or better 72.6% versus 56%). In these latter MRD negativity by NGS at level of 10^{-5} was documented in 41% of patients treated with IsaKd versus 23% with Kd.

IRRs occurred mostly during the first infusion and were grade ≥ 3 in less than 1% of patients. Grade 3–4 adverse events are summarized in Table 1.

As well as for daratumumab, an ongoing phase II study (NCT04287855) is evaluating isatuximab plus pomalidomide, carfilzomib and dexamethasone. Moreover, a phase Ib study (NCT04045795) is assessing safety and tolerability of isatuximab administered subcutaneously versus intravenously.

In Figures 1 and 2, we pictured the results of main phase III clinical trials including elotuzumab, daratumumab and isatuximab.

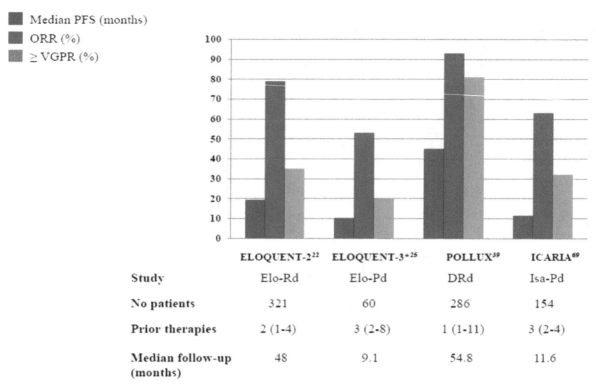

Study	ELOQUENT-2[22]	ELOQUENT-3*[25]	POLLUX[39]	ICARIA[69]
	Elo-Rd	Elo-Pd	DRd	Isa-Pd
No patients	321	60	286	154
Prior therapies	2 (1-4)	3 (2-8)	1 (1-11)	3 (2-4)
Median follow-up (months)	48	9.1	54.8	11.6

Figure 1. Results of Phase III and randomized phase II* trials with elotuzumab, daratumumab and isatuximab plus IMiDs. Elo-Rd: elotuzumab, lenalidomide, dexamethasone; Elo-Pd: elotuzumab, pomalidomide, dexamethasone; DRd: daratumumab, lenalidomide, dexamethasone; Isa-Pd: isatuximab, pomalidomide, dexamethasone.

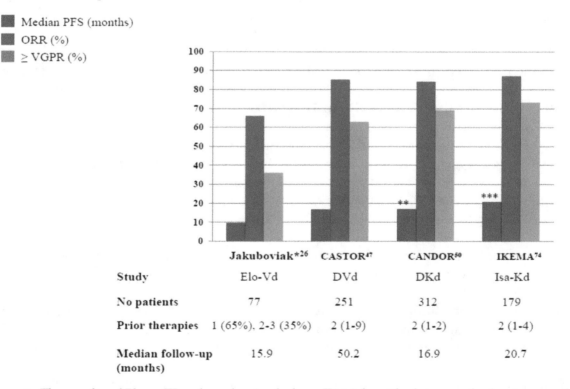

Study	Jakuboviak*[26]	CASTOR[47]	CANDOR[50]	IKEMA[74]
	Elo-Vd	DVd	DKd	Isa-Kd
No patients	77	251	312	179
Prior therapies	1 (65%), 2-3 (35%)	2 (1-9)	2 (1-2)	2 (1-4)
Median follow-up (months)	15.9	50.2	16.9	20.7

Figure 2. The results of Phase III and randomized phase II* trials with elotuzumab, daratumumab and isatuximab plus PIs. Elo-Vd: elotuzumab, bortezomib, dexamethasone; DVd: daratumumab, bortezomib, dexamethasone; DKd: daratumumab, carfilzomib, dexamethasone; Isa-Kd: isatuximab, carfilzomib, dexamethasone ** Not reached after a median follow-up of 16.9 months *** Not reached after a median follow-up of 20.7 months.

5. Conclusions and Perspectives

Immunotherapies like as MoAbs are becoming the major players in the treatment of MM patients. In the RRMM patients triplets, including elotuzumab and daratumumab were found to be superior to doublet standard regimens and they are bound to rapidly change the outcome of RRMM patients. Although, the overall survival data are still immature for mostly phase III studies, in the ELOQUENT-2 trial elotuzumab, in combination with lenalidomide and dexamethasone, demonstrated significant improvement in overall survival after a median follow-up of almost six years. A third monoclonal antibody, isatuximab, was recently approved for RRMM setting by FDA. The benefit given by the triplet containing MoAbs, compared with doublet drug combinations, is also consistent in the subset of patients with high-risk cytogenetics, advanced ISS stage and in older patients. Monoclonal antibodies have shown a good safety profile and recent approval of subcutaneous daratumumab will improve quality of life for many patients. However, the increasing use of MoAbs upfront will probably make the treatment of RRMM more problematic but novel immunotherapeutic approaches as CAR-T cells, bispecific antibodies (BiTEs) and antibody-drug conjugates are coming into play and the outcome of MM patients is expected to continue to improve.

Author Contributions: Conceptualization, M.O., M.T.P. and A.O.; Investigation, L.C., S.M., F.F.; writing—original draft preparation, L.C., S.M., F.F.; review and editing, M.O., M.T.P. and A.O. All authors have read and agreed to the published version of the manuscript.

References

1. Kumar, S.K.; Rajkumar, S.V.; Dispenzieri, A.; Hayman, S.R.; Buadi, S.K.; Zeldenrust, S.R.; Dingli, D.; Russel, S.J.; Lust, J.S.; Greipp, P.R.; et al. Improved survival in multiple myeloma and the impact of novel therapies. *Blood* **2008**, *111*, 2516–2520. [CrossRef]
2. Brenner, H.; Gondos, A.; Pulte, D. Recent major improvement in long-term survival of younger patients with multiple myeloma. *Blood* **2008**, *111*, 2521–2526. [CrossRef] [PubMed]
3. Kumar, S.K.; Dispenzieri, A.; Lacy, M.Q.; Gertz, M.A.; Buadi, F.K.; Pandey, S.; Kapoor, P.; Dingli, D.; Hayman, S.R.; Leung, N.; et al. Continued improvement in survival in multiple myeloma: Changes in early mortality and outcomes in older patients. *Leukemia* **2014**, *28*, 1122–1128. [CrossRef] [PubMed]
4. Tacchetti, P.; Patriarca, F.; Petrucci, M.T.; Galli, M.; Pantani, L.; Dozza, L.; Raimondo, F.D.; Boccadoro, M.; Offidani, M.; Montefusco, V.; et al. A triplet bortezomib- and immunomodulator-based therapy before and after double ASCT improves overall survival of newly diagnosed MM patients: Final analysis of phase 3 GIMEMA-MMY-3006 study. *HemaSphere* **2018**, *2*, abstract S105.
5. Nandakumar, B.; Binder, M.; Dispenzieri, A.; Kapoor, P.; Buadi, F.; Gertz, M.A.; Buadi, F.K.; Pandey, S.; Dingli, D.; Haymen, S.R.; et al. Continued improvement in survival in multiple myeloma including high-risk patients. *J. Clin. Oncol.* **2019**, *37*, abstract 8039. [CrossRef]
6. Kumar, S.K.; Dimopoulos, M.A.; Kastritis, E.; Terpos, E.; Hahi, H.; Goldschmidt, H.; Hillengass, J.; Leleu, X.; Beksac, M.; Alsina, M.; et al. Natural history of relapsed myeloma, refractory to immunomodulatory drugs and proteasome inhibitors: A multicenter IMWG study. *Leukemia* **2017**, *31*, 2443–2448. [CrossRef] [PubMed]
7. Neuse, C.J.; Lomas, O.C.; Schliemann, C.; Shen, Y.J.; Manier, S.; Bustoros, M.; Gobrial, I.M. Genome instability in multiple myeloma. *Leukemia* **2020**, *34*, 2887–2897. [CrossRef] [PubMed]
8. Kumar, S.J.; Therneau, T.M.; Gertz, M.A.; Lacy, M.Q.; Dispenzieri, A.; Rajkumar, S.V.; Fonseca, R.; Witzig, T.E.; Lust, J.A.; Larson, D.R.; et al. Clinical course of patients with relapsed multiple myeloma. *Mayo Clin. Proc.* **2004**, *79*, 867–874. [CrossRef]
9. Jagannath, S.; Rifkin, R.M.; Gasparetto, C.; Toomey, K.; Durie, B.G.M.; Hardin, J.W.; Terebelo, H.; Lynne, W.; Narang, M.; Srinivasan, S.; et al. Development of a predictive model of multiple myeloma patients outcomes based on treatment sequencing using data from the Connect MM patients registry. *HemaSphere* **2018**, *2*, abstract PF570.

10. Raab, M.S.; Cavo, M.; Delforge, M.; Driessen, C.; Fink, L.; Flinois, A.; McQuire-Gonzalez, S.; Safaei, R.; Karlin, L.; Mateos, M.-V.; et al. Multiple Myeloma: Practice patterns across Europe. *Br. J. Haematol.* **2016**, *175*, 66–76. [CrossRef]

11. Rajkumar, S.V.; Harousseau, J.L.; Durie, B.; Anderson, K.C.; Dimopoulos, M.; Kyle, R.; Blade, J.; Richarson, P.; Orlowaski, R.; Siegel, D.; et al. Consensus recommendations for the uniform reporting of clinical trials: Report of the International Myeloma Workshop Consensus Panel 1. *Blood* **2011**, *117*, 4691–4695. [CrossRef] [PubMed]

12. Sonneveld, P.; Broijl, A. Treatment of relapsed and refractory multiple myeloma. *Haematologica* **2016**, *101*, 396–406. [CrossRef] [PubMed]

13. Offidani, M.; Boccadoro, M.; di Raimondo, F.; Petrucci, M.T.; Tosi, P.; Cavo, M. Expert panel consensus statement for proper evaluation of first relapse in multiple myeloma. *Current. Hematol. Malig. Rep.* **2019**, *14*, 187–196. [CrossRef] [PubMed]

14. Coiffier, B.; Thieblemont, C.; van den Neste, E.; Lepeu, G.; Plantier, I.; Castaigne, I.; Castaigne, S.; Lefort, S.; Marit, G.; Sebban, C.; et al. Long-term outcome of patients in the LNH-98.5 trial, the first randomized study comoparing ritiximab-CHOP to standard CHOP chemotherapy in DLBCL patients: A study by the Groupe d'Etudes des Lymphomes de l'Adulte. *Blood* **2010**, *116*, 2040–2045. [CrossRef] [PubMed]

15. Connors, J.M.; Jurczak, W.; Strauss, D.J.; Ansell, S.M.; Kim, W.S.; Gallamini, A.; Younes, A.; Alekseev, S.; Illes, A.; Picardi, M.; et al. Brentuximab vedotin with chemotherapy for stage III or IV Hodgkin's lymphoma. *N. Engl. J. Med.* **2018**, *378*, 331–344. [CrossRef] [PubMed]

16. Magen, H.; Muchtar, E. Elotuzumab: The first approved monoclonal antibody for multiple myeloma. *Ther. Advanc. Hematol.* **2016**, *7*, 187–195. [CrossRef]

17. Zonder, J.A.; Mohrbacher, A.F.; Singhal, S.; van Rhee, F.; Bensinger, W.I.; Ding, H.; Fry, J.; Afar, D.E.H.; Singhal, A.K. A phase 1, multicenter, open-label, dose escalation study of elotuzumab in patients with advanced multiple myeloma. *Blood* **2012**, *120*, 552–559. [CrossRef]

18. Mateos, M.-V.; Granell, M.; Oriol, A.; Martinez-Lopez, J.; Blade, J.; Hernandez, M.T.; Martin, J.; Gironella, M.; Lynch, M.; Bleickardt, E.; et al. Elotuzumab in combination with thalidomide and low-dose dexamethasone: A phase 2 single-arm safety study in patients with relapsed/refractory multiple myeloma. *Br. J. Haematol.* **2016**, *175*, 448–456. [CrossRef]

19. Lonial, S.; Vij, R.; Harousseau, J.L.; Facon, T.; Moreau, P.; Mazumder, A.; Kaufman, J.L.; Leleu, X.; Tsao, L.C.; Westland, C.; et al. Elotuzumab in combination with lenalidomide and low-dose dexamethasone in relapsed or refractory multiple myeloma. *J. Clin. Oncol.* **2012**, *30*, 1953–1959. [CrossRef]

20. Richardson, P.G.; Jagannath, S.; Moreau, P.; Jakubowiak, A.J.; Raab, M.S.; Facon, T.; Vij, R.; White, D.; Reece, D.E.; Benboubker, L.; et al. Elotuzumab in combination with lenalidomide and dexamethasone in patients with relapsed multiple myeloma: Final phase 2 results from the randomised, open-label, phase 1b-2 dose-escalation study. *Lancet Haematol.* **2015**, *2*, e516–e527. [CrossRef]

21. Lonial, S.; Dimopoulos, M.A.; Palumbo, A.; White, D.; Grosicki, S.; Spicka, I.; Walter-Croneck, A.; Moreau, P.; Mateos, M.-V.; Magen, H.; et al. Elotuzumab therapy for relapsed or refractory multiple myeloma. *N. Engl. J. Med.* **2015**, *373*, 621–631. [CrossRef] [PubMed]

22. Dimopoulos, M.A.; Lonial, S.; Betts, K.A.; Chen, C.; Zichlin, M.L.; Brun, A.; Signorovitch, J.E.; Makenbaeva, D.; Mekan, S.; Sy, O.; et al. Elotuzumab plus lenalidomide and dexamethasone in relapsed/refractory multiple myeloma: Extended 4-year follow-up and analysis of relative progression-free survival from the randomized ELOQUENT-2 trial. *Cancer* **2018**, *124*, 4032–4043. [CrossRef] [PubMed]

23. Dimopoulos, M.A.; Lonial, S.; White, D.; Moreau, P.; Weisel, K.; San-Miguel, J.; Shpilberg, O.; Grosicki, S.; Špička, I.; Walter-Croneck, A.; et al. Elotuzumab, lenalidomide and dexamethasone in RRMM: Final overall survival results from the phase 3 randomized ELOQUENT-2 study. *Blood Cancer J.* **2020**, *10*, 91. [CrossRef] [PubMed]

24. Gentile, M.; Specchia, G.; Derudas, D.; Galli, M.; Botta, C.; Rocco, S.; Conticello, C.; Califano, C.; Giuliani, N.; Mangiacavalli, S.; et al. Elotuzumab, lenalidomide, and dexamethasone as salvage therapy for patients with multiple myloma: Italian, multicentre, retrospective clinical experience with 300 cases outside of controlled clinical trials. *Haematologica* **2020**. [CrossRef] [PubMed]

25. Dimopoulos, M.A.; Dytfeld, D.; Grosicki, S.; Moreau, P.; Takezako, N.; Hori, M.; Leleu, X.; LeBlanc, R.; Suzuki, K.; Hori, M.; et al. Elotuzumab plus pomalidomide and dexamethasone for multiple myeloma. *N. Engl. J. Med.* **2018**, *379*, 1811–1822. [CrossRef] [PubMed]

26. Jakubowiak, A.J.; Offidani, M.; Pegourie, B.; de La Rubia, J.; Garderet, L.; Laribi, K.; Bosi, A.; Marasca, R.; Laubach, J.; Mohrbacher, L.; et al. Randomized phase 2 study: Elotuzumab plus bortezomib/dexamethasone vs. bortezomib/dexamethasone for relapsed/refractory MM. *Blood* **2016**, *127*, 2833–2840. [CrossRef]

27. Dimopoulos, M.A.; Oriol, A.; Nahi, H.; San-Miguel, J.; Bahlis, N.J.; Usmani, S.Z.; Rabin, N.; Orlowaski, R.Z.; Komarnicki, M.; Suzuki, K.; et al. Daratumumab, lenalidomide, and dexamethasone for multiple myeloma. *N. Engl. J. Med.* **2016**, *375*, 1319–1331. [CrossRef] [PubMed]

28. Palumbo, A.; Chanan-Khan, A.; Weisel, K.; Nooka, A.K.; Masszi, T.; Beksac, M.; SPICKA, I.; Hungria, V.; Munder, M.; Mateos, M.; et al. Daratumumab, bortezomib, and dexamethasone for multiple myeloma. *N. Engl. J. Med.* **2016**, *375*, 754–766. [CrossRef]

29. Dimopoulos, M.; Quach, H.; Mateos, M.-V.; Landgren, O.; Leleu, X.; Siegel, D.; Weisel, K.; Yang, H.; Klippel, Z.; Zahlten-Kumeli, A.; et al. Carfilzomib, dexamethasone, and daratumumab versus carfilzomib and dexamethasone for patients with relapsed or refractory multiple myeloma (CANDOR): Results from a randomized, multicenter, open-label, phase 3 trial. *Lancet* **2020**, *396*, 186–197. [CrossRef]

30. Mikhael, J.; Richardson, P.; Usmani, S.Z.; Raje, N.; Bensinger, W.; Karanes, C.; Campana, F.; Kanagavel, D.; Dubin, F.; Liu, Q.; et al. A phase 1b study of isatuximab plus pomalidomide/dexamethasone in relpased/refractory multiple myeloma. *Blood* **2019**, *134*, 123–133. [CrossRef]

31. Chari, A.; Richter, J.R.; Shah, N.; Wong, S.W.K.; Jagannath, S.; Cho, H.J.; Biran, N.; Wolf, J.; Parekh, S.S.; Munster, P.N.; et al. Phase I-b study of isatuximab + carfilzomib in relapsed and refractory multiple myeloma. *J. Clin. Oncol.* **2018**, *36*, abstract 8014. [CrossRef]

32. Silvennoinen, R.H.; Tsallos, D.; Nahi, H.; Antilla, P.; Koskenvesa, P.; Lievonen, J.; Rasanen, A.; Varmavuo, V.; Anttila, P.; Koskenvesa, P.; et al. A phase 2 study of carfilzomib plus elotuzumab plus dexamethasone for myeloma patients relapsed after 1–3 prior treatment lines. *Blood* **2018**, *132*, abstract 1975. [CrossRef]

33. Yee, A.J.; Laubach, J.P.; Campagnaro, E.L.; Lipe, B.C.; Nadeem, O.; Friedman, R.S.; Cole, C.E.; O'Donnell, E.K.; Bianchi, G.; Branagan, A.R.; et al. A phase II study of elotuzumab in combination with pomalidomide, bortezomib, and dexamethasone in relapsed and refractory multiple myeloma. *Blood* **2019**, *134*, abstract 3169. [CrossRef]

34. Lokhorst, H.M.; Plesner, T.; Laubach, J.P.; Nahi, H.; Gimsing, P.; Hansson, M.; minnema, M.C.; Lassen, U.; Krejcik, J.; Palumbo, A.; et al. Targeting CD38 with daratumumab monotherapy in multiple myeloma. *N. Engl. J. Med.* **2015**, *373*, 1207–1219. [CrossRef] [PubMed]

35. Lonial, S.; Weiss, B.M.; Usmani, S.Z.; Singhal, S.; Chari, A.; Bahlis, N.J.; Belch, A.; Krishnan, A.; Vescio, R.A.; Mateos, M.V.; et al. Daratumumab monotherapy in patients with treatment-refractory multiple myeloma (SIRIUS): An open-label, randomised, phase 2 trial. *Lancet* **2016**, *387*, 1551–1560. [CrossRef]

36. Usmani, S.Z.; Weiss, B.M.; Plesner, T.; Bahlis, N.J.; Belch, A.; Lonial, S.; Lokhorst, H.M.; Voorhesss, P.M.; Richardson, P.G.; Chari, A.; et al. Clinical efficacy of daratumumab monotherapy in patients with heavily pretreated relapsed or refractory multiple myeloma. *Blood* **2016**, *128*, 37–44. [CrossRef] [PubMed]

37. Usmani, S.Z.; Nahi, H.; Plesner, T.; Weiss, B.M.; Bahlis, N.J.; Belch, A.; Voorhees, P.M.; Laubach, J.P.; van de Donk, N.W.C.J.; Ahmadi, T.; et al. Daratumumab monotherapy in patients with heavily pretreated relapsed or refractory multiple myeloma: Final results from the phase 2 GEN501 and SIRIUS trial. *Lancet Hematol.* **2020**, *7*, e447–e455. [CrossRef]

38. Chari, A.; Lonial, S.; Mark, T.M.; Krishnan, A.Y.; Stockerl-Goldstein, K.E.; Usmani, S.Z.; Lodhe, A.; Etheredge, D.; Fleming, S.; Liu, B.; et al. Results of an early access treatment protocol of daratumumab in United States patients with relapsed or refractory multiple myeloma. *Cancer* **2018**, *124*, 4342–4349. [CrossRef]

39. Alegre, A.; de la Rubia, J.; Sureda Balari, A.; Encinas Rodriguez, C.; Suarez, A.; Blanchard, M.J.; Lieonart, J.B.; Rodriguez-Otero, P.; Insunza, A.; Palomera, L.; et al. Results of an early access treatment protocol of daratumumab monotherapy in Spanish patients with relapsed or refractory multiple myeloma. *HemaSphere* **2020**, *4*, e380. [CrossRef]

40. Jullien, M.; Trudel, S.; Tessoulin, B.; Mahé, B.; Dubruille, V.; Blin, N.; Gastinne, T.; Bonnet, A.; Lok, A.; Lebourgeois, A.; et al. Single-agent daratumumab in very advanced relapsed and refractory multiple myeloma patients: A real-life single center retrospective study. *Ann. Hematol.* **2019**, *98*, 1435–1440. [CrossRef]

41. Van der Veer, M.S.; de Weers, M.; van Kessel, B.; Bakker, J.M.; Wittebol, S.; Parren, P.W.; Lokhorst, H.M.; Mutis, T. Towards effective immunotherapy of myeloma: Enhanced elimination of myeloma cells by combination of lenalidomide with the human CD38 monoclonal antibody daratumumab. *Haematologica* **2011**, *96*, 284–290. [CrossRef] [PubMed]

42. Plesner, T.; Arkenau, H.-T.; Gimsing, P.; Krejcik, J.; Lemech, C.; Minnema, M.C.; Lassen, U.; Laubach, J.P.; Palumbo, A.; Lisby, S.; et al. Phase 1/2 study of daratumumab, lenalidomide, and dexamethasone for relapsed multiple myeloma. *Blood* **2016**, *128*, 1821–1828. [CrossRef] [PubMed]

43. Plesner, T.; Arkenau, H.-T.; Gay, F.; Minnema, M.C.; Boccadoro, M.; Moreau, P.; Cavenagh, J.; Perrot, A.; Laubach, J.P.; Krejcik, J.; et al. Enduring efficacy and tolerability of daratumumab in combination with lenalidomide and dexamethasone in patients with relapsed or relapsed/refractory multiple myeloma (GEN503): Final results of an open-label, phase 1/2 study. *Br. J. Haematol.* **2019**, *186*, e35–e39. [CrossRef] [PubMed]

44. Kaufman, J.L.; Usmani, S.Z.; San-Miguel, J.; Bahlis, N.; White, D.J.; Benboubker, L.; Cook, G.; Leiba, M.; Ho, P.J.; Kim, K.; et al. Four-year follow-up of the phase 3 POLLUX study of daratumumab plus lenalidomide and dexamethasone (D-Rd) versus lenalidomide and dexamethasone (Rd) alone in relapsed or refractory multiple myeloma. *Blood* **2019**, *134*, abstract 1866. [CrossRef]

45. Mateos, M.-V.; Spencer, A.; Nooka, A.K.; Pour, L.; Weisel, K.; Cavo, M.; Laubach, J.P.; Cook, G.; Lida, S.; Benboubker, L.; et al. Daratumumab-based regimens are highly effective and well tolerated in relapsed or refractory multiple myeloma regardless of patient age: Subgroup analysis of the phase 3 CASTOR and POLLUX studies. *Haematologica* **2020**, *105*, 468–477. [CrossRef]

46. Chari, A.; Suvannasankha, A.; Fay, J.W.; Arnulf, B.; Kaufman, J.L.; Ifthikharuddin, J.J.; Weiss, B.M.; Krishnan, A.; Lentzsch, S.; Comenzo, R.; et al. Daratumumab plus pomalidomide and dexamethasone in relapsed and/or refractory multiple myeloma. *Blood* **2017**, *130*, 974–981. [CrossRef]

47. Facon, T.; Lonial, S.; Weiss, B.M.; Suvannasankha, A.; Fay, J.; Arnulf, B.; Ifthikharuddin, J.J.; Boer, C.; Wang, J.; Wu, K.; et al. Daratumumab in combination with pomalidomide and dexamethasone for relapsed and/or refractory multiple myeloma patients with ≥2 prior lines of therapy: Updated analysis of MMY1001. *Blood* **2017**, *130*, abstract 1824.

48. Siegel, D.S.; Schiller, G.J.; Samaras, C.; Sebag, M.; Berdeja, J.; Ganguly, S.; Matous, J.; Song, K.; Seet, C.S.; Talamo, G.; et al. Pomalidomide, dexamethasone, and daratumumab in relapsed refractory multiple myeloma after lenalidomide treatment. *Leukemia* **2020**, *34*, 3286–3297. [CrossRef]

49. Pierceall, W.E.; Amatangelo, M.; Bahlis, N.J.; Siegel, D.S.; Rahman, A.; van Oekelen, O.; Neri, P.; Young, M.; Chung, W.; Serbina, N.; et al. Immunomodulation in pomalidomide, dexamethasone, dexamethasone, and daratumumab-treated relapsed/refractory multiple myeloma patients. *Clin. Cancer Res.* **2020**, *26*, 5895–5902. [CrossRef]

50. Nooka, A.K.; Joseph, N.S.; Kaufman, J.L.; Heffner, L.T.; Gupta, V.A.; Gleason, C.; Boise, L.H.; Lonial, S. Clinical efficacy of daratumumab, pomalidomide, and dexamethasone in patients with relapsed or refractory myeloma: Utility of re-treatment with daratumumab among refractory patients. *Cancer* **2019**, *125*, 2991–3000. [CrossRef]

51. Weisel, K.C.; Sonneveld, P.; Mateos, M.-V.; Hungria, V.T.M.; Spencer, A.; Estell, J.; Narreto, W.G.; Corradini, P.; Min, C.-K.; Medvedova, E.; et al. Efficacy and safety of daratumumab, bortezomib, and dexamethasone (D-Vd) versus bortezomib and dexamethasone (Vd) in first relapse patients with multiple myeloma: Four-year update of CASTOR. *Blood* **2019**, *134*, abstract 3192. [CrossRef]

52. Chari, A.; Martinez-Lopez, J.; Mateos, M.-V.; Bladè, J.; Benboubker, L.; Oriol, A.; Arnulf, B.; Rodriguez-Otero, P.; Pineiro, L.; Jakubowiak, A.; et al. Daratumumab plus carfilzomib and dexamethasone in patients with relapsed or refractory multiple myeloma. *Blood* **2019**, *134*, 421–431. [CrossRef] [PubMed]

53. Weisel, K.; Quach, H.; Nooka, A.; Venner, C.P.; Kim, K.; Facon, T. Carfilzomib, dexamethasone, and daratumumab (KdD) versus Kd in relapsed or refractory multiple myeloma: Subgroup analysis of the phase 3 CANDOR study by number of prior lines of therapy and prior therapies. *HemaSphere* **2020**, *4*, abstract EP938.

54. Terpos, E.; Gavriatopoulou, M.; Katodritou, E.; Dialoupi, I.; Hatjiharissi, E.; Verrou, E.; Leonidakis, A.; Migkou, M.; Delimpasi, S.; Symeonidis, A.; et al. Daratuimumab with ixazomib and dexamethasone in multiple myeloma patients who have received prior treatment with a lenalidomide-based regimen: Design and first results of the phase 2 Daria study. *HemaSphere* **2020**, *4*, abstract EP973.

55. Costello, C.L.; Padilla, M.; Ball, E.D.; Mulroney, C. Phase II study of the combination daratumumab, ixazomib, pomalidomide, and dexamethasone as salvage therapy in relapsed/refractory multiple myeloma: Results of a safety run-in analysis. *Blood* **2019**, *134*, abstract 3117. [CrossRef]

56. Kumar, S.; Harrison, S.J.; Cavo, M.; de La Rubia, J.; Popat, R.; Gasparetto, C.; Hungria, V.; Salwender, H.; Suzuki, K.; Kim, I.; et al. Updated results from BELLINI, a phase III study of venetoclax or placebo in combination with bortezomib and dexamethasone in relapsed/refractory multiple myeloma. *J. Clin. Oncol.* **2020**, *38*, abstract 8538. [CrossRef]

57. Kaufman, J.L.; Baz, R.C.; Harrison, S.J.; Quach, H.; Ho, S.-J.; Vangsted, A.J.; Moreau, P.; Gibbs, S.D.J.; Salem, A.H.; Coppola, S.; et al. Updated analysis of a phase I/II study of venetoclax in combination with daratumumab and dexamethasone, ± bortezomib, in patients with relapsed/redractory multiple myeloma. *J. Clin. Oncol.* **2020**, *38*, abstract 8511. [CrossRef]

58. Chari, A.; Vogl, D.T.; Gavriatopoulou, M.; Nooka, A.K.; Yee, A.J.; Huff, C.A.; Moreau, P.; Dingli, D.; Cole, C.; Lonial, S.; et al. Oral selinexor-dexamethasone for triple-class refractory multiple myeloma. *N. Engl. J. Med.* **2019**, *381*, 727–738. [CrossRef] [PubMed]

59. Gasparetto, C.; Lentzsch, S.; Schiller, G.J.; Callander, N.S.; Tuchman, S.; Bahlis, N.J.; White, D.; Chen, C.; Baljevic, M.; Sutherland, H.J.; et al. Selinexor, daratumumab, and dexamethasone in patients with relapsed/refractory multiple myeloma. *J. Clin. Oncol.* **2020**, *38*, abstract 8510. [CrossRef]

60. Usmani, S.Z.; Nahi, H.; Mateos, M.-V.; van de Donk, N.W.C.J.; Hari, A.; Kaufman, J.L.; Moreau, P.; Oriol, A.; Plesner, T.; Benboubker, L.; et al. Subcutaneous delivery of daratumumab in relapsed or refractory multiple myeloma. *Blood* **2019**, *134*, 668–677. [CrossRef] [PubMed]

61. San-Miguel, J.; Usmani, S.Z.; Mateos, M.-V.; van de Donk, N.W.C.J.; Kaufman, J.L.; Moreau, P.; Oriol, A.; Plesner, T.; Benboubker, L.; Liu, K.; et al. Subcutaneous daratumumab in patients with relapsed or refractory multiple myeloma: Part 2 of the open-label, multicenter, dose-escalation phase 1b study (PAVO). *Hematologica* **2020**. [CrossRef]

62. Mateos, M.-V.; Nahi, H.; Legiec, W.; Grosicki, S.; Vorobyev, V.; Spicka, I.; Hungria, V.; Korenkova, S.; Bahlis, N.; Flogegard, M.; et al. Subcutaneous versus intravenous daratumumab in patients with relapsed or refractory multiple myeloma (COLUMBA): A multicentre, open-label, non-inferiority, randomised, phase 3 trial. *Lancet Haematol.* **2020**, *7*, e370–e380. [CrossRef]

63. Chari, A.; Goldschmidt, H.; San-Miguel, J.; McCarthy, H.; Suzuki, K.; Hungria, V.; Balari, A.S.; Perrot, A.; Hulin, C.; Magen, H.; et al. Subcutaneous daratumumab in combination with standard multiple myeloma standard treatment regimens: An open-label, multicenter pghase 2 study (PLEIADES). *Clin. Lymphoma Myeloma Leuk.* **2019**, *19*, e16–e17. [CrossRef]

64. Martin, T.; Corzo, K.; Chiron, M.; van de Velde, K.; Abbadessa, G.; Campana, F.; Solanki, M.; Meng, R.; Lee, H.; Wiederschain, D.; et al. Therapeutic Opportunities with Pharmacological Inhibition of CD38 with Isatuximab. *Cells* **2019**, *8*, 1522. [CrossRef] [PubMed]

65. Deckert, J.; Wetzel, M.C.; Bartle, L.M.; Skaletskaya, A.; Goldmacher, V.S.; Vallée, F.; Zhou-Liu, Q.; Ferrari, P.; Pouzieux, S.; Lahoute, C.; et al. SAR650984, a novel humanized CD38-targeying antibody, demonstrates potent antitumor activity in models of multiple myeloma and other CD38+ hematologic malignancies. *Clin. Cancer Res.* **2014**, *20*, 4574–4583. [CrossRef]

66. Martin, T.; Strickland, S.; Glenn, M.; Charpentier, E.; Guillemin, H.; Hsu, K.; Mikhael, J. Phase I trial of isatuximab monotherapy in the treatment of refractory multiple myeloma. *Blood Cancer J.* **2019**, *9*, 41. [CrossRef] [PubMed]

67. Mikhael, J.; Richter, J.; Vij, R.; Cole, C.; Zonder, J.; Kaufman, J.L.; Bensinger, W.; Dimopoulos, M.; Lendvai, N.; Hari, P.; et al. A dose-finding phase 2 study of single agent isatuximab (anti-CD38 mAb) in relapsed/refractory multiple myeloma. *Leukemia* **2020**, *34*, 3298–3309. [CrossRef] [PubMed]

68. Dimopoulos, M.; Bringhen, S.; Anttila, P.; Capra, M.; Cavo, M.; Cole, C.; Gasparetto, C.; de Moraes Hungria, V.T.; Jenner, M.W.; Vorobyev, V.I.; et al. Isatuximab as monotherapy and combined with dexamethasone in patients with relapsed/refractory multiple myeloma. *Blood* **2020**. [CrossRef]

69. Martin, T.; Baz, R.; Benson, D.M.; Lendvai, N.; Wolf, J.; Munster, P.; Lesokhin, A.M.; Wack, C.; Charpentier, E.; Campana, F.; et al. A phase 1b study of isatuximab plus lenalidomide and dexamethasone for relapsed/refractory multiple myeloma. *Blood* **2017**, *129*, 3294–3303. [CrossRef]

70. Attal, M.; Richardson, P.G.; Rajkumar, S.V.; San-Miguel, J.; Beksac, M.; Spicka, I.; Leleu, X.; Schjesvold, F.; Moreau, P.; Dimopoulos, M.A.; et al. Isatuximab plus pomalidomide and low-dose dexamethasone versus pomalidomide and low-dose dexamethasone in patients with relapsed and refractory multiple myeloma (ICARIA-MM): A randomised, multicentre, open-label, phase 3 study. *Lancet* **2019**, *394*, 2096–2107. [CrossRef]

71. Schjesvold, F.H.; Richardson, P.G.; Facon, T.; Alegre, A.; Spencer, A.; Jurczyszyn, A.; Sunami, K.; Frenzel, L.; Min, C.-K.; Guillonneau, S.; et al. Isatuximab plus pomalidomide and dexamethasone in elderly patients with relapsed/refractory multiple myeloma: ICARIA-MM subgroup analysis. *Haematologica* **2020**. [CrossRef] [PubMed]

72. Dimopoulos, M.A.; Leleu, X.; Moreau, P.; Richardson, P.G.; Liberati, A.M.; Harrison, S.J.; Prince, H.M.; Ocio, E.M.; Assadourian, S.; Campana, F.; et al. Isatuximab plus pomalidomide and dexamethasone in relapsed/refractory multiple myeloma patients with renal impairment: ICARIA-MM subgroup analysis. *Leukemia* **2020**. [CrossRef] [PubMed]

73. Richardson, P.; Harrison, S.; Facon, T.; Yong, K.; Raje, N.; Alegre, A.; Simpson, D.; Wang, M.-C.; Andrew, S.; Vlummens, P.; et al. Isatuximab plus pomalidomide and dexamethasone in relapsed/refractory multiple myeloma patients with 1q21 gain: Insight from phase 1 and phase 3 studies. *HemaSphere* **2020**, *4*, abstract EP1017.

74. Moreau, P.; Dimopoulos, M.A.; Mikhael, J.; Yong, K.; Capra, M.; Facon, T.; Roman, H.; Spicka, I.; Risse, M.-L.; Asset, G.; et al. Isatuximab plus carfilzomib and dexamethasone vs carfilzomib and dexamethasone in relapsed/refractory multiple myeloma (IKEMA): Interim analysis of a phase 3 randomized, open-label study. *HemaSphere* **2020**, *4*, abstract LB2603.

Monoclonal Antibodies and Airway Diseases

Annina Lyly [1,2,*][iD], Anu Laulajainen-Hongisto [2][iD], Philippe Gevaert [3], Paula Kauppi [4][iD] and Sanna Toppila-Salmi [1,5][iD]

[1] Inflammation Centre, Skin and Allergy Hospital, Helsinki University Hospital, University of Helsinki, P.O. Box 160, 00029 HUS Helsinki, Finland; sanna.salmi@helsinki.fi

[2] Department of Otorhinolaryngology—Head and Neck Surgery, Helsinki University Hospital, University of Helsinki, 00029 HUS Helsinki, Finland; anu.laulajainen-hongisto@hus.fi

[3] Department of Otorhinolaryngology, Upper Airway Research Laboratory, Ghent University Hospital, 9000 Ghent, Belgium; philippe.gevaert@ugent.be

[4] Heart and Lung Center, Pulmonary Department, University of Helsinki and Helsinki University Hospital, 00029 HUS Helsinki, Finland; paula.kauppi@hus.fi

[5] Medicum, Haartman Institute, University of Helsinki, 00029 HUS Helsinki, Finland

* Correspondence: annina.lyly@hus.fi

Abstract: Monoclonal antibodies, biologics, are a relatively new treatment option for severe chronic airway diseases, asthma, allergic rhinitis, and chronic rhinosinusitis (CRS). In this review, we focus on the physiological and pathomechanisms of monoclonal antibodies, and we present recent study results regarding their use as a therapeutic option against severe airway diseases. Airway mucosa acts as a relative barrier, modulating antigenic stimulation and responding to environmental pathogen exposure with a specific, self-limited response. In severe asthma and/or CRS, genome–environmental interactions lead to dysbiosis, aggravated inflammation, and disease. In healthy conditions, single or combined type 1, 2, and 3 immunological response pathways are invoked, generating cytokine, chemokine, innate cellular and T helper (Th) responses to eliminate viruses, helminths, and extracellular bacteria/fungi, correspondingly. Although the pathomechanisms are not fully known, the majority of severe airway diseases are related to type 2 high inflammation. Type 2 cytokines interleukins (IL) 4, 5, and 13, are orchestrated by innate lymphoid cell (ILC) and Th subsets leading to eosinophilia, immunoglobulin E (IgE) responses, and permanently impaired airway damage. Monoclonal antibodies can bind or block key parts of these inflammatory pathways, resulting in less inflammation and improved disease control.

Keywords: airways; asthma; chronic rhinosinusitis; biologicals; monoclonal antibody

1. Introduction

Chronic inflammatory airway diseases include several overlapping morbidities, such as asthma and chronic obstructive pulmonary disease (COPD) in the lower airways; and allergic rhinitis (AR), nonallergic rhinitis (NAR), and chronic rhinosinusitis (CRS) in the upper airways. AR has a prevalence of 20–30%, NAR has a prevalence of 10%, and CRS has a prevalence of 10–20%, and these common diseases cause remarkable suffering and costs [1–3]. They can be subdivided based on such as age of onset, presence of allergy (skin prick test or systemic allergen specific immunoglobulin E (IgE)), with or without nasal polyps and/or T helper (Th) cell 2 prominent inflammation. Exposure to environmental irritants (such as smoking and occupational exposure), recurrent infections, lifestyle factors (such as obesity, stress), co-existing diseases, and genetic/epigenetic factors play a role in disease onset and progression [4,5]. The diagnostic methods include clinical examination, lung function tests, allergy tests, and paranasal sinus computed tomography scans [5–7]. Symptom control of mild cases can be well achieved by the basic treatment such as inhaled/intranasal corticosteroids, inhaled beta agonists, antihistamines, and nasal lavage [5,6].

Patients with moderate to severe forms often suffer from recurrent infective exacerbations and disease recurrence/progression despite maximal baseline therapy and surgeries. Hence, they require advanced diagnostic methods and therapeutics. Antibodies are an important part of humoral adaptive immunity and homeostasis. They also play a role in airway diseases such as IgE in allergy and CRS with nasal polyps (CRSwNP), antibody deficiency in CRS, and aberrant antiviral IgG responses in asthma exacerbations [5,8]. Since their introduction about five decades ago, a wide range of monoclonal antibodies are nowadays commercially available and have been largely used in basic and clinical science of airways. This review focuses on presenting two main airway pathologies of human adults: asthma and CRS. We first introduce monoclonal antibodies and their role in biomarker diagnostics of adult asthma and CRS. Secondly, we present the role of monoclonal antibodies as advanced therapeutics of asthma/CRS.

2. Monoclonal Antibodies

Antibodies (immunoglobulin (Ig) A, IgD, IgE, IgG, IgM) are secreted by B-cells that are activated to plasma cells after antigen presentation in regional lymph nodes or secondary lymphoid organs (Figure 1) [9].

Monoclonal antibodies (mAbs) come from a single B-cell parent clone and recognize specifically a single epitope per antigen [10]. Antibodies are crucial to make leukocytes (such as T killer cells) to detect and destroy pathogens and infected host cells. MAbs are made for laboratory and therapeutic use by various techniques. The first technique described in 1975 was based on creating a hybridoma by combining an activated B-cell from an immunized animal spleen and immortalized myeloma cell, resulting in a stable hybrid cell line producing monoclonal antibody [11]. The first mAbs used in therapeutic purposes were of murine origin, which generated unwanted immunogenic reactions and human anti-mouse antibody formation [12].

The revolution of molecular biology techniques has enabled the production of humanized and fully human mAbs that have helped to tackle this problem, although anti-drug antibodies are still one of the outcomes of immunogenicity [12 For research and laboratory use, there are exponential numbers of commercially available specific monoclonal antibodies for immunoassays such as immunohistochemistry, immunofluorescence and]. enzyme-linked immunosorbent assay (ELISA) [13]. Since their invention about 50 years ago, there has been a large interest to use monoclonal antibodies in experiments to discover relevant proteins and pathways behind airway pathologies [14,15].

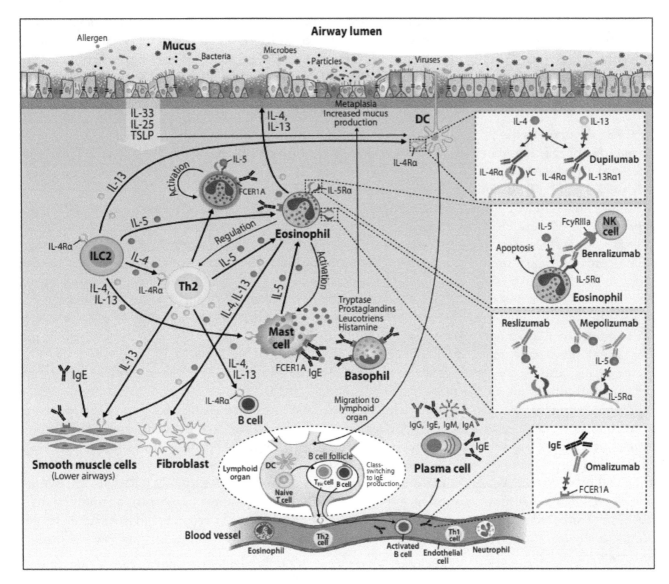

Figure 1. Monoclonal antibodies in the treatment of airway diseases, with their postulated pathways. Abbreviations: DC = dendritic cell, FCER1A = Fc fragment of Immunoglobulin E receptor 1A, FcγRIIIa = Fc fragment of IgG low affinity IIIa receptor, IgA = Immunoglobulin A, IgE = Immunoglobulin E, IgG = Immunoglobulin G, IgM = Immunoglobulin M, IL(-4, -4Rα, -5, -5Rα, -13, -13Rα, -25, -33) = Interleukin(-type), ILC2 = Group 2 innate lymphoid cells, NK cell = Natural killer cell, TFH cell = T follicular helper cell, Th1 = T helper type 1, Th2 = T helper type 2, TSLP = Thymic stromal lymphopoietin.

3. Chronic Inflammatory Airway Diseases

3.1. Asthma and Airway Allergy

Asthma is characterized by reversible lower airway obstruction [6]. Reversible obstruction can be resolved spontaneously by time but also by bronchodilators. Typical asthma symptoms include recurrent or prolonged (over 8 weeks) cough, wheezing, dyspnea, nighttime symptoms, and an overproduction of mucus. Reversible airway obstruction can be diagnosed by spirometry and peak expiratory flow (PEF) monitoring, and bronchial hyperresponsiveness is detected with methacholine or mannitol challenge or by exercise test [6,16,17]. This reversible obstruction is caused by inflammation of bronchus epithelia and is associated with Th2 type inflammation and cytokines in approximately 50% of adult asthma patients. The prevalence of asthma varies, being up to 10% in adults [16]. Severe asthma has been defined as needing drug therapy at Global Initiative for Asthma (GINA) step level 4 or 5 and having recurrent per oral corticosteroid courses or maintenance treatment with per oral corticosteroid or having recurrent exacerbations or at least one severe exacerbation in the last 12 months [6]. Severe uncontrolled asthma is reported in 2.3–3.6% of patients with chronic asthma. Severe uncontrolled eosinophilic asthma has been estimated to form less than 1% of all asthma [18].

3.2. CRS

CRS is defined as the presence of two or more symptoms, one of which is either nasal obstruction or nasal discharge, together with facial pain/pressure or loss of smell, for more than 12 weeks [5]. The overall prevalence of CRS has been estimated to be 10.9%, with wide variation between countries (6.9% to 27.1%) [2]. Traditionally, CRS has been classified into two subtypes: CRS with nasal polyps (CRSwNP) and without nasal polyps (CRSsNP), which is diagnosed after endoscopic evaluation of the presence of bilateral polyps in the middle meatus. Data on the overall prevalence of CRSwNP are limited, but it is estimated to be approximately 2–3% [5,19,20]. However, the inflammatory profile of CRS has proven to be more complex than whether or not polyps are present [21]. Therefore, the new European Position Paper on Rhinosinusitis and Nasal polyps (EPOS) guidelines propose a new clinical classification, which is based first on the etiology (primary vs. secondary) and then the localization of the disease (unilateral vs. bilateral), followed by the evidence of either type 2 or non-type 2 inflammation [5]. The diagnostics of CRS consist of clinical examination including nasal endoscopy, computed tomography imaging, validated patient symptom questionnaires (for example, the sinonasal outcome test SNOT-22), olfactory tests, and histopathologic examination of inflamed tissue [5]. The symptoms are caused by chronic inflammation of the upper airway mucosa, and the prolonged inflammation may cause tissue remodeling [5]. In CRS, the remodeling of sinonasal tissues consists mostly of polyp formation, goblet cell hyperplasia, and epithelial barrier abnormalities. Barrier remodeling results in greater permeability, facilitating prolonged or recurrent CRS [5]. All of these changes are usually seen in type 2 CRS and, despite being only a minority of the cases, the most severe forms of CRS leading to high use of oral corticosteroids/antibiotics and recurrent surgeries are often type 2 CRS [5]. To evaluate the endotype, the combination of phenotype (e.g., CRSwNP, non-steroidal anti-inflammatory drugs (NSAID) exacerbated respiratory disease (N-ERD), co-morbid asthma), response to treatment (surgery, systemic corticosteroids, antibiotics) and also markers such as polyp eosinophilia are key instruments to estimate it [5,22,23].

3.3. Co-Morbid Asthma and CRS

Asthma, CRS, and AR are all multifactorial chronic airway diseases that have partly overlapping pathogenetic mechanisms and risk factors [24]. These environmental risk factors, such as exposure to pollution and tobacco smoke, are linked to asthma and CRS pathogenesis and disease aggravation via the disruption of interplay of epithelial barriers with particles, allergens, and microbes [25,26]. In CRS, the most commonly discussed microbial agent is *Staphylococcus aureus*, but some evidence also implicates dysbiosis of the microbial community as a whole rather than a specific dominant pathogen [5,27].

CRS, AR, and asthma all have several subforms. The main phenotypes of CRS are CRSsNP and CRSwNP [5], yet there are additional subtypes of CRS such as allergic fungal rhinosinusitis, isolated sinusitis, eosinophilic CRS, central compartment allergic disease, and non-eosinophilic CRS. In AR, there is evidence that the sensitization profile and/or allergic multimorbidity are associated with morbidity in children [28] and adults [29]. In asthma, differences are seen between different asthma types in their genetic backgrounds, association with AR and CRS, and possibly also in microbe–host interactions [26]. Childhood-onset asthma is, more often than adult-onset asthma, associated with genetic predisposition, whereas the background of adult-onset asthma is often multifactorial. In adult-onset asthma, the activation of inflammatory molecular pathways leads to persistent mucosal inflammation, variable airway obstruction, and tissue remodeling [30].

Up to 40% of patients with CRSwNP and asthma are hypersensitive to acetylsalicylic acid (ASA) and/or other non-steroidal anti-inflammatory drugs (NSAID) [31]. NSAID exacerbated respiratory disease (N-ERD) usually includes a triad of CRSwNP, asthma, and hypersensitivity to ASA and/or other NSAIDs. Abnormalities of the cyclooxygenase (COX) pathway, severe eosinophilic hyperplastic inflammation, and tissue remodeling with fibrosis in both paranasal sinuses and lower airways are characteristics of N-ERD [32–35]. The treatment of N-ERD consists of conventional asthma and CRS medications; however, repeated oral corticosteroid courses are often also needed [36,37]. The CRSwNP of N-ERD patients is often resistant to medical treatments and may lead to repeated paranasal surgeries.

Oral ASA treatment after desensitization (ATAD) has shown to be effective in improving quality of life (QOL) and total nasal symptom score in patients with N-ERD [5,38]. However, the treatment is associated with adverse effects (typically gastrointestinal) and should be continued strictly on a daily basis [5]. Studies with ATAD show high discontinuation rates, and not all patients benefit from it [5,39]. Monoclonal antibodies have shown efficacy in patients with severe CRS + N-ERD [40–42].

3.4. Mechanisms behind Airway Diseases

The airway epithelium secretes cytokines such as thymic stromal lymphopoietin (TSLP), interleukin 33 (IL-33), and IL-25 in response to tissue damage, pollutants, pathogen recognition, or allergen exposure [43] (Figure 1). These cytokines are involved in the activation of innate lymphoid cells type 2 (ILC2). The activation of ILC2 leads to the release of IL-9, IL-4, IL-13, and IL-5, and to Th2 type inflammation both in asthma and CRS [44–46]. IL-9 has a role in mast cell involvement and airway hyperreactivity [47]. IL-4 and IL-13 are involved in B-cell maturation and IgE production [43]. IL-5 is a growth factor important for the proliferation, maturation, and activation of eosinophils, which associate both with asthmatic inflammation and with (IgE-dependent) allergic inflammation. Eosinophilia, IgE production, and goblet cell hyperplasia result from the Th2 type cytokines [48,49]. Eosinophilic inflammation is found both in allergic and non-allergic conditions. Allergen sensitization is developed when naïve T lymphocytes are differentiated into Th2 type cells and further allergen-specific IgE producing B-cells [7].

CRS is often associated with mucociliary dysfunction [50,51]. Microbial agents, especially S. aureus, and microbiome dysbiosis seem to play an important role in CRS pathogenesis. S. aureus can directly affect mucosal barrier function leading to type 2 inflammation via serine protease-like protein (Spl), TSPL and IL-33 [52,53]. S. aureus colonization is especially common in patients with CRSwNP, but S. aureus-specific IgE has been associated with both CRSwNP and asthma [22,52,53]. Type 2 cytokines inhibit t-PA (tissue plasminogen activator), which results in fibrin mesh deposition to form the nasal polyp tissue matrix [54].

4. The Role of Antibodies in Airway Diseases

Allergic asthma/AR/allergic conjunctivitis are characterized by a type 2 dominated immune response associated with increased serum IgE levels in response to inhaled allergen. Specific IgE for several allergens has been shown to be a risk factor of asthma in children and young adults [55]. There is also evidence that AR is a predisposing factor of adult-onset of asthma [29]. There is no clear evidence of an association between airway allergy and CRS [5].

4.1. IgE

Specific IgE to allergens and pathogens (such as S. aureus superantigens) have been demonstrated in the nasal polyp tissue of CRSwNP patients as well as in the bronchial tissue of asthma patients [56–58]. Local IgE production might play a role in CRSwNP pathogenesis and polyp regrowth after sinus surgery [59]. The mechanisms by which S. aureus leads to type 2 cytokine signaling in airways is not fully understood. S. aureus colonization might benefit from type 2 inflammation, as it may suppress normal immune responses against it. S. aureus secretes superantigenic toxins that modify host immune responses toward the production of local polyclonal IgE [22]. It has been suggested that type 2 inflammation is triggered by *S. aureus* via Toll-like receptor 2, which is a pattern recognition receptor [60–62]. Studies have also been shown that the Asian CRSwNP population has more type 2 low inflammation, and CRSwNP tissue of Asian patients present lower superantigen effects [63,64].

4.2. Other Antibodies

Other antibodies have been less studied in asthma/CRS. Primary antibody deficiencies have been shown to be related to CRS, such as common variable immune deficiency (CVID), selective IgA deficiency, IgG subclass deficiency, and specific antibody deficiency [65]. Airway infections are very frequently involved in triggering asthma or CRS exacerbations [5]. The anti-virus effects of monoclonal antibodies are indirect—for example, improvement of the antiviral capacity of dendritic cells [66]. Antiviral mAb therapy usually directly and rapidly targets the infectious agent, yet evidence has revealed that antiviral mAbs may be used to recruit the endogenous immune systems of infected organisms to induce long-lasting vaccine-like effects [67]. A study of French adult asthmatics has shown that patients hospitalized for asthma exacerbations with a positive virus sample had lower serum IgG level than did their virus negative counterparts [68]. Moreover, longer hospital stays and longer duration of oral steroids were linked to lower serum IgG concentrations, suggesting that severe exacerbations could be related to aberrant antiviral IgG production; however, more studies are needed to confirm this.

5. Monoclonal Antibodies and Diagnostics of Airway Diseases

Monoclonal antibodies are widely used for research purposes of airway diseases and are in clinical use in allergy diagnostics. Blood tests remain an important component in asthma diagnostics; the detection of elevated IgE levels and eosinophils can be used to help identify allergen sensitivity.

5.1. Measurement of Total and Specific IgE in Airway Diseases

Specific IgE (i.e., IgE directed against a specific allergen) and eosinophil counts were confirmed as the most consistent biomarkers to measure the risk of asthma in children [69]. The measurement of specific and total serum IgE levels can be useful to distinguish between allergic and non-allergic asthma, although reports suggest that about 30% of asthmatic patients with a negative skin prick test results have high total circulating IgE (>150 U/mL) [8]. If specific IgEs are considered for selecting an appropriate biologic agent, screening for perennial allergens such as dust mite would have the best rationale [69].

5.2. Potential Biomarkers for Airway Diseases

In order to predict outcomes and therapeutic responses of asthma and/or CRS, there is active research on biomarkers, such as type 1, 2, and 3-related cytokines. Type 1, 2, and 3 responses are evoked by natural mucosal immune responses against viruses/bacteria, parasites, and bacteria/fungi correspondingly, and they are characterized by certain cytokine profiles: IFN-γ and IL-12 in type 1, IL-4, IL-5, and IL-13 in type 2, and IL-17A and IL-22 in type 3 [5]. In pathogen penetration, single or combined type 1, 2, and 3 immunological responses are invoked to eliminate the pathogen, whereas in asthma and CRS, aberrant type 2 responses (and to a lesser extent also type 1 and 3) play a role in airway disease severity and therapeutic responses [70,71].

Patients selected by biomarkers might obtain a greater benefit from therapy with anti-IL-13 mAbs [72]. Elevated bronchial expression of IL-5 and IL-13 has been shown to be associated with sputum and blood eosinophilia and moderate-to-severe asthma [72]. IL-13 and IL-4 regulate the synthesis of IgE and are thus important biomarkers of Th2 cell activation. As a result of IgE binding with the high-affinity receptor (FcεRI) found in basophils and mast cells, there is a cellular activation that ends in the liberation of various inflammatory mediators including cytokines such as IL-5, IL-4, and IL-13. IL-13 and IL-4 also induce periostin. Periostin binds to several integrin molecules on the epithelial cell surface to support the adhesion and migration of epithelial cells, and elevated airway mucosal periostin may be useful in detecting type 2 CRSwNP [73–75] and asthma [76]. Automated immunoassays have been shown to be a potent test for measuring human serum IL-13 [77] and periostin [78] concentrations for clinical purposes. De Schryver et al. have shown that methylprednisolone and omalizumab significantly reduce serum periostin levels and that the periostin expression is in accordance with clinical outcome [79]. However, serum levels of biomarkers are not specific for asthma or CRS. Elevated periostin levels have been detected for example in pulmonary fibrosis and lung carcinoma, and elevated type 2 cytokines or serum IgE in helminth infections and atopic dermatitis [27,80].

6. Monoclonal Antibodies and Treatment of Airway Diseases

Unraveling the pathogenesis of diseases has provided the basis for the pharmaceutical industry to develop protein drugs, or "biologics", with higher specificity and mechanism of action than small molecule drugs. In 2015, monoclonal antibodies were the most important class of biologics approved by the United States Food and Drug Administration (FDA) [81], and their utilization in therapy has rapidly increased since. Personalized medicine is addressing the issue of providing targeted treatment for the right patient [82]. The endotype-driven treatment approach requires careful selection of the patient population who might benefit from a treatment by advanced therapies [83,84]. In the following chapter, mAbs used to treat asthma and CRSwNP are introduced; their main mechanisms of actions are illustrated in Figure 1.

6.1. Commercially Available Monoclonal Antibodies and Their Mechanisms of Action

6.1.1. Omalizumab—Anti-IgE

In the fast phase of allergic reaction, allergen-specific IgE produced by B-cells binds to high affinity FcR (FcεRI) expressed on immune cells such as basophils and mast cells. Then, allergen exposure can lead to antigen cross-linking IgE molecules on the same mast cell, receptor aggregation, and initiation of the intracellular signal cascade leading to degranulation and the release of histamine, prostaglandins, and cytokines that mediate the clinical manifestations of atopy [85]. Omalizumab, a humanized IgG1/k monoclonal antibody, targets the Fc region of IgE, and by binding to free IgE in blood and body fluids, it neutralizes the ability of IgE to bind to its receptor (FcεRI, high-affinity receptor and FcεRII, low-affinity receptor) [86]. On top of inhibiting the cross-linking on mast cells, this induces the down-regulation of IgE receptor expression on other immune cells such as basophils and dendritic cells [87,88]. Omalizumab was the first biological therapy developed for asthma, and it has now been used for 15 years. During these years, the functions of IgE in bronchial asthma have proven to be more complex than that of the classical role in allergy and anaphylaxis (reviewed in [89]). For example, smooth muscle cells in lung tissue have receptors for IgE, and it is involved in their proliferation, independent of the presence of allergens. IgE also plays a role in non-allergic diseases such as chronic idiopathic urticaria and CRSwNP and is involved in eosinophilic inflammation [89].

6.1.2. Mepolizumab and Reslizumab—Anti-IL-5

Type 2 inflammation present in asthma and CRSwNP is featured with airway eosinophilic infiltration, particularly in nasal polyps. Eosinophils are also frequently elevated in peripheral blood in type 2 asthma. High eosinophil levels are associated with exacerbations and bronchial obstruction [90]. The key mediator of eosinophils is interleukin-5 (IL5), being responsible for their differentiation, growth, activation, and survival as well as recruitment to airways [91,92]. Mepolizumab is a humanized IgG1/k monoclonal antibody toward IL-5, binding to it with high affinity and preventing its linkage to IL-5Rα [93,94]. Reslizumab is a humanized IgG4/κ monoclonal antibody specifically interacting with the epitope IL-5 uses to bind its receptor IL-5Ra, thereby blocking its bioactivity [95].

6.1.3. Benralizumab—Anti-IL-5Ralpha

Different from mepolizumab and reslizumab, benralizumab binds to IL-5-receptor instead of its ligand. Benralizumab is an afucosylated humanized IgG1/κ monoclonal antibody, selectively recognizing the IL-5Rα subunit [96]. The interaction of benralizumab with IL-5Rα prevents IL-5 binding to target cells and impedes the heterodimerization of IL-5Rα and βc subunits, thus inhibiting the activation of IL-5-dependent signaling cascades. In addition, benralizumab binds to the FcγRIIIa membrane receptor expressed by natural killer cells through the constant Fc region. FcγRIIIa activation induces the eosinophil apoptosis mechanism called antibody-dependent cell-mediated cytotoxicity, which is amplified by afucosylation [97], resulting in depletion of the blood eosinophils. A recent study describes also reduction in the number of basophiles after treatment with benralizumab [98].

6.1.4. Dupilumab—Anti IL-4Ralpha

Dupilumab is a fully human monoclonal antibody to the interleukin-4 receptor α subunit, IL-4Ralpha, which is utilized by two cytokines IL-4 and IL-13 [99]. IL-4 mediates its biological effects by binding to IL-4Rα, which is followed by the recruitment of either gamma c or IL-13 receptor alpha 1 (IL-13Rα1) to form a signaling complex [100]. IL-13 binds to IL-13Rα1 and then forms a signaling complex by recruiting IL-4Rα [100]. Altogether, IL-4Ralpha is involved in three different combinations of receptor complexes, and the intracellular response potencies are varied between the binding ligand, IL-4 vs. IL-13 [100,101].

Due to the shared receptor, IL-4 and IL-13 also have overlapping functions, and these sister cytokines act both cooperatively as well as independently in type 2 inflammation cascades. Both interleukins promote B-cell proliferation and class switch to IgG4 and IgE [102]. IL-13 is a cytokine secreted by activated Th2 cells, and it acts as an important mediator of allergic inflammation pathogenesis. Distinct functions for IL-13 include tissue remodeling, goblet cell mucus hypersecretion, subepithelial fibrosis, and emphysematous changes [103]. IL-4 and IL-13 can both induce Th2 cells and epithelial cells to produce eosinophil-promoting factors (i.e., IL-5 and eotaxins) and stimulate eosinophils to migrate to sites of inflammation from blood [104]. However, a recent murine model study shows that only dual IL-4/IL-13 blockade prevented type 2 inflammation broadly enough to prevent lung-function impairment—blocking only IL-4 or IL-13 alone was not enough to provide major clinical benefits [105]. This has been seen also in clinical experiments with IL-4 and IL-13 blockers for the treatment of type 2 diseases [106]. Dual blockade of IL-4/IL-13 with dupilumab halted eosinophil infiltration into lung tissue in mouse model without affecting circulating eosinophils, demonstrating that tissue, but not circulating eosinophils, contribute to disease pathology [105].

6.2. Monoclonal Antibodies in Asthma Treatment

Monoclonal antibodies are considered as a treatment option for severe asthma [107]. First, the patient's symptoms are carefully assessed in order to estimate if the patient truly has asthma, if the current symptoms are associated with asthma, if the current asthma drug therapy is adequate, if the patient is adherent for the drug therapy, and that there are no environmental factors that should be considered [17,107]. Poor symptom control, frequent yearly exacerbations or serious exacerbations, and diminished lung function are signs of uncontrolled asthma and an indication for biologicals if the situation is not controlled with other maximal medication [107]. Controlled asthma that deteriorates if high-dose inhaled corticosteroids or systemic corticosteroids are tapered is another indication for biologicals [107].

The selection of a suitable drug is based both on allergy (whether the patient has allergic asthma to perennial allergens) but also on eosinophils (whether the patient has high or low blood eosinophils) [108]. Contradictory to biologicals in rheumatic diseases, the biologicals targeting IgE or Th2 cytokines have been well tolerated and safe to use [109,110]. The commercially available antibodies and their therapeutic use is summarized in Table 1.

Table 1. Monoclonal antibodies in the treatment of different airway diseases.

Therapy (Target)	Asthma	CRSwNP	Dose	Response
Omalizumab (anti-IgE)	Severe allergic asthma with perennial allergy	Approved as add-on therapy for adults with severe CRSwNP by EMA in August 2020 Pending FDA approval [41]	According to weight and total S-IgE value, every 2–4 weeks s.c.	Asthma: Reduction in exacerbations, improvement in symptoms, asthma related QoL↑, FEV1↑ CRSwNP: Reduction in symptom score and nasal polyp score
Mepolizumab (anti-IL5)	Severe eosinophilic asthma with B-eos>300cells/ul	Ongoing studies for use in CRSwNP [41]	100 or 300 mg s.c. every four weeks	Asthma: Reduction in exacerbations, improvement in symptoms, B-eos ↓, asthma related QoL↑, FEV1↑
Reslizumab (anti-IL5)	Severe eosinophilic asthma with B-eos>400cells/ul	Ongoing studies	According to weight every four weeks i.v.	Asthma: Reduction in exacerbations, improvement in symptoms, B-eos↓, Asthma related QoL↑, FEV1↑
Benralizumab (anti-IL5R)	Severe eosinophilic asthma with B-eos>300cells/ul	Ongoing studies for use in CRSwNP [41]	30 mg every 4 weeks s.c. three times and then 30 mg every 8 weeks s.c.	Asthma: Reduction in exacerbations, improvement in symptoms, B-eos↓
Dupilumab (anti-IL4Ralpha)	Severe eosinophilic asthma with B-eos>300cells/ul	Severe CRSwNP (approved by EMA and FDA)	First dose of 400 mg/600 mg s.c. according to weight, then 200 mg/300 mg every 2 weeks s.c.	Asthma: Reduction in exacerbations, improvement in symptoms, B-eos ↓, Asthma related QoL↑, FEV1↑ CRSwNP: polyp size reduction, reduction in OCS and surgeries, improvement in symptom score

Abbreviations: B-eos = blood eosinophils, CRSwNP = chronic rhinosinusitis with nasal polyps, EMA = European Medicines Agency, FDA = U.S. Food and Drug Administration, FEV1 = forced expiratory volume in one second, i.v. = intravenous, NO = nitric oxide, OCS = oral corticosteroids, s.c. = subcutaneous, QoL = Quality of Life.

The first monoclonal antibody treatment for lower airway diseases was anti-IgE therapy with omalizumab. After that, anti-IL5-, anti-IL-5Ralpha- and anti-IL-4R-treatment have been introduced for the treatment of asthma. These monoclonal antibodies are humanized IgG antibodies and selective for their binding capacity. Both anti-IL-5 and anti-IL-5Ralpha-antibody treatment may be associated with anti-drug-antibody development [12].

Omalizumab is indicated as an add-on therapy in adults and children over six years for inadequately controlled severe asthma. Omalizumab reduces asthma exacerbations by OR 0.55 (95% CI 0.42–0.60) and hospitalizations by OR 0.16 (95% CI 0.06–0.42) [111,112]. Furthermore, it is beneficial in the reduction of inhaled corticosteroids [111].

Mepolizumab, reslizumab (anti-IL-5), and benralizumab (anti-IL-5Ra) are used for severe eosinophilic asthma. Mepolizumab reduces exacerbations by approximately 50% in patients with eosinophils at least 150 cells/uL at screening or at least 300 cells/uL in the previous year and high-dose inhaled corticosteroids and at least one additional controller medication [113]. In addition, improvement in QOL, asthma control measures with asthma control questionnaire, and lung function (FEV1) have been reported [113]. Furthermore, mepolizumab has been shown to reduce oral corticosteroid need [113]. Reslizumab reduces asthma exacerbations by OR0.50 (95% CI 0.37–0.67) in patients with medium-to-high dose inhaled corticosteroids and blood eosinophils at least 400 cells per uL and one or more exacerbations in the previous year [114,115].

Benralizumab reduces exacerbations and the need of per oral glucocorticosteroids, and it improves QOL and lung function not only in clinical trials but also in real-world studies [110,116,117]. Benralizumab has been reported to reduce asthma exacerbations from 4.9 to 1.3 per year and to reduce daily prednisolone dose from a median 10 to 0 mg [117].

Dupilumab (anti IL-4Ralpha) reduces asthma exacerbations and improves lung function in patients with moderate to severe asthma [118]. Furthermore, with dupilumab treatment dose of maintenance, oral glucocorticoids can be reduced. Reduction in the oral glucocorticoid dose and elimination of per oral glucocorticoids is more likely in the asthma patients with the baseline level of eosinophils at least 300 cells/mm^3 [118]. A transient rise in eosinophils is seen more often in the dupilumab-treated patients when compared to placebo-treated patients [118]. In addition, injection-site reactions were more common in the dupilumab-treated patients.

6.3. Monoclonal Antibodies in CRS Treatment

Targeted monoclonal antibody therapies have shown encouraging results in the management of severe CRSwNP. As type 2 CRSwNP and asthma largely overlap, also therapeutics are in some cases targeted to both severe asthma and severe CRSwNP. According to the European Position Paper on Rhinosinusitis and Nasal polyps 2020 (EPOS 2020) guidelines, the indications for using biological treatment for CRSwNP include bilateral polyps and at least one previous endoscopic sinus surgery, together with at least three of the following criteria: evidence of type 2 inflammation, need for systemic corticosteroids (or contraindication for it), significantly impaired quality of life, significant loss of smell, or diagnosis of comorbid asthma. The effect of the treatment should be evaluated after 4 months and 1 year, and in case there is no response, treatment should be discontinued [5].

Anti-IgE therapy (omalizumab) is the second and latest biologic therapy approved for CRSwNP by the European Medicines Agency (EMA) in August 2020, and it is pending FDA approval for CRSwNP [41]. A study by Gevaert et al. has shown a decrease of symptom score for nasal congestion, anterior rhinorrhoea, loss of sense of smell, wheeze and dyspnea, and a significant reduction of endoscopic nasal polyp score, radiologic Lund–MacKay score, and asthma symptoms [119]. Another randomized controlled trial (RCT) by Pinto et al. showed improvement in symptoms, but no significant improvement in Lund–Mackay score or other endpoints [120]. In a recent study on patients with N-ERD, both nasal and lung symptoms improved significantly with omalizumab treatment [121]. However, these studies were small, with only around 20 patients in each group. Recent results from two bigger phase 3 RCTs of 265 patients has shown that omalizumab significantly reduced endoscopic nasal polyp score, nasal congestion score, and SNOT-22 score compared to placebo at week 24 [122]. Patients with comorbid asthma reported significant improvement in Asthma Quality of Life Questionnaire scores [122].

Anti-IL-5 treatment with reslizumab was found to decrease nasal polyp scores in an RCT, in which patients received a single injection of reslizumab ($n = 16$) or placebo ($n = 8$) [123]. Studies with mepolizumab have shown a significant reduction in patients' need for surgery and an improvement in symptoms [5,124,125]. A Cochrane review summarized that mepolizumab may improve both disease-specific and generic health-related quality of life (HRQL), yet its effect to reduce surgery or improve nasal polyp score is uncertain [126]. At the moment, phase 3 RCTs are ongoing for both benralizumab and mepolizumab, altogether with over 800 patients with severe CRSwNP [41]. More information about the efficacy of anti-IL-5-treatments will be available after they are finished. However, preliminary results of RCT of 407 patients has shown that mepolizumab significantly reduced endoscopic nasal polyp score, nasal obstruction VAS score, VAS (overall, composite, loss of smell), SNOT22 score, and the need for surgery [127]. Nasopharyngitis was the most common adverse event in this study (23–25%) [127].

An anti-IL-4/IL-13 drug, dupilumab, is the first monoclonal antibody approved for the treatment of CRSwNP in 2019 [5]. Before that, it has been used for the treatment of asthma since 2018 and atopic dermatitis since 2017. In a double-blind RCT (DBRCT) with 276 patients with severe CRSwNP using regular topical nasal steroids, dupilumab reduced polyp size, sinus opacification, and severity of symptoms (nasal congestion and obstruction, sense of smell) compared with placebo. It also diminished the need for rescue treatment with systemic corticosteroids and sinus surgery [128]. A Cochrane review summarizes that dupilumab has been shown to improve disease-specific HRQL compared to placebo, and it might improve symptoms and generic HRQL and reduce the need for further surgery [126]. Moreover, there is no evidence of an increased risk of serious adverse events; however, there may be little or no difference in the risk of nasopharyngitis [126]. Among dupilumab-treated atopic dermatitis patients, conjunctivitis is the most common side effect [129]. However, in patients with asthma and CRSwNP, the incidence of conjunctivitis was very low, similar as for placebo [129].

6.4. Future Monoclonal Antibody Treatments for Airway Diseases

6.4.1. Anti-TSLP

Thymic stromal lymphopoietin (TSLP) is produced by fibroblasts and epithelium and plays a role in T cell maturation. TSLP enhances IL type2 cytokine production in mast cells and activates ILC2s together with IL-33 or IL-25. TSLP has shown to associate with asthma and CRSwNP after virus challenge [130]. Tezepelumab (AMG-157/MEDI9929) is a human anti-TSLP antibody. A DBRCT of 31 mild asthmatics has shown that AMG-157 attenuated allergen-induced early and late asthmatic responses, and it decreased blood and sputum eosinophils [131]. Anti-OX40L promotes regulatory T (Treg) cells and suppresses T-cell mediated inflammation, and hence, it might be a potential therapeutic target for severe asthma [132]. Yet, in a study that used a combination of anti-OX40L and anti-TSLP, the expected effects on Treg-mediated inflammation was not observed [133]. Tezepelumab (anti-TSLP) decreases exacerbations and improves lung function measured by FEV1 (forced expiratory volume in one second) statistically significantly compared to placebo in patients with medium-to-high dose inhaled corticosteroids and long-acting beta-2-agonist [134]. The exacerbation rates were 61–71% lower than in the placebo group depending on the dose of the tezepelumab [134]. A reduction in asthma exacerbations was found irrespective of eosinophil level.

6.4.2. Anti-TNF

Type 2 low pathways might also comprise future targets for monoclonal antibody therapy [135]. Anti-TNF could have potential in patients with neutrophilic non-infectious COPD [136] and in severe asthma with mixed type 1/type2 [137,138]. ILC3s secrete IL-17, which leads to airway mucosal neutrophilia in some forms of asthma and CRS. A randomized, placebo-controlled double-blind trial was performed in 300 patients with moderate to severe asthma by using anti-IL-17, brodalumab, and it did not show a remarkable effect [139].

6.4.3. Anti-IL-8

Neutrophils have surface IL-8 receptors and are the main target cells for IL-8 responses. Anti-IL-8R, CXCR2, has been shown to reduce airway neutrophilia [140]. Two placebo-controlled studies with CXCR2 antagonists have been performed in severe (neutrophilic) asthma patients [141,142]. The results did not show clinical effectiveness; however, in one of the studies, a reduction in sputum and blood neutrophils was observed [141].

6.4.4. CRTH2 Antagonists

In addition to monoclonal antibodies, other molecules are also under investigation for future therapeutics of airway diseases. An example of these are chemoattractant receptor-homologous molecule (CRTH2) antagonists. Prostaglandin D2 (PGD2) is an arachidonic acid metabolite of the cyclooxygenase (COX) pathway. It plays a role in the pathophysiology of allergic rhinitis, CRS, and asthma [143]. PGD2 acts via DP1 and DP2 receptors, and CRTH2. PGD2 links adaptive and innate immune pathways via DP2 receptors located on Th2 cells, ILC2s, and eosinophils. Hence, PGD2 might be a good target for type 2 disorders [144,145]. CRTH2 antagonists represent a category of small molecules that have been discovered to have therapeutic potential for asthma [146,147]. CRTH2 antagonists have decreased the allergen-mediated airway responses of the upper [148] and lower airways [149,150]. CRTH2 antagonist has been given as monotherapy or in combination with standard therapy to patients with mild to moderate asthma, and it has shown a modest effectiveness on symptom scores, disease control, lung function, and inflammatory markers [151–154]. CRTH2 antagonists are proposed to have therapeutic effectiveness similar to antihistamines [148] and leukotriene receptor antagonists [5,154]. Dual DP/CRTH2 antagonist (AMG853) treatment for 12 weeks failed to show clinical effectiveness in patients with moderate to severe asthma [155]. Another CRTH2 receptor antagonist, fevipiprant, for 12 weeks, has shown to improve clinical and physiological parameters and to reduce airway eosinophils in patients with moderate-severe asthma [154], and it reduced asthma exacerbations moderately, but not significantly, in 52-week phase 3 trials in patients with severe asthma [156].

7. Conclusions

Taken together, monoclonal antibodies have several physiological and pathomechanistic roles in asthma, allergic rhinitis, and chronic rhinosinusitis. Local IgE production has been mostly studied. Future studies of other antibodies and their role in the pathomechanisms of inflammatory airway diseases are needed. Several monoclonal antibody treatments have indication for severe type 2 asthma; these are anti-IgE omalizumab, anti-IL-5 mepolizumab/reslizumab, anti-IL-5R benralizumab and anti-IL-4Ralpha dupilumab. Studies show that these treatments have an effect in patients with co-morbid severe type 2 asthma and CRS. For the treatment of severe CRSwNP, dupilumab and omalizumab are currently approved, and more are probably to come in the future. In addition to ongoing trials of the above-mentioned monoclonal antibodies, several other monoclonal antibodies are under active investigation. In addition to type 2 diseases, there is a high need to investigate therapeutic targets also for type 2 low asthma and CRS.

Author Contributions: Conceptualization and methodology, S.T.-S. and P.K.; resources, S.T.-S.; writing—original draft preparation, A.L., A.L-H., P.K. and S.T.-S.; writing—review and editing, P.G.; visualization, A.L., and A.L.-H.; supervision, P.G.; project administration, S.T.-S. All authors have read and agreed to the published version of the manuscript.

Acknowledgments: We thank Helena Schmidt for the illustration.

Abbreviations

CRS	Chronic rhinosinusitis
CRSwNP	Chronic rhinosinusitis with nasal polyps
N-ERD	NSAID-exacerbated respiratory disease
mAb	Monoclonal antibody
RCT	Randomized controlled trial

References

1. Dierick, B.J.; Van Der Molen, T.; Flokstra-de-Blok, B.M.J.; Muraro, A.; Postma, M.J.; Kocks, J.W.; Van Boven, J.F. Burden and socioeconomics of asthma, allergic rhinitis, atopic dermatitis and food allergy. *Expert Rev. Pharm. Outcomes Res.* **2020**, 1–17. [CrossRef] [PubMed]

2. Hastan, D.; Fokkens, W.; Bachert, C.; Newson, R.B.; Bislimovska, J.; Bockelbrink, A.; Bousquet, P.J.; Brozek, G.; Bruno, A.; Dahlén, S.E.; et al. Chronic rhinosinusitis in Europe—An Underestimated Disease. A GA2LEN study. *Allergy* **2011**, *66*, 1216–1223. [CrossRef] [PubMed]

3. Settipane, R.A.; Kaliner, M. Nonallergic Rhinitis. *Am. J. Rhinol. Allergy* **2013**, *27*, S48–S51. [CrossRef] [PubMed]

4. Toskala, E.; Kennedy, D.W. Asthma risk factors. *Int. Forum Allergy Rhinol.* **2015**, *5*, S11–S16. [CrossRef] [PubMed]

5. Fokkens, W.J.; Lund, V.J.; Hopkins, C.; Hellings, P.W.; Kern, R.; Reitsma, S.; Toppila-Salmi, S.; Bernal-Sprekelsen, M.; Mullol, J.; Alobid, I.; et al. European Position Paper on Rhinosinusitis and Nasal Polyps 2020. *Rhinology* **2020**, *58*, 1–464. [CrossRef] [PubMed]

6. Global Strategy for Asthma Management and Prevention. Available online: www.ginasthma.org (accessed on 20 April 2020).

7. Bousquet, J.; Anto, J.M.; Bachert, C.; Baiardini, I.; Bosnic-Anticevich, S.; Canonica, G.W.; Melen, E.; Palomares, O.; Scadding, G.K.; Togias, A.; et al. Allergic rhinitis. *Nat. Rev.* **2020**, *6*, 1–17.

8. Barnes, P.J. Intrinsic asthma: Not so different from allergic asthma but driven by superantigens? *Clin. Exp. Allergy* **2009**, *39*, 1145–1151. [CrossRef]

9. Panda, S.; Ding, J.L. Natural Antibodies Bridge Innate and Adaptive Immunity. *J. Immunol.* **2014**, *194*, 13–20. [CrossRef]

10. Marshall, J.S.; Warrington, R.; Watson, W.; Kim, H.L. An introduction to immunology and immunopathology. *Allergy Asthma Clin. Immunol.* **2018**, *14*, 1–10. [CrossRef]

11. Köhler, G.; Milstein, C. Continuous cultures of fused cells secreting antibody of predefined specificity. *Nature* **1975**, *256*, 495–497. [CrossRef]

12. Vaisman-Mentesh, A.; Gutierrez-Gonzalez, M.; DeKosky, B.J.; Wine, Y. The Molecular Mechanisms That Underlie the Immune Biology of Anti-drug Antibody Formation Following Treatment with Monoclonal Antibodies. *Front. Immunol.* **2020**, *11*, 11. [CrossRef] [PubMed]

13. Wang, L.L.; Moshiri, A.S.; Novoa, R.; Simpson, C.L.; Takeshita, J.; Payne, A.S.; Chu, E.Y. Comparison of C3d immunohistochemical staining to enzyme-linked immunosorbent assay and immunofluorescence for diagnosis of bullous pemphigoid. *J. Am. Acad. Dermatol.* **2020**, *83*, 172–178. [CrossRef] [PubMed]

14. Black, C.A. A brief history of the discovery of the immunoglobulins and the origin of the modern immunoglobulin nomenclature. *Immunol. Cell Biol.* **1997**, *75*, 65–68. [CrossRef] [PubMed]

15. Platts-Mills, T.A.; Heymann, P.W.; Commins, S.P.; Woodfolk, J.A. The discovery of IgE 50 years later. *Ann. Allergy Asthma Immunol.* **2016**, *116*, 179–182. [CrossRef]

16. McCracken, J.L.; Veeranki, S.P.; Ameredes, B.T.; Calhoun, W.J. Diagnosis and management of asthma in adults a review. *JAMA—J. Am. Med. Assoc.* **2017**, *318*, 279–290. [CrossRef]
17. Porsbjerg, C.; Ulrik, C.; Skjold, T.; Backer, V.; Laerum, B.; Lehman, S.; Janson, C.; Sandstrøm, T.; Bjermer, L.; Dahlen, B.; et al. Nordic consensus statement on the systematic assessment and management of possible severe asthma in adults. *Eur. Clin. Respir. J.* **2018**, *5*, 1440868. [CrossRef]
18. Kerkhof, M.; Tran, T.N.; Soriano, J.B.; Golam, S.; Gibson, D.; Hillyer, E.V.; Price, D. Healthcare resource use and costs of severe, uncontrolled eosinophilic asthma in the UK general population. *Thorax* **2017**, *73*, 116–124. [CrossRef]
19. Larsen, K.; Tos, M. The Estimated Incidence of Symptomatic Nasal Polyps. *Acta Oto-Laryngol.* **2002**, *122*, 179–182. [CrossRef]
20. Johansson, L.; Åkerlund, A.; Melén, I.; Holmberg, K.; Bende, M. Prevalence of Nasal Polyps in Adults: The Skovde Population-Based Study. *Ann. Otol. Rhinol. Laryngol.* **2003**, *112*, 625–629. [CrossRef]
21. McCormick, J.P.; Thompson, H.M.; Cho, D.-Y.; Woodworth, B.A.; Grayson, J.W. Phenotypes in Chronic Rhinosinusitis. *Curr. Allergy Asthma Rep.* **2020**, *20*, 1–8. [CrossRef]
22. Tomassen, P.; Vandeplas, G.; Van Zele, T.; Cardell, L.; Arebro, J.; Olze, H.; Förster-Ruhrmann, U.; Kowalski, M.L.; Olszewska-Ziąber, A.; Holtappels, G.; et al. Inflammatory endotypes of chronic rhinosinusitis based on cluster analysis of biomarkers. *J. Allergy Clin. Immunol.* **2016**, *137*, 1449–1456.e4. [CrossRef] [PubMed]
23. Lyly, A.; Laulajainen-Hongisto, A.; Turpeinen, H.; Vento, S.I.; Myller, J.; Numminen, J.; Sillanpää, S.; Sahlman, J.; Kauppi, P.; Toppila-Salmi, S. Factors affecting upper airway control of NSAID-exacerbated respiratory disease: A real-world study of 167 patients. *Immun. Inflamm. Dis.* **2020**, in press. [CrossRef]
24. Jarvis, D.; Newson, R.; Lotvall, J.; Hastan, D.; Tomassen, P.; Keil, T.; Gjomarkaj, M.; Forsberg, B.; Gunnbjornsdottir, M.; Minov, J.; et al. Asthma in adults and its association with chronic rhinosinusitis: The GA2LEN survey in Europe. *Allergy* **2012**, *67*, 91–98. [CrossRef] [PubMed]
25. Bashiardes, S.; Zilberman-Schapira, G.; Elinav, E. Use of Metatranscriptomics in Microbiome Research. *Bioinform. Biol. Insights* **2016**, *10*, BBI.S34610–25. [CrossRef] [PubMed]
26. Laulajainen-Hongisto, A.; Toppila-Salmi, S.K.; Luukkainen, A.; Kern, R. Airway Epithelial Dynamics in Allergy and Related Chronic Inflammatory Airway Diseases. *Front. Cell Dev. Biol.* **2020**, *8*, 204. [CrossRef] [PubMed]
27. Gause, W.C.; Rothlin, C.; Loke, P. Heterogeneity in the initiation, development and function of type 2 immunity. *Nat. Rev. Immunol.* **2020**, *20*, 603–614. [CrossRef] [PubMed]
28. Gough, H.; Grabenhenrich, L.; Reich, A.; Eckers, N.; Nitsche, O.; Schramm, D.; Beschorner, J.; Hoffmann, U.; Schuster, A.; Bauer, C.; et al. Allergic multimorbidity of asthma, rhinitis and eczema over 20 years in the German birth cohort MAS. *Pediatric Allergy Immunol.* **2015**, *26*, 431–437. [CrossRef] [PubMed]
29. Toppila-Salmi, S.; Chanoine, S.; Karjalainen, J.; Pekkanen, J.; Bousquet, J.; Siroux, V. Risk of adult-onset asthma increases with the number of allergic multimorbidities and decreases with age. *Allergy* **2019**, *74*, 2406–2416. [CrossRef]
30. Willis-Owen, S.A.; Cookson, W.O.; Moffatt, M.F. The Genetics and Genomics of Asthma. *Annu. Rev. Genom. Hum. Genet.* **2018**, *19*, 223–246. [CrossRef]
31. Stevenson, D.D.; Szczeklik, A. Clinical and pathologic perspectives on aspirin sensitivity and asthma. *J. Allergy Clin. Immunol.* **2006**, *118*, 773–786. [CrossRef]
32. White, A.A.; Stevenson, D.D. Aspirin-Exacerbated Respiratory Disease. *N. Engl. J. Med.* **2018**, *379*, 1060–1070. [CrossRef] [PubMed]
33. Kowalski, M.L.; Agache, I.; Bavbek, S.; Bakirtas, A.; Blanca, M.; Bochenek, G.; Bonini, M.; Heffler, E.; Klimek, L.; Laidlaw, T.M.; et al. Diagnosis and Management of NSAID-Exacerbated Respiratory Disease (N-ERD)—A EAACI Position Paper. *Allergy* **2018**, *74*, 28–39. [CrossRef] [PubMed]
34. Mascia, K.; Haselkorn, T.; Deniz, Y.M.; Miller, D.P.; Bleecker, E.R.; Borish, L. Aspirin sensitivity and severity of asthma: Evidence for irreversible airway obstruction in patients with severe or difficult-to-treat asthma. *J. Allergy Clin. Immunol.* **2005**, *116*, 970–975. [CrossRef] [PubMed]
35. Roca-Ferrer, J.; Perez-Gonzalez, M.; Garcia-Garcia, F.J.; Pereda, J.; Pujols, L.; Alobid, I.; Mullol, J.; Picado, C. Low prostaglandin E2 and cyclooxygenase expression in nasal mucosa fibroblasts of aspirin-intolerant asthmatics. *Respirology* **2013**, *18*, 711–717. [CrossRef]

36. Velazquez, J.R.; Teran, L.M. Aspirin-Intolerant Asthma: A Comprehensive Review of Biomarkers and Pathophysiology. *Clin. Rev. Allergy Immunol.* **2012**, *45*, 75–86. [CrossRef]

37. Fokkens, W.J.; Lund, V.J.; Mullol, J.; Bachert, C.; Alobid, I.; Baroody, F.; Cohen, N.; Cervin, A.; Douglas, R.; Gevaert, P.; et al. EPOS 2012: European position paper on rhinosinusitis and nasal polyps 2012. A summary for otorhinolaryngologists. *Rhinol. J.* **2012**, *50*, 1–12. [CrossRef]

38. Stevenson, D.D.; Simon, R.A.; Mathison, D.A. Aspirin-sensitive asthma: Tolerance to aspirin after positive oral aspirin challenges. *J. Allergy Clin. Immunol.* **1980**, *66*, 82–88. [CrossRef]

39. Laulajainen-Hongisto, A.; Turpeinen, H.; Vento, S.I.; Numminen, J.; Sahlman, J.; Kauppi, P.; Virkkula, P.; Hytönen, M.; Toppila-Salmi, S. High Discontinuation Rates of Peroral ASA Treatment for CRSwNP: A Real-World Multicenter Study of 171 N-ERD Patients. *J. Allergy Clin. Immunol. Pract.* **2020**, *8*, 3565–3574. [CrossRef]

40. Iqbal, I.Z.; Kao, S.S.; Ooi, E.H. The role of biologics in chronic rhinosinusitis: A systematic review. *Int. Forum Allergy Rhinol.* **2019**, *10*, 165–174. [CrossRef]

41. Kim, C.; Han, J.; Wu, T.; Bachert, C.; Fokkens, W.; Hellings, P.; Hopkins, C.; Lee, S.; Mullol, J.; Lee, J.T. Role of Biologics in Chronic Rhinosinusitis with Nasal Polyposis: State of the Art Review. *Otolaryngol. Neck Surg.* **2020**. [CrossRef]

42. Laidlaw, T.M.; Buchheit, K.M. Biologics in chronic rhinosinusitis with nasal polyposis. *Ann. Allergy Asthma Immunol.* **2020**, *124*, 326–332. [CrossRef] [PubMed]

43. Eyerich, S.; Metz, M.; Bossios, A.; Eyerich, K. New biological treatments for asthma and skin allergies. *Allergy* **2020**, *75*, 546–560. [CrossRef] [PubMed]

44. Licona-Limon, P.; Kim, L.K.; Palm, N.W.; Flavell, R. TH2, allergy and group 2 innate lymphoid cells. *Nat. Immunol.* **2013**, *14*, 536–542. [CrossRef] [PubMed]

45. Scadding, G. Cytokine profiles in allergic rhinitis topical collection on rhinitis. *Curr. Allergy Asthma Rep.* **2014**, *14*, 326–332. [CrossRef]

46. Toppila-Salmi, S.; Van Drunen, C.M.; Fokkens, W.J.; Golebski, K.; Mattila, P.; Joenväärä, S.; Renkonen, J.; Renkonen, R. Molecular mechanisms of nasal epithelium in rhinitis and rhinosinusitis. *Curr. Allergy Asthma Rep.* **2015**, *15*, 495. [CrossRef]

47. Cheng, G.; Arima, M.; Honda, K.; Hirata, H.; Eda, F.; Yoshida, N.; Fukushima, F.; Ishii, Y.; Fukuda, T. Anti–Interleukin-9 Antibody Treatment Inhibits Airway Inflammation and Hyperreactivity in Mouse Asthma Model. *Am. J. Respir. Crit. Care Med.* **2002**, *166*, 409–416. [CrossRef]

48. Whitsett, J.A.; Alenghat, T. Respiratory epithelial cells orchestrate pulmonary innate immunity. *Nat. Immunol.* **2015**, *16*, 27–35. [CrossRef]

49. Athari, S.S. Targeting cell signaling in allergic asthma. *Signal Transduct. Target. Ther.* **2019**, *4*, 1–19. [CrossRef]

50. Cutting, G.R. Modifier Genetics: Cystic Fibrosis. *Annu. Rev. Genom. Hum. Genet.* **2005**, *6*, 237–260. [CrossRef]

51. Gudis, D.; Zhao, K.-Q.; Cohen, N.A. Acquired Cilia Dysfunction in Chronic Rhinosinusitis. *Am. J. Rhinol. Allergy* **2012**, *26*, 1–6. [CrossRef]

52. Ryu, G.; Kim, D.W. Th2 inflammatory responses in the development of nasal polyps and chronic rhinosinusitis. *Curr. Opin. Allergy Clin. Immunol.* **2020**, *20*, 1–8. [CrossRef] [PubMed]

53. Stentzel, S.; Teufelberger, A.; Nordengrün, M.; Kolata, J.; Schmidt, F.; Van Crombruggen, K.; Michalik, S.; Kumpfmüller, J.; Tischer, S.; Schweder, T.; et al. Staphylococcal serine protease–like proteins are pacemakers of allergic airway reactions to Staphylococcus aureus. *J. Allergy Clin. Immunol.* **2017**, *139*, 492–500.e8. [CrossRef] [PubMed]

54. Takabayashi, T.; Kato, A.; Peters, A.T.; Hulse, K.E.; Suh, L.A.; Carter, R.; Norton, J.; Grammer, L.C.; Cho, S.H.; Tan, B.K.; et al. Excessive Fibrin Deposition in Nasal Polyps Caused by Fibrinolytic Impairment through Reduction of Tissue Plasminogen Activator Expression. *Am. J. Respir. Crit. Care Med.* **2013**, *187*, 49–57. [CrossRef] [PubMed]

55. Siroux, V.; Ballardini, N.; Soler, M.; Lupinek, C.; Boudier, A.; Pin, I.; Just, J.; Nadif, R.; Antó, J.-M.; Melen, E.; et al. The asthma-rhinitis multimorbidity is associated with IgE polysensitization in adolescents and adults. *Allergy* **2018**, *73*, 1447–1458. [CrossRef] [PubMed]

56. Bachert, C.; Humbert, M.; Hanania, N.A.; Zhang, N.; Holgate, S.; Buhl, R.; Bröker, B.M. Staphylococcus aureus and its IgE-inducing enterotoxins in asthma: Current knowledge. *Eur. Respir. J.* **2020**, *55*, 1901592. [CrossRef] [PubMed]

57. Bachert, C.; Zhang, N.; Holtappels, G.; De Lobel, L.; Van Cauwenberge, P.; Liu, S.; Lin, P.; Bousquet, J.; Van Steen, K. Presence of IL-5 protein and IgE antibodies to staphylococcal enterotoxins in nasal polyps is associated with comorbid asthma. *J. Allergy Clin. Immunol.* **2010**, *126*, 962–968.e6. [CrossRef] [PubMed]

58. Tomassen, P.; Jarvis, D.; Newson, R.; Van Ree, R.; Forsberg, B.; Howarth, P.; Janson, C.; Kowalski, M.L.; Krämer, U.; Matricardi, P.M.; et al. *Staphylococcus aureus* enterotoxin-specific IgE is associated with asthma in the general population: A GA(2)LEN study. *Allergy* **2013**, *68*, 1289–1297. [CrossRef]

59. Bachert, C.; Marple, B.; Hosemann, W.; Cavaliere, C.; Wen, W.; Zhang, N. Endotypes of Chronic Rhinosinusitis with Nasal Polyps: Pathology and Possible Therapeutic Implications. *J. Allergy Clin. Immunol. Pract.* **2020**, *8*, 1514–1519. [CrossRef]

60. Lan, F.; Zhang, N.; Holtappels, G.; De Ruyck, N.; Krysko, O.; Van Crombruggen, K.; Braun, H.; Johnston, S.L.; Papadopoulos, N.G.; Zhang, L.; et al. Staphylococcus aureusInduces a Mucosal Type 2 Immune Response via Epithelial Cell–derived Cytokines. *Am. J. Respir. Crit. Care Med.* **2018**, *198*, 452–463. [CrossRef]

61. Bachert, C.; Holtappels, G.; Merabishvili, M.; Meyer, T.C.; Murr, A.; Zhang, N.; Van Crombruggen, K.; Gevaert, E.; Völker, U.; Bröker, B.M.; et al. Staphylococcus aureus controls interleukin-5 release in upper airway inflammation. *J. Proteom.* **2018**, *180*, 53–60. [CrossRef]

62. Takeda, K.; Sakakibara, S.; Yamashita, K.; Motooka, D.; Nakamura, S.; El Hussien, M.A.; Katayama, J.; Maeda, Y.; Nakata, M.; Hamada, S.; et al. Allergic conversion of protective mucosal immunity against nasal bacteria in patients with chronic rhinosinusitis with nasal polyposis. *J. Allergy Clin. Immunol.* **2019**, *143*, 1163–1175.e15. [CrossRef] [PubMed]

63. Cheng, K.-J.; Wang, S.-Q.; Xu, Y.-Y. Different roles of Staphylococcus aureus enterotoxin in different subtypes of nasal polyps. *Exp. Ther. Med.* **2016**, *13*, 321–326. [CrossRef] [PubMed]

64. Ba, L.; Zhang, N.; Meng, J.; Zhang, J.; Lin, P.; Zhou, P.; Liu, S.; Bachert, C. The association between bacterial colonization and inflammatory pattern in Chinese chronic rhinosinusitis patients with nasal polyps. *Allergy* **2011**, *66*, 1296–1303. [CrossRef] [PubMed]

65. Ocampo, C.J.; Peters, A.T. Antibody Deficiency in Chronic Rhinosinusitis: Epidemiology and Burden of Illness. *Am. J. Rhinol. Allergy* **2013**, *27*, 34–38. [CrossRef] [PubMed]

66. Yu, X.; Cragg, M.S. Engineered antibodies to combat viral threats. *Nature* **2020**. [CrossRef] [PubMed]

67. Pelegrin, M.; Naranjo-Gomez, M.; Piechaczyk, M. Antiviral Monoclonal Antibodies: Can They Be More Than Simple Neutralizing Agents? *Trends Microbiol.* **2015**, *23*, 653–665. [CrossRef] [PubMed]

68. Verduyn, M.; Botto, G.; Jaubert, J.; Lier, C.; Flament, T.; Guilleminault, L. Serum IgG Concentrations in Adult Patients Experiencing Virus-Induced Severe Asthma Exacerbations. *J. Allergy Clin. Immunol. Pract.* **2019**, *7*, 1507–1513.e1. [CrossRef]

69. Kim, H.; Ellis, A.K.; Fischer, D.A.; Noseworthy, M.; Olivenstein, R.; Chapman, K.R.; Lee, J. Asthma biomarkers in the age of biologics. *Allergy Asthma Clin. Immunol.* **2017**, *13*, 1–17. [CrossRef]

70. Fahy, J.V. Type 2 Inflammation in Asthma—Present in Most, Absent in Many. *Nat. Rev. Immunol.* **2015**, *15*, 57–65. [CrossRef]

71. Robinson, D.; Humbert, M.; Buhl, R.; Cruz, A.A.; Inoue, H.; Korom, S.; Hanania, N.A.; Nair, P. Revisiting Type 2-high and Type 2-low airway inflammation in asthma: Current knowledge and therapeutic implications. *Clin. Exp. Allergy* **2017**, *47*, 161–175. [CrossRef]

72. Barranco, P.; Phillips-Angles, E.; Dominguez-Ortega, J.; Quirce, S. Dupilumab in the management of moderate-to-severe asthma: The data so far. *Ther. Clin. Risk Manag.* **2017**, *13*, 1139–1149. [CrossRef] [PubMed]

73. Xu, M.; Chen, D.; Zhou, H.; Zhang, W.; Xu, J.; Chen, L. The Role of Periostin in the Occurrence and Progression of Eosinophilic Chronic Sinusitis with Nasal Polyps. *Sci. Rep.* **2017**, *7*, 1–9. [CrossRef] [PubMed]

74. Wang, M.; Wang, X.; Zhang, N.; Wang, H.; Li, Y.; Fan, E.; Zhang, L.; Zhang, L.; Bachert, C. Association of periostin expression with eosinophilic inflammation in nasal polyps. *J. Allergy Clin. Immunol.* **2015**, *136*, 1700–1703.e9. [CrossRef] [PubMed]

75. Ebenezer, J.A.; Christensen, J.M.; Oliver, B.G.; Oliver, R.A.; Tjin, G.; Ho, J.; Habib, A.R.; Rimmer, J.; Sacks, R.; Harvey, R.J. Periostin as a marker of mucosal remodelling in chronic rhinosinusitis. *Rhinol. J.* **2017**, *55*, 234–241. [CrossRef] [PubMed]

76. Carpagnano, G.E.; Scioscia, G.; Lacedonia, D.; Soccio, P.; Lepore, G.; Saetta, M.; Barbaro, M.P.F.; Barnes, P.J. Looking for Airways Periostin in Severe Asthma: Could it Be Useful for Clustering Type 2 Endotype? *Chest* **2018**, *154*, 1083–1090. [CrossRef] [PubMed]

77. Ledger, K.S.; Agee, S.J.; Kasaian, M.T.; Forlow, S.B.; Durn, B.L.; Minyard, J.; Lu, Q.A.; Todd, J.; Vesterqvist, O.; Burczynski, M.E. Analytical validation of a highly sensitive microparticle-based immunoassay for the quantitation of IL-13 in human serum using the Erenna®immunoassay system. *J. Immunol. Methods* **2009**, *350*, 161–170. [CrossRef]

78. Jeanblanc, N.M.; Hemken, P.M.; Datwyler, M.J.; Brophy, S.E.; Manetz, T.S.; Lee, R.; Liang, M.; Chowdhury, P.S.; Varkey, R.; Grant, E.P.; et al. Development of a new ARCHITECT automated periostin immunoassay. *Clin. Chim. Acta* **2017**, *464*, 228–235. [CrossRef]

79. Schryver, E.D.; Derycke, L.; Calus, L.; Holtappels, G.; Hellings, P.W.; Van Zele, T.; Bachert, C.; Gevaert, P. The effect of systemic treatments on periostin expression reflects their interference with the eosinophilic inflammation in chronic rhinosinusitis with nasal polyps. *Rhinology* **2017**, *55*, 152–160. [CrossRef]

80. Weidinger, S.; Novak, N. Atopic dermatitis. *Lancet* **2016**, *387*, 1109–1122. [CrossRef]

81. Kinch, M.S. An overview of FDA-approved biologics medicines. *Drug Discov. Today* **2015**, *20*, 393–398. [CrossRef]

82. De Greve, G.; Hellings, P.; Fokkens, W.; Pugin, B.; Callebaut, I.; Seys, S.F. Endotype-driven treatment in chronic upper airway diseases. *Clin. Transl. Allergy* **2017**, *7*, 1–14. [CrossRef] [PubMed]

83. Cardell, L.; Stjärne, P.; Jonstam, K.; Bachert, C. Endotypes of chronic rhinosinusitis: Impact on management. *J. Allergy Clin. Immunol.* **2020**, *145*, 752–756. [CrossRef] [PubMed]

84. Manka, L.A.; Wechsler, M.E. Selecting the right biologic for your patients with severe asthma. *Ann. Allergy Asthma Immunol.* **2018**, *121*, 406–413. [CrossRef] [PubMed]

85. Geha, R.S.; Jabara, H.H.; Brodeur, S.R. The regulation of immunoglobulin E class-switch recombination. *Nat. Rev. Immunol.* **2003**, *3*, 721–732. [CrossRef] [PubMed]

86. Pelaia, C.; Calabrese, C.; Terracciano, R.; De Blasio, F.; Vatrella, A.; Pelaia, G. Omalizumab, the first available antibody for biological treatment of severe asthma: More than a decade of real-life effectiveness. *Ther. Adv. Respir. Dis.* **2018**, *12*, 12. [CrossRef] [PubMed]

87. Beck, L.A.; Marcotte, G.V.; MacGlashan, D.M., Jr.; Togias, A.; Saini, S.S. Omalizumab-induced reductions in mast cell FcεRI expression and function. *J. Allergy Clin. Immunol.* **2004**, *114*, 527–530. [CrossRef] [PubMed]

88. MacGlashan, D.W.; Bochner, B.S.; Adelman, D.C.; Jardieu, P.M.; Togias, A.; McKenzie-White, J.; Sterbinsky, S.A.; Hamilton, R.G.; Lichtenstein, L.M. Down-regulation of Fc(epsilon)RI expression on human basophils during in vivo treatment of atopic patients with anti-IgE antibody. *J. Immunol.* **1997**, *158*, 1438–1445.

89. Novosad, J.; Krčmová, I. Evolution of our view on the IgE molecule role in bronchial asthma and the clinical effect of its modulation by omalizumab: Where do we stand today? *Int. J. Immunopathol. Pharmacol.* **2020**, *34*. [CrossRef]

90. Bousquet, J.; Chanez, P.; Lacoste, J.Y.; Barnéon, G.; Ghavanian, N.; Enander, I.; Venge, P.; Ahlstedt, S.; Simony-Lafontaine, J.; Godard, P.; et al. Eosinophilic Inflammation in Asthma. *N. Engl. J. Med.* **1990**, *323*, 1033–1039. [CrossRef]

91. Fulkerson, P.C.; Rothenberg, M.E. Targeting eosinophils in allergy, inflammation and beyond. *Nat. Rev. Drug Discov.* **2013**, *12*, 117–129. [CrossRef]

92. Pelaia, C.; Paoletti, G.; Puggioni, F.; Racca, F.; Pelaia, G.; Canonica, G.W.; Heffler, E. Interleukin-5 in the Pathophysiology of Severe Asthma. *Front. Physiol.* **2019**, *10*, 1514. [CrossRef] [PubMed]

93. Gnanakumaran, G.; Babu, K.S. Technology evaluation: Mepolizumab, GlaxoSmithKline. *Curr. Opin. Mol. Ther.* **2003**, *5*, 321–325. [PubMed]

94. Fainardi, V.; Pisi, G.; Chetta, A. Mepolizumab in the treatment of severe eosinophilic asthma. *Immunotherapy* **2016**, *8*, 27–34. [CrossRef] [PubMed]

95. Zhang, J.; Kuvelkar, R.; Murgolo, N.J.; Taremi, S.S.; Chou, C.-C.; Wang, P.; Billah, M.M.; Egan, R.W. Mapping and characterization of the epitope(s) of Sch 55700, a humanized mAb, that inhibits human IL-5. *Int. Immunol.* **1999**, *11*, 1935–1944. [CrossRef] [PubMed]

96. Kolbeck, R.; Kozhich, A.; Koike, M.; Peng, L.; Andersson, C.K.; Damschroder, M.M.; Reed, J.L.; Woods, R.; Dall'Acqua, W.W.; Stephens, G.L.; et al. MEDI-563, a humanized anti–IL-5 receptor α mAb with enhanced antibody-dependent cell-mediated cytotoxicity function. *J. Allergy Clin. Immunol.* **2010**, *125*, 1344–1353.e2. [CrossRef]

97. Ghazi, A.; Trikha, A.; Calhoun, W.J. Benralizumab—A Humanized Mab to IL-5rα with Enhanced Antibody-Dependent Cell-Mediated Cytotoxicity—A Novel Approach for the Treatment of Asthma. *Expert Opin. Biol. Ther.* **2012**, *12*, 113–118. [CrossRef]

98. Lommatzsch, M.; Marchewski, H.; Schwefel, G.; Stoll, P.; Virchow, J.C.; Bratke, K. Benralizumab strongly reduces blood basophils in severe eosinophilic asthma. *Clin. Exp. Allergy* **2020**, *50*, 1267–1269. [CrossRef]

99. Wenzel, S.E.; Ford, L.; Pearlman, D.; Spector, S.; Sher, L.; Skobieranda, F.; Wang, L.; Kirkesseli, S.; Rocklin, R.; Bock, B.; et al. Dupilumab in Persistent Asthma with Elevated Eosinophil Levels. *N. Engl. J. Med.* **2013**, *368*, 2455–2466. [CrossRef]

100. Laporte, S.L.; Juo, Z.S.; Vaclavikova, J.; Colf, L.A.; Qi, X.; Heller, N.M.; Keegan, A.D.; Garcia, K.C. Molecular and Structural Basis of Cytokine Receptor Pleiotropy in the Interleukin-4/13 System. *Cell* **2008**, *132*, 259–272. [CrossRef]

101. Gandhi, N.A.; Bennett, B.L.; Graham, N.M.H.; Pirozzi, G.; Stahl, N.; Yancopoulos, G.D. Targeting key proximal drivers of type 2 inflammation in disease. *Nat. Rev. Drug Discov.* **2016**, *15*, 35–50. [CrossRef]

102. Poulsen, L.K.; Hummelshoj, L. Triggers of IgE class switching and allergy development. *Ann. Med.* **2007**, *39*, 440–456. [CrossRef] [PubMed]

103. Wynn, T.A. IL-13 effector functions. *Annu. Rev. Immunol.* **2003**, *21*, 425–456. [CrossRef] [PubMed]

104. Rosenberg, H.F.; Phipps, S.; Foster, P.S. Eosinophil trafficking in allergy and asthma. *J. Allergy Clin. Immunol.* **2007**, *119*, 1303–1310. [CrossRef] [PubMed]

105. Le Floc'H, A.; Allinne, J.; Nagashima, K.; Scott, G.; Birchard, D.; Asrat, S.; Bai, Y.; Lim, W.K.; Martin, J.; Huang, T.; et al. Dual blockade of IL-4 and IL-13 with dupilumab, an IL-4Rα antibody, is required to broadly inhibit type 2 inflammation. *Allergy* **2020**, *75*, 1188–1204. [CrossRef] [PubMed]

106. May, R.D.; Fung, M. Strategies targeting the IL-4/IL-13 axes in disease. *Cytokine* **2015**, *75*, 89–116. [CrossRef] [PubMed]

107. Chung, K.F.; Wenzel, S.E.; Brozek, J.L.; Bush, A.; Castro, M.; Sterk, P.J.; Adcock, I.M.; Bateman, E.D.; Bel, E.H.; Bleecker, E.R.; et al. International ERS/ATS guidelines on definition, evaluation and treatment of severe asthma. *Eur. Respir. J.* **2013**, *43*, 343–373. [CrossRef]

108. Bousquet, J.J.; Brusselle, G.; Buhl, R.; Busse, W.W.; Cruz, A.A.; Djukanovic, R.; Domingo, C.; Hanania, N.A.; Humbert, M.; Gow, A.M.; et al. Care pathways for the selection of a biologic in severe asthma. *Eur. Respir. J.* **2017**, *50*, 1701782. [CrossRef]

109. Boyman, O.; Kaegi, C.; Akdis, M.; Bavbek, S.; Bossios, A.; Chatzipetrou, A.; Eiwegger, T.; Firinu, D.; Harr, T.; Knol, E.F.; et al. EAACI IG Biologicals task force paper on the use of biologic agents in allergic disorders. *Allergy* **2015**, *70*, 727–754. [CrossRef]

110. Kotisalmi, E.; Hakulinen, A.; Mäkelä, M.; Toppila-Salmi, S.; Kauppi, P. A Comparison of Biologicals in the Treatment of Adults with Severe Asthma—Real-Life Experiences. *Asthma Res. Pract.* **2020**, *6*, 1–11. [CrossRef]

111. Normansell, R.; Walker, S.; Milan, S.J.; Walters, E.H.; Nair, P. Omalizumab for asthma in adults and children. *Cochrane Database Syst. Rev.* **2014**, CD003559. [CrossRef]

112. Humbert, M.; Taillé, C.; Mala, L.; Le Gros, V.; Just, J.; Molimard, M. Omalizumab effectiveness in patients with severe allergic asthma according to blood eosinophil count: The STELLAIR study. *Eur. Respir. J.* **2018**, *51*, 1702523. [CrossRef] [PubMed]

113. Pavord, I.; Bleecker, E.R.; Buhl, R.; Chanez, P.; Bel, E.H.; Howarth, P.; Bratton, D.J.; Albers, F.C.; Yancey, S. Response to mepolizumab treatment is sustained across 4-weekly dosing periods. *ERJ Open Res.* **2020**, *6*, 00068–02020. [CrossRef] [PubMed]

114. Castro, M.; Zangrilli, J.; Wechsler, M.E.; Bateman, E.D.; Brusselle, G.; Bardin, P.; Murphy, K.; Maspero, J.F.; O'Brien, C.; Korn, S. Reslizumab for inadequately controlled asthma with elevated blood eosinophil counts: Results from two multicentre, parallel, double-blind, randomised, placebo-controlled, phase 3 trials. *Lancet Respir. Med.* **2015**, *3*, 355–366. [CrossRef]

115. Bjermer, L.; Lemiere, C.; Maspero, J.; Weiss, S.; Zangrilli, J.; Germinaro, M. Reslizumab for Inadequately Controlled Asthma with Elevated Blood Eosinophil Levels: A Randomized Phase 3 Study. *Chest* **2016**, *150*, 789–798. [CrossRef]

116. Bleecker, E.R.; Fitzgerald, J.M.; Chanez, P.; Papi, A.; Weinstein, S.F.; Barker, P.; Sproule, S.; Gilmartin, G.; Aurivillius, M.; Werkström, V.; et al. Efficacy and safety of benralizumab for patients with severe asthma uncontrolled with high-dosage inhaled corticosteroids and long-acting β2-agonists (SIROCCO): A randomised, multicentre, placebo-controlled phase 3 trial. *Lancet* **2016**, *388*, 2115–2127. [CrossRef]

117. Kavanagh, J.E.; Hearn, A.P.; Dhariwal, J.; D'Ancona, G.; Douiri, A.; Roxas, C.; Fernandes, M.; Green, L.; Thomson, L.; Nanzer, A.M.; et al. Real-World Effectiveness of Benralizumab in Severe Eosinophilic Asthma. *Chest* **2020**. [CrossRef]

118. Rabe, K.F.; Nair, P.; Brusselle, G.; Maspero, J.F.; Castro, M.; Sher, L.; Zhu, H.; Hamilton, J.D.; Swanson, B.N.; Khan, A.; et al. Efficacy and Safety of Dupilumab in Glucocorticoid-Dependent Severe Asthma. *N. Engl. J. Med.* **2018**, *378*, 2475–2485. [CrossRef]

119. Gevaert, P.; Calus, L.; Van Zele, T.; Blomme, K.; De Ruyck, N.; Bauters, W.; Hellings, P.; Brusselle, G.; De Bacquer, D.; Van Cauwenberge, P.; et al. Omalizumab is effective in allergic and nonallergic patients with nasal polyps and asthma. *J. Allergy Clin. Immunol.* **2013**, *131*, 110–116.e1. [CrossRef]

120. Pinto, J.; Mehta, N.; DiTineo, M.; Wang, J.; Baroody, F.; Naclerio, R. A randomized, double-blind, placebo-controlled trial of anti-IgE for chronic rhinosinusitis. *Rhinol. J.* **2010**, *48*, 318–324. [CrossRef]

121. Forster-Ruhrmann, U.; Stergioudi, D.; Pierchalla, G.; Fluhr, J.; Bergmann, K.-C.; Olze, H. Omalizumab in patients with NSAIDs-exacerbated respiratory disease. *Rhinology* **2020**, *58*, 226–232. [CrossRef]

122. Gevaert, P.; Omachi, T.A.; Corren, J.; Mullol, J.; Han, J.; Lee, S.E.; Kaufman, D.; Ligueros-Saylan, M.; Howard, M.; Zhu, R.; et al. Efficacy and safety of omalizumab in nasal polyposis: 2 randomized phase 3 trials. *J. Allergy Clin. Immunol.* **2020**, *146*, 595–605. [CrossRef] [PubMed]

123. Gevaert, P.; Lang-Loidolt, D.; Lackner, A.; Stammberger, H.; Staudinger, H.; Van Zele, T.; Holtappels, G.; Tavernier, J.; Van Cauwenberge, P.; Bachert, C. Nasal IL-5 levels determine the response to anti–IL-5 treatment in patients with nasal polyps. *J. Allergy Clin. Immunol.* **2006**, *118*, 1133–1141. [CrossRef] [PubMed]

124. Bachert, C.; Sousa, A.R.; Lund, V.J.; Scadding, G.; Gevaert, P.; Nasser, S.M.; Durham, S.R.; Cornet, M.E.; Kariyawasam, H.H.; Gilbert, J.; et al. Reduced need for surgery in severe nasal polyposis with mepolizumab: Randomized trial. *J. Allergy Clin. Immunol.* **2017**, *140*, 1024–1031.e14. [CrossRef] [PubMed]

125. Gevaert, P.; Van Bruaene, N.; Cattaert, T.; Van Steen, K.; Van Zele, T.; Acke, F.; De Ruyck, N.; Blomme, K.; Sousa, A.R.; Marshall, R.P.; et al. Mepolizumab, a humanized anti–IL-5 mAb, as a treatment option for severe nasal polyposis. *J. Allergy Clin. Immunol.* **2011**, *128*, 989–995.e8. [CrossRef]

126. Chong, L.Y.; Piromchai, P.; Sharp, S.; Snidvongs, K.; Philpott, C.; Hopkins, C.; Burton, M.J. Biologics for chronic rhinosinusitis. *Cochrane Database Syst. Rev.* **2020**, *2020*. [CrossRef]

127. Hopkins, C.; Bachert, C.; Fokkens, W.; Desrosiers, M.; Wagenmann, M.; Lee, S.; Sousa, A.; Smith, S.; Martin, N.; Mayer, B.; et al. Late Breaking Abstract—Add-on mepolizumab for chronic rhinosinusitis with nasal polyps: SYNAPSE study. *Eur. Respir. J.* **2020**, *56*, 4616.

128. Bachert, C.; Han, J.K.; Desrosiers, M.; Hellings, P.W.; Amin, N.; Lee, S.E.; Mullol, J.; Greos, L.S.; Bosso, J.V.; Laidlaw, T.M.; et al. Efficacy and safety of dupilumab in patients with severe chronic rhinosinusitis with nasal polyps (LIBERTY NP SINUS-24 and LIBERTY NP SINUS-52): Results from two multicentre, randomised, double-blind, placebo-controlled, parallel-group phase 3 trials. *Lancet* **2019**, *394*, 1638–1650. [CrossRef]

129. Akinlade, B.; Guttman-Yassky, E.; De Bruin-Weller, M.; Simpson, E.; Blauvelt, A.; Cork, M.; Prens, E.; Asbell, P.; Akpek, E.; Corren, J.; et al. Conjunctivitis in dupilumab clinical trials. *Br. J. Dermatol.* **2019**, *181*, 459–473. [CrossRef]

130. Golebski, K.; Van Tongeren, J.; Van Egmond, D.; De Groot, E.J.; Fokkens, W.J.; Van Drunen, C.M. Specific Induction of TSLP by the Viral RNA Analogue Poly(I:C) in Primary Epithelial Cells Derived from Nasal Polyps. *PLoS ONE* **2016**, *11*, e0152808. [CrossRef]

131. Gauvreau, G.M.; O'Byrne, P.M.; Boulet, L.-P.; Wang, Y.; Cockcroft, D.; Bigler, J.; Fitzgerald, J.M.; Boedigheimer, M.; Davis, B.E.; Dias, C.; et al. Effects of an Anti-TSLP Antibody on Allergen-Induced Asthmatic Responses. *N. Engl. J. Med.* **2014**, *370*, 2102–2110. [CrossRef]

132. Catley, M.C.; Coote, J.; Bari, M.; Tomlinson, K.L. Monoclonal antibodies for the treatment of asthma. *Pharmacol. Ther.* **2011**, *132*, 333–351. [CrossRef] [PubMed]

133. Baatjes, A.J.; Smith, S.G.; Dua, B.; Watson, R.; Gauvreau, G.M.; O'Byrne, P.M. Treatment with anti-OX40L or anti-TSLP does not alter the frequency of T regulatory cells in allergic asthmatics. *Allergy* **2015**, *70*, 1505–1508. [CrossRef] [PubMed]

134. Corren, J.; Parnes, J.R.; Wang, L.; Mo, M.; Roseti, S.L.; Griffiths, J.M.; Van Der Merwe, R. Tezepelumab in Adults with Uncontrolled Asthma. *N. Engl. J. Med.* **2017**, *377*, 936–946. [CrossRef] [PubMed]

135. Michel, O.; Dinh, P.H.D.; Doyen, V.; Corazza, F. Anti-TNF inhibits the Airways neutrophilic inflammation induced by inhaled endotoxin in human. *BMC Pharmacol. Toxicol.* **2014**, *15*, 60. [CrossRef] [PubMed]

136. Antoniu, S.A.; Mihaltan, F.; Ulmeanu, R. Anti-TNF-α therapies in chronic obstructive pulmonary diseases. *Expert Opin. Investig. Drugs* **2008**, *17*, 1203–1211. [CrossRef] [PubMed]

137. Cazzola, M.; Polosa, R. Anti-TNF-α and Th1 cytokine-directed therapies for the treatment of asthma. *Curr. Opin. Allergy Clin. Immunol.* **2006**, *6*, 43–50. [CrossRef]

138. Antoniu, S.A. Infliximab for chronic obstructive pulmonary disease: Towards a more specific inflammation targeting? *Expert Opin. Investig. Drugs* **2006**, *15*, 181–184. [CrossRef]

139. Busse, W.W.; Holgate, S.; Kerwin, E.; Chon, Y.; Feng, J.; Lin, J.; Lin, S.-L. Randomized, Double-Blind, Placebo-controlled Study of Brodalumab, a Human Anti–IL-17 Receptor Monoclonal Antibody, in Moderate to Severe Asthma. *Am. J. Respir. Crit. Care Med.* **2013**, *188*, 1294–1302. [CrossRef]

140. Nair, P.; Aziz-Ur-rehman, A.; Radford, K. Therapeutic implications of "neutrophilic asthma". *Curr. Opin. Pulm. Med.* **2015**, *21*, 33–38. [CrossRef]

141. Nair, P.; Gaga, M.; Zervas, E.; Alagha, K.; Hargreave, F.E.; O'Byrne, P.M.; Stryszak, P.; Gann, L.; Sadeh, J.; Chanez, P.; et al. Safety and efficacy of a CXCR2 antagonist in patients with severe asthma and sputum neutrophils: A randomized, placebo-controlled clinical trial. *Clin. Exp. Allergy* **2012**, *42*, 1097–1103. [CrossRef]

142. O'Byrne, P.M.; Metev, H.; Puu, M.; Richter, K.; Keen, C.; Uddin, M.; Larsson, B.; Cullberg, M.; Nair, P. Efficacy and safety of a CXCR2 antagonist, AZD5069, in patients with uncontrolled persistent asthma: A randomised, double-blind, placebo-controlled trial. *Lancet Respir. Med.* **2016**, *4*, 797–806. [CrossRef]

143. Ricciotti, E.; Fitzgerald, G.A. Prostaglandins and Inflammation. *Arter. Thromb. Vasc. Biol.* **2011**, *31*, 986–1000. [CrossRef] [PubMed]

144. Barnes, P.J. Cellular and molecular mechanisms of asthma and COPD. *Clin. Sci.* **2017**, *131*, 1541–1558. [CrossRef] [PubMed]

145. Mjösberg, J.; Trifari, S.; Crellin, N.K.; Peters, C.P.; Van Drunen, C.M.; Piet, B.; Fokkens, W.J.; Cupedo, T.; Spits, H. Human IL-25- and IL-33-responsive type 2 innate lymphoid cells are defined by expression of CRTH2 and CD161. *Nat. Immunol.* **2011**, *12*, 1055–1062. [CrossRef]

146. Diamant, Z.; Aalders, W.; Parulekar, A.; Bjermer, L.; Hanania, N.A. Targeting lipid mediators in asthma: Time for reappraisal. *Curr. Opin. Pulm. Med.* **2019**, *25*, 121–127. [CrossRef]

147. Roth-Walter, F.; Adcock, I.M.; Benito-Villalvilla, C.; Bianchini, R.; Bjermer, L.; Caramori, G.; Cari, L.; Chung, K.F.; Diamant, Z.; Eguiluz-Gracia, I.; et al. Comparing biologicals and small molecule drug therapies for chronic respiratory diseases: An EAACI Taskforce on Immunopharmacology position paper. *Allergy* **2019**, *74*, 432–448. [CrossRef]

148. Ratner, P.; Andrews, C.P.; Hampel, F.C.; Martin, B.; Mohar, D.E.; Bourrelly, D.; Danaietash, P.; Mangialaio, S.; Dingemanse, J.; Hmissi, A.; et al. Efficacy and safety of setipiprant in seasonal allergic rhinitis: Results from Phase 2 and Phase 3 randomized, double-blind, placebo- and active-referenced studies. *Allergy, Asthma Clin. Immunol.* **2017**, *13*, 1–15. [CrossRef]

149. Diamant, Z.; Sidharta, P.N.; Singh, D.; O'Connor, B.J.; Zuiker, R.; Leaker, B.R.; Silkey, M.; Dingemanse, J. Setipiprant, a selective CRTH2 antagonist, reduces allergen-induced airway responses in allergic asthmatics. *Clin. Exp. Allergy* **2014**, *44*, 1044–1052. [CrossRef]

150. Singh, D.; Cadden, P.; Hunter, M.; Collins, L.P.; Perkins, M.; Pettipher, R.; Townsend, E.; Vinall, S.; O'Connor, B. Inhibition of the asthmatic allergen challenge response by the CRTH2 antagonist OC000459. *Eur. Respir. J.* **2012**, *41*, 46–52. [CrossRef]

151. Barnes, N.; Pavord, I.; Chuchalin, A.; Bell, J.; Hunter, M.; Lewis, T.; Parker, D.; Payton, M.; Collins, L.P.; Pettipher, R.; et al. A randomized, double-blind, placebo-controlled study of the CRTH2 antagonist OC000459 in moderate persistent asthma. *Clin. Exp. Allergy* **2012**, *42*, 38–48. [CrossRef]

152. Hall, I.P.; Fowler, A.V.; Gupta, A.; Tetzlaff, K.; Nivens, M.C.; Sarno, M.; Finnigan, H.A.; Bateman, E.D.; Sutherland, E.R. Efficacy of BI 671800, an oral CRTH2 antagonist, in poorly controlled asthma as sole controller and in the presence of inhaled corticosteroid treatment. *Pulm. Pharmacol. Ther.* **2015**, *32*, 37–44. [CrossRef] [PubMed]

153. Erpenbeck, V.J.; Popov, T.A.; Miller, D.; Weinstein, S.F.; Spector, S.; Magnusson, B.; Osuntokun, W.; Goldsmith, P.; Weiss, H.M.; Beier, J. The oral CRTh2 antagonist QAW039 (fevipiprant): A phase II study in uncontrolled allergic asthma. *Pulm. Pharmacol. Ther.* **2016**, *39*, 54–63. [CrossRef] [PubMed]

154. Bateman, E.D.; Guerreros, A.G.; Brockhaus, F.; Holzhauer, B.; Pethe, A.; Kay, R.A.; Townley, R.G. Fevipiprant, an oral prostaglandin DP2receptor (CRTh2) antagonist, in allergic asthma uncontrolled on low-dose inhaled corticosteroids. *Eur. Respir. J.* **2017**, *50*, 1700670. [CrossRef] [PubMed]

155. Busse, W.W.; Wenzel, S.E.; Meltzer, E.O.; Kerwin, E.M.; Liu, M.C.; Zhang, N.; Chon, Y.; Budelsky, A.L.; Lin, J.; Lin, S.-L. Safety and efficacy of the prostaglandin D2 receptor antagonist AMG 853 in asthmatic patients. *J. Allergy Clin. Immunol.* **2013**, *131*, 339–345. [CrossRef]

156. Brightling, C.; Gaga, M.; Inoue, H.; Li, J.; Maspero, J.; Wenzel, S.; Maitra, S.; Lawrence, D.; Brockhaus, F.; Lehmann, T.; et al. Effectiveness of fevipiprant in reducing exacerbations in patients with severe asthma (LUSTER-1 and LUSTER-2): Two phase 3 randomised controlled trials. *Lancet Respir. Med.* **2020**. [CrossRef]

3

Pharmacokinetic and Pharmacodynamic Considerations for the Use of Monoclonal Antibodies in the Treatment of Bacterial Infections

Shun Xin Wang-Lin and Joseph P. Balthasar *

Department of Pharmaceutical Sciences, University at Buffalo, State University of New York, Buffalo, NY 14214, USA; sl256@buffalo.edu
* Correspondence: jb@buffalo.edu

Abstract: Antibiotic-resistant bacterial pathogens are increasingly implicated in hospital- and community-acquired infections. Recent advances in monoclonal antibody (mAb) production and engineering have led to renewed interest in the development of antibody-based therapies for treatment of drug-resistant bacterial infections. Currently, there are three antibacterial mAb products approved by the Food and Drug Administration (FDA) and at least nine mAbs are in clinical trials. Antibacterial mAbs are typically developed to kill bacteria or to attenuate bacterial pathological activity through neutralization of bacterial toxins and virulence factors. Antibodies exhibit distinct pharmacological mechanisms from traditional antimicrobials and, hence, cross-resistance between small molecule antimicrobials and antibacterial mAbs is unlikely. Additionally, the long biological half-lives typically found for mAbs may allow convenient dosing and vaccine-like prophylaxis from infection. However, the high affinity of mAbs and the involvement of the host immune system in their pharmacological actions may lead to complex and nonlinear pharmacokinetics and pharmacodynamics. In this review, we summarize the pharmacokinetics and pharmacodynamics of the FDA-approved antibacterial mAbs and those are currently in clinical trials. Challenges in the development of antibacterial mAbs are also discussed.

Keywords: bacterial infections; monoclonal antibodies; pharmacokinetics; pharmacodynamics

---

1. Introduction

The clinical application of antibodies for the treatment of infectious diseases was first introduced in the form of serum therapy in early 1890s by Emil von Behring and Shibasaburo Kitasato [1]. Serum therapy was then widely applied to treat infections caused by several bacterial pathogens, including *Corynebacterium diphtheria*, *Streptococcus pneumoniae*, *Neisseria meningitides*, *Haemophilus influenzae*, Group A *Streptococcus*, and *Clostridium tetani* [2]. Although serum therapy became the standard-of-care for several infectious diseases in the pre-antibiotic era, treatment with polyclonal antisera poses several drawbacks, including "serum sickness" or immune complex hypersensitivity that can occur in 10–50% patients, lot-to-lot variation in efficacy, low content of specific antibodies, and potential hazards in the transmission of infectious diseases [2–5]. In 1937, the discovery of sulfonamides led to a boom in the development of antimicrobial chemotherapy [6], and the significant advantages associated with antimicrobials, such as less toxicity and cost, higher efficacy, and broad spectrum activity, resulted in the abandonment of serum therapy. Drug resistance, which has been a concern from the onset of antibacterial chemotherapy, has become a major clinical problem within the past few decades. It has been suggested that broad spectrum antimicrobial activity contributes to the widespread development of resistant strains, and specific mechanisms of resistance can either exist before, or emerge rapidly after, the clinical launch of new antibiotics [7]. In 2004/5, pan-drug resistant strains (i.e., resistant to all antimicrobials currently approved by FDA) of *Acinetobacter* and *Pseudomonas* were identified [7]. Unfortunately, as drug resistance has been increasing, the rate of approval of new antibiotics has been decreasing. The number of new antibacterial drugs approved has decreased from an average of five per year in the 1980s to less than one per year in the 2000s [7].

The discovery of hybridoma technology in 1975 and recent advances in monoclonal antibody (mAb) engineering, which make production of unlimited amount of human mAbs possible [8,9], have renewed interest in the development of antibacterial antibody therapies. Monoclonal antibodies are widely used to treat immune deficiencies, cancers, multiple sclerosis, rheumatoid arthritis, and psoriasis, but the application of mAbs for bacterial infections has progressed slowly. Currently, there are only three mAbs approved by the FDA for use in the treatment of bacterial infections (Table 1). All three mAbs are indicated as adjuvant therapies to antibiotics and do not have bactericidal activity. They are directed against bacterial exotoxins and protect host cells from toxin-mediated cytotoxicity through neutralization of exotoxin activities. As of December 2017, there are nine mAb products in clinical trials (Table 2). Of these, six are 'naked' mAbs, two are mAb cocktails containing two mAbs that bind to different targets (ASN100 and Shigamab), and one is an antibody-antibiotic conjugate (DSTA4637S) that kills intracellular bacteria through the intracellular delivery of a potent antibiotic. Of note, five of the nine mAb products in clinical testing bind to the bacterial cell surface and have shown bactericidal activity in preclinical studies (DSTA4637S, 514G3, MEDI3902, Aerumab, and Aerucin); the other four target exotoxins and protect against infections via toxin neutralization (MEDI4893, ASN100, Salvecin, and Shigamab).

In this review, we discuss important considerations of mAb-based therapies for the treatment of bacterial infections, including unique challenges, pharmacokinetic (PK) properties, and pharmacodynamic (PD) mechanisms of action. The PK/PD characteristics of FDA-approved antibacterial mAbs and those in clinical trial are also summarized.

2. Pharmacokinetic Considerations

All FDA-approved antibacterial mAbs and the majority of those in clinical trials are of the immune gamma globulin (IgG) isotype. IgG is the predominant immunoglobulin isotype, comprising approximately 80% of immunoglobulin in human serum. An intact IgG has a molecular weight of ~150 kDa, with two antigen binding domains and a highly conserved crystallizable region (Fc) that is responsible for binding to Fc gamma receptors (FcγRs) on immune cells and activating Fc-mediated effector functions. IgG typically exhibits linear pharmacokinetics (i.e., area under the drug concentration-time curve (AUC) is directly proportional to the dose) in healthy human subjects, with small volumes of distribution (3–9 L), relatively slow clearance (8–12 mL/h), and long half-lives (20–25 days) [10]. The long biological persistence of IgG is partially attributed to Brambell receptor (FcRn) mediated salvage of IgG from lysosomal catabolism [11]. In contrast to the pharmacokinetics of pooled endogenous IgG, therapeutic mAbs often demonstrate nonlinear PK (i.e., AUC is not proportional to the dose), depending on the total body load of the pharmacological target (i.e., the quantity of bacteria, in the case of antimicrobial mAb), the accessibility of the targets, mAb-target affinity, and mAb doses. Key PK considerations for antibacterial mAbs are summarized below, including a discussion of determinants of target mediated drug disposition (TMDD) and mAb distribution in infected organs.

Table 1. Food and Drug Administration (FDA)-approved monoclonal antibodies (mAbs) for use in bacterial infection.

Antibody	Company	Format	Pathogen/Target	First Approved Indication	Reported Mechanism of Action	Approval Year
Raxibacumab	GlaxoSmith Kline	Human IgG1(λ)	*Bacillus anthracis*/Protective antigen	Treatment and prophylaxis of inhalational anthrax	Toxin neutralization	2012
Obiltoxaximab	Elusys	Chimeric IgG1(κ)	*Bacillus anthracis*/Protective antigen	Treatment and prophylaxis of inhalational anthrax	Toxin neutralization	2016
Bezlotoxumab	Merck & Co.	Human IgG1	*Clostridium difficile*/Enterotoxin B	Prevention of *Clostridium difficile* infection recurrence	Toxin neutralization	2016

Table 2. mAbs currently in clinical trials.

Antibody	Sponsor	Format	Pathogen	Target	Reported Mechanism of Action	Current Status
MEDI4893	MedImmune	Human IgG1(κ)	*Staphylococcus aureus*	Alpha toxin	Toxin neutralization	Phase 2
ASN100	Arsanis	Human IgG1(κ)	*Staphylococcus aureus*	Alpha toxin and five leukocidins	Toxin neutralization	Phase 2
DSTA4637S	Genentech	Human IgG1	*Staphylococcus aureus*	β-O-linked N-acetylglucosamine on wall teichoic acids	Antibody-antibiotic conjugate	Phase 1
Salvecin (AR-301)	Aridis	Human IgG1	*Staphylococcus aureus*	Alpha toxin	Toxin neutralization	Phase 1/2a
514G3	XBiotech	Human IgG3	*Staphylococcus aureus*	Protein A	Opsonophagocytosis	Phase 1/2
MEDI3902	MedImmune	Human bispecific IgG1	*Pseudomonas aeruginosa*	PsI and PcrV	Opsonophagocytosis; inhibition of cell attachment and cytotoxicity	Phase 2
Aerumab (AR-101)	Aridis	Human IgM(κ)	*Pseudomonas aeruginosa*	O-antigen (serotype O11)	Opsonophagocytosis; complement-mediated bacterial killing	Phase 2b
Aerucin	Aridis	Human IgG1	*Pseudomonas aeruginosa*	Alginate (surface polysaccharide)	Opsonophagocytosis; complement-mediated bacterial killing	Phase 2
Shigamab	Bellus Health	Chimeric IgG1(κ)	*Escherichia coli*	Shiga toxin 1 and 2	Toxin neutralization	Phase 2

2.1. Target Mediated Drug Disposition

Target mediated drug disposition describes the phenomenon where binding of a high affinity drug to its pharmacological target affects the PK characteristics of the drug (i.e., kinetics of distribution and clearance) [12]. At relatively low doses (compared to the amount of target), high affinity mAb-target binding results in drug accumulation at the sites of action (i.e., target-expressing tissue or site of infection), which may lead to a large apparent volume of distribution of the mAb. With increased doses and increased mAb concentrations, the target sites become increasingly saturated, which may decrease tissue to plasma mAb concentration ratios, decreasing the apparent volume of distribution. Additionally, mAb-target binding may trigger receptor-mediated endocytosis, in which mAb-target complexes are engulfed and degraded in lysosomes. This target-mediated elimination accelerates the clearance of mAbs and thereby shortens their biological persistence and half-life. Due to the effect of the drug in enhancing the elimination of the target, the volume of distribution and clearance of the drug may decrease during the course of repeated dosing.

All marketed antibacterial mAbs and those in clinical trials were developed to kill bacteria or attenuate bacterial pathological activity via antibody-mediated effector functions or toxin neutralization (Tables 1 and 2). Antibody-toxin and antibody-bacteria complexes may be cleared by phagocytic cells through Fc engagement with FcγRs, and via subsequent endocytosis and catabolism in phagolysosomes. Thus, antibacterial mAbs may be expected to exhibit TMDD characteristics. However, the pharmacokinetics of antibacterial mAbs have not been well evaluated to date. Obiltoxaximab, a chimeric IgG1 targeting the protective antigen of *Bacillus anthracis*, showed ~2-fold faster clearances in rabbits and monkeys challenged with *B. anthracis* spores compared to those in non-infected animals [13]. Similarly, a mAb directed against *Staphylococcus aureus* also demonstrated significantly increased clearance (12.1–15.8 mL/day/kg) and decreased half-life (3.74–5.28 days) in *S. aureus* infected mice compared to those in non-infected mice (4.69–5.19 mL/day/kg and 16.4–18.0 days, respectively) [14]. In contrast, pulmonary infection with *Acinetobacter baumannii* did not impact the PK of an anti-K2 capsule mAb in mouse blood, although a substantial accumulation of mAb (5.64–36.1 fold higher amount) was observed in tissues (i.e., lung, liver, and spleen) with high bacterial load compared to values found in non-infected mice [15]. Further investigations are needed, as TMDD results in nonlinear PK, which impacts the design of efficacious dosing regimens, and contributes to potential intra- and inter-patient PK variability (e.g., due to differences in bacterial burden and immune status).

2.2. Distribution of mAbs in Infected Tissues

The tissue disposition of anti-bacterial mAbs may be complex, involving extravasation of mAb molecules from blood to tissue interstitial fluids, diffusion of the molecule in the interstitial fluids to bacterial targets, binding to bacterial targets, and elimination of mAbs from tissue via convective drainage through the lymphatics and via catabolism. Extravasation of IgG antibodies is typically thought to be governed by both diffusion and convection (i.e., bulk movement of molecules through paracellular pores in the vascular endothelium), but convection has been estimated to contribute more than 98% of the total transport [16–18]. Bacterial invasion and dissemination normally accompany disruption of the vascular endothelial integrity due to bacterial toxin-mediated cytotoxicity. This vascular damage may lead to increased antibody extravasation within infected tissues. Once bacterial cells seed in the tissue, rapid bacterial growth and release of exotoxins stimulate immune responses, including recruitment of effector cells (i.e., lymphocytes, polymorphonuclear leukocytes, and phagocytes) and massive release of cytokines and chemokines. These reactions on one hand result in increased fluid infiltration and increased vascular permeability that facilitate mAb extravasation; but, on the other hand, build up fluid pressure within tissue that hampers antibody distribution (by decreasing the hydrostatic pressure gradient driving convective transport of mAb from blood to tissue interstitial fluid) [19,20]. In addition, antibody-dependent phagocytosis accelerates the elimination of mAbs (i.e., target-mediated elimination) in the tissue. Bacterial infections in visceral organs may also result in formation of abscesses, which enclose bacteria by pseudocapsules and protect them from immune cells and mAbs. Furthermore, many pathogenic bacteria generate biofilms that are comparatively inaccessible to antibodies, immune cells, and even small molecule antibiotics. Another concern is that biofilms may mediate a near continuous release of virulence factors, such as exopolysaccharides of *Staphylococcus epidermis*, that act as decoys to reduce mAb molecules reaching the bacteria [21]. Therefore, formation of both abscesses and biofilms create barriers to mAb distribution, and hence adversely affect the antibody-mediated clearance of bacteria.

3. Pharmacodynamic Mechanisms of Action

Antibacterial mAbs have been developed against a variety of bacterial cell surface targets (i.e., proteins and polysaccharides) and soluble exotoxins (Tables 1 and 2). The potential pharmacodynamic mechanism of action depends on the nature of the target, its role in bacterial pathogenesis, and mAb isotype and structure (i.e., intact IgG mAb or IgG fragments, immunoconjugates, bispecific antibodies, etc.). Anti-exotoxin mAbs typically attenuate bacterial pathological activity via neutralization of exotoxins. Monoclonal antibodies targeting bacterial surface epitopes are expected to increase bacterial clearance through enhancing antibody-dependent phagocytosis, and/or complement-mediated bactericidal activity, or via immune system-independent bacterial killing. In addition, there has been increasing interest in the development of immunoconjugates and immunomodulatory mAbs that either carry potent antimicrobials or stimulate exhausted immune effector functions to augment bactericidal activity.

3.1. Toxin Neutralization

Antibacterial mAbs that act through the mechanism of neutralization are typically directed against exotoxins. mAb binding to soluble exotoxins leads to the formation of antibody-toxin complexes, which are primarily cleared by the reticuloendothelial system. All three marketed antibacterial mAbs achieve effects via toxin neutralization (Table 1). The efficacy of neutralizing mAbs has been shown to be directly correlated with mAb binding affinity. Anti-protective antigen (PA) mAb with higher binding affinity showed superior protection against anthrax lethal toxin challenge in macrophage cytotoxicity assays and in a rat infection model, when compared to mAbs with relatively low affinities [22]. Additionally, antibody-FcγR engagement was found to be required for anti-PA mAb neutralization activity, where mAb-mediated protection against anthrax infection was only shown in wild-type mice but not FcγR-deficient mice [23]. However, FcγR engagement may not be required for all anti-toxin mAb. For example, MAb166, an anti-PcrV (type III secretion injectisome) antibody, blocks the delivery of *Pseudomonas aeruginosa* type III toxins to host cells [24]. A single dose of 10 μg of MAb166 Fab fragments, which lack an Fc domain, was able to confer similar protection (≥80% survival) as intact MAb166 against clinical isolates of *P. aeruginosa* in a mouse pneumonia infection model [24,25].

3.2. Opsonophagocytosis

Opsonophagocytosis has been considered as one of the key bactericidal mechanisms of the innate immune system. Antibody-mediated opsonophagocytosis involves antibody binding to bacterial surface antigens, followed by the engagement of FcγRs on the surface of professional phagocytes (i.e., monocytes/macrophages, neutrophils and dendritic cells), which in turn trigger actin-myosin driven endocytosis of antibody-bacteria complexes [26]. Phagosome vacuoles fuse with lysosomes, which leads to formation of phagolysosomes where bacteria are catabolized. Antibody-dependent phagocytosis is readily activated at the presence of phagocytes and antibody-bacteria complexes. It has been estimated that a surface density of only 5.33–26.7 antibodies/μm^2 (i.e., IgG density on the surface of targeted particles) is required to trigger antibody-dependent phagocytosis [27]. In one example of the significance of opsonophagocytosis for mAb treatment of bacterial infection, Russo et al. developed a mAb 13D6 against K1 capsular polysaccharide of *Acinetobacter baumannii*, which showed potent inhibitory effects on bacterial growth in a rat soft tissue infection model. Antibody-dependent phagocytic killing has been found to be the primary bactericidal mechanism in this study [28].

3.3. Complement-Dependent Cytotoxicity

Antibody-dependent (i.e., classical) complement activation is another important bactericidal mechanism of the innate immune system. Binding of antibodies on the bacterial surface enhances the recruitment and binding of soluble complement factors, including C1q, to the Fc domain of the mAb, which leads to the activation of the complement cascade (i.e., complement fixation), formation of the membrane attack complex, thus leading to bacterial killing. Activation of the antibody-dependent pathway requires interaction of C1q with at least two IgG molecules [29]. Based on the molecular size of C1q, it is estimated that the surface density of IgG must be such that IgG molecules are separated by no greater than ~40 nm to fix C1q [30]. In contrast, IgM is much more efficient in complement activation, as a single IgM molecule is able to fix C1q [29]. An anti-keratin antibody IgM (3B4) directed against Methicillin-resistant *Staphylococcus aureus* (MRSA) was generated by An et al. with strong binding to MRSA and mannose-binding lectin (MBL), which in turn activated the classical and MBL complement pathways and led to potent bactericidal activity [31]. Passive immunization with 3B4 significantly decreased bacterial burden in organs and improved animal survival in a mouse bacteremia model [31].

3.4. Direct Bactericidal mAbs

In addition to the mechanisms of action discussed above, antibacterial mAbs showing direct bactericidal activity have been occasionally identified. Binding of these mAbs may trigger lysis of bacterial cells directly (i.e., without requirement for fixation of complement of engagement of other components of the host immune system). For instance, LaRocca et al. developed an IgG1 mAb (CB2) that targets outer surface protein B (OspB) of *Borrelia burgdorferi* for the treatment of Lyme disease [32]. CB2 exhibited complement-independent pore forming when bound to *B. burgdorferi*, which resulted in osmotic lysis of bacterial cells. However, this bactericidal effect was not transferable to *Escherichia coli* expressing recombinant OspB, suggesting a unique interaction between CB2 and *B. burgdorferi* [32]. The underlying mechanism of action is unclear, but it was found to be correlated with cholesterol glycolipids in the *B. burgdorferi* outer membrane that exist as temperature-sensitive lipid raft-like microdomains [33].

3.5. Immunoconjugates

The use of mAbs to deliver highly potent payloads has been successfully applied in cancer treatment [34]. This strategy, on one hand, does not require the mAb itself to be protective; on the other hand, it increases the half-life and specificity of the payload and, hence, decreases off-target toxicity. However, application of this approach to bacterial infection is still in its infancy. In 2015, Lehar and colleagues for the first time adapted the immunoconjugate strategy to antimicrobials and developed a novel THIOMAB™ (Genentech, South San Francisco, CA, USA) antibody antibiotic conjugate (AAC) against *Staphylococcus aureus* [35]. The antibody module opsonizes *S. aureus* and mediates uptake into phagolysosomes, where a potent antibiotic payload is released, allowing efficient killing of intracellular bacteria [35]. This AAC strategy demonstrated promising bactericidal activity against vancomycin-resistant *S. aureus*, and it was especially efficacious for bacteria with an intracellular life cycle [36]. Antibody-antibiotic conjugates may be expected to demonstrate favorable pharmacokinetics (i.e., long half-lives), and decreased off-site toxicity. For example, the AAC strategy ameliorated antibiotic-mediated disruption to the normal flora, and may decrease selective pressure that enhances the development of cross resistance, due to the specificity provided by the antibody carrier. The advantages provided by antibody conjugation may allow for reconsideration of antimicrobials that failed in development due to unfavorable PK or toxicity.

Radioimmunoconjuates, which link radionuclides to mAbs, may allow targeted delivery of bactericidal radiation to bacteria. As a proof-of-principle, Dadachova et al. developed a radioimmunoconjugate with Bismuth-213 linked to a mAb (D11) targeting the pneumococcal capsular polysaccharide [37]. Administration of [213]Bi-D11 showed dose-dependent bacterial killing in vitro and in a mouse bacteremia model, without detectable hematological toxicity [37]. In addition, radioimmunotherapy has also shown to confer protection against human immunodeficiency virus (HIV) in severe combined immunodeficiency (SCID) mice, and to selectively kill HIV-infected human T cells and human peripheral blood mononuclear cells in vitro [38]. These data suggest that radioimmunoconjugates may provide protection in immunocompromised patients and may be efficacious against infected host cells that express bacterial antigens on cell surfaces, which could be a novel approach to clear latent intracellular bacteria.

3.6. Immunomodulatory mAbs

Immunomodulatory mAbs, such as T-cell engaging antibodies and antibodies targeting programmed cell death protein 1 (PD-1) or cytotoxic T lymphocyte-associated protein 4 (CRLA-4), have gained great success in the treatment of cancer. However, their application in bacterial infections has not been well explored. Akin to cancer, chronic exposure of antigens to T-cells during persistent infections leads to cellular exhaustion of effector functions [39]. Thus, immunomodulatory mAbs theoretically may aid in the clearance of bacteria through stimulating the host immune system. Recently, evidence from the literature supports the potential benefit of anti-PD-1 mAb for the treatment of tuberculosis (TB) infection. PD-1 and its ligands (PD-L1 and PD-L2) were found to be significantly decreased in CD4$^+$ and CD8$^+$ T cells in TB patients after standard-of-care therapy [40]. Treatment with anti-PD-1 mAb has been shown to restore cytokine secretion and antigen responsiveness of T cells isolated from TB patients ex vivo [41].

4. Challenges in the Development of mAbs for the Treatment of Bacterial Infections

Development of antibacterial mAbs has been progressing relatively slowly. Only three antibacterial mAbs have been marketed in the United States (Table 1), and nine mAb products are in Phase 1–2 clinical trials (Table 2). Although modest success in this area may be partly due to a real or perceived lack of economic incentive to the pharmaceutical industry, limited development of antibacterial mAbs may also relate to a host of scientific challenges. Some of the complexities include difficulties in the selection of accessible and conserved bacterial targets, risk for antibody-dependent enhancement of bacterial infection, and various bacterial countermeasures against antibodies.

4.1. Difficulties in Selection of Bacterial Targets

Antibacterial mAbs have been primarily developed to target either bacterial cell surface targets or secreted exotoxins. Although anti-exotoxin antibodies have been successful, these mAbs only attenuate bacterial pathological activity though neutralization of toxins, and are not expected to provide bactericidal activities. Anti-exotoxin mAbs, therefore, are typically indicated for prophylaxis or as adjunctive therapies to antibiotics. Antibacterial mAbs directed against bacterial surface epitopes have primarily been developed for binding to outer membrane proteins (OMPs) or exopolysaccharides (i.e., capsules or O-antigens of lipopolysaccharides) as shown in Table 2. OMPs are attractive therapeutic targets for vaccination and passive immunization due to the high conservation of OMPs among clinical isolates. Outer membrane protein A (OmpA)-like proteins, for instance, are conserved across all sequenced clinical isolates with high protein homology in many Gram-negative bacteria such as *Escherichia coli*, *Pseudomonas aeruginosa*, and *Acinetobacter baumannii* [42,43]. However, a concern for mAbs targeting OMPs are reports that exopolysaccharides mask these conserved targets, impede mAb binding, and hinder opsonization [44–48]. In contrast, exopolysaccharides are readily accessible to antibody binding. Several of the mAbs in development are directed against exopolysaccharides, such as DSTA4637S, MEDI3902, Aerumab, and Aerucin (Table 2). However, exopolysaccharide epitopes are not typically conserved. Large numbers of capsular serotypes have been identified for many bacterial pathogens. For example, at least 18 and 90 capsular serotypes have been described for *Staphylococcus aureus* and *Streptococcus pneumoniae*, respectively [49,50]. A single mAb thus may only provide protection against a specific capsular serotype. For instance, Aerumab binds only to serotype

O11 of *P. aeruginosa* (Table 2) and, therefore, mAb cocktails that recognize different serotypes may be required to confer meaningful antibacterial efficacy. In addition, exopolysaccharides may shed from bacterial cells and act as decoys, which may reduce the amount of unbound antibody reaching the bacterial surface. Capsular polysaccharides shed from *Klebsiella pneumoniae, Streptococcus pneumoniae,* and *P. aeruginosa* have been shown to increase the resistance to antimicrobial peptides (e.g., polymyxin B and neutrophil α-defensin 1) of an unencapsulated strains (i.e., 3-fold increase in minimum inhibitory concentrations). Incubation with these antimicrobial peptides also stimulated the release of capsular polysaccharide [51]. Shed capsular polysaccharides from *A. baumannii* appear to neutralize free anti-capsule mAb molecules and may contribute to the lack of efficacy of mAb treatment in an *A. baumannii* mouse pneumonia infection model [15].

4.2. Antibody-Dependent Enhancement of Infection

Although the role of immunoglobulin in host defense against invading microorganisms via activation of effector cells and complement is undisputed, accumulating evidence supports that, in some instances, antibody augments microorganism infection via assisting in their colonization and invasion to host cells. Antibody-dependent enhancement (ADE) of infection was first discovered in Murray Valley encephalitis virus by Hawkes [52], and it was found to also have relevance for other viruses, such as Dengue virus, human immunodeficiency virus, Ebola virus, and Zika virus [53–57]. ADE of viral infection is mainly due to the intracellular viability of viruses, where binding with mAb facilitates viral adherence and entry to host cells through interaction with Fc receptors or complement receptors [58,59]. ADE of bacterial infection has been reported less frequently; however, striking mechanisms have been identified. IgA1-dependent enhancement of pneumococcal adherence to Detroit 562 pharyngeal epithelial cells found by Weiser et al. is a particular example. IgA1 protease secreted by *Streptococcus pneumoniae* cleave the anti-capsule IgA1 mAb that is bound on the bacterial exopolysaccharide. Positive charges on the IgA1 Fab fragments neutralize the negative charges on the polysaccharide, which unmasks phosphorylcholine underneath the capsular polysaccharide, thus enhancing *S. pneumoniae* binding to epithelial cells [60]. The increase in *S. pneumoniae* adherence was found to be directly correlated with the isoelectric points of the IgA1 Fab fragments [60]. Recently, antibodies obtained from persons with latent tuberculosis were found to be protective, whereas antibodies obtained from those with active tuberculosis promote *Mycobacterium tuberculosis* infection of human lung epithelial cells and promote bacterial replication in macrophages [61]. Additionally, the activity of anti-*M. tuberculosis* mAbs (protective vs. non-protective) was shown to be correlated with both antibody isotype and glycosylation patterns [62,63]. Monoclonal antibodies directed against capsule epitopes of *Acinetobacter baumannii*, one of the three top priority pathogens listed by World Health Organization, also demonstrated ADE of infection. Our laboratory had shown that an anti-capsule mAb IgG3 enhances *A. baumannii* adherence/invasion to macrophages and human lung epithelial cells through IgG engagement of FcγRs, and this ADE of infection leads to a significant increase of animal mortality in a mouse pneumonia infection model [64].

4.3. Countermeasures against Antibacterial mAbs

Although antibacterial mAbs exploit pharmacological mechanisms that are distinct from those of antimicrobials and hence cross-resistance with small-molecule antibiotics is unlikely, host immunoglobulin has applied "selection pressure" to bacteria for millennia, which has led to the evolution of a variety of bacterial defense mechanisms. Countermeasures against host immunoglobulin may, in many cases, provide defense against therapeutic monoclonal antibacterial antibodies. Antibody neutralizing proteins, for instance, protein A of *S. aureus* and protein G of *Streptococcus*, are membrane proteins that bind antibody Fc domain and thus impede opsonophagocytosis and complement activation [65–67]. Additionally, binding of serum IgG via the Fc region decorates the bacterial surface, decreasing bacterial recognition by the immune system. Many bacteria also secrete proteinases that degrade antibodies and therefore inactivate antibody effector functions. *Streptococcus pyogenes,* for example, secrete IdeS (Immunoglobulin G-degrading enzyme of *S. pyogenes*) that specifically cleaves the γ-chain of human IgG in the hinge region, and SpeB (*Streptococcal* erythrogenic toxin B) that has a broad immunoglobulin-degrading activity toward IgG, IgA, IgM, IgD, and IgE [68,69]. Following IgG cleavage, the resultant antibody fragments (e.g., Fab or F(ab')$_2$) may compete for binding with intact antibodies and further impede antibody-mediated bactericidal activities [70]. Similar proteinases are also found in *S. aureus*, *P. aeruginosa*, *Streptococcus pneumoniae*, and *Haemophilus influenzae* [71–74]. Antibody-based therapies that rely on antibody effector functions are likely to be affected by these antibody neutralizing proteins and proteinases. Additionally, some bacteria can survive and replicate inside phagocytes, which then turn into "Trojan horses" that contribute to the systemic dissemination of bacteria and recurrence of infection. *M. tuberculosis*, for instance, inhibits fusion of lysosomes with phagosomes in macrophages, which protects bacteria from killing mediated by lysosomal constituents [75]. *Rickettsia prowazekii* escapes from phagosome vacuoles before the phagosome-lysosome fusion, likely via phospholipase-mediated dissolution of phagosome membrane [76]. *S. aureus* is resistant to killing by phagolysosomal catabolism through neutralization of toxic oxygen radicals by released catalase, superoxide dismutase, and carotenoids [36,77,78]. Thus, passive immunization that depends on opsonophagocytosis alone may be ineffective against these bacteria, and antibody-antibiotic conjugates that release potent antibiotic molecules intracellularly may be an effective strategy to kill these intracellular bacteria [35].

5. Currently Marketed mAbs for the Treatment of Bacterial Infections

5.1. Raxibacumab

Raxibacumab (Abthrax) is an anti-protective antigen (PA) mAb that has been approved for the treatment of adult and pediatric patients with inhalational anthrax due to *Bacillus anthracis*. Raxibacumab is approved for use in combination with appropriate antibacterial drugs, and for prophylaxis of inhalational anthrax when alternative therapies are not available or are not appropriate. Raxibacumab binds free PA with a high affinity (equilibrium dissociation constant K_d = 2.78 nM), which inhibits engagement of PA to its cellular receptors on macrophages. The antibody impedes intracellular entry of anthrax lethal factor and edema factor, which contribute substantially to the pathogenic effects of anthrax toxin [79,80]. Raxibacumab demonstrated linear PK in the dose range of 1–40 mg/kg following single IV doses in healthy human volunteers with a half-life of 20–22 days [81,82]. Co-administration with ciprofloxacin, a standard-of-care (SoC) antibiotic for *B. anthracis* bacteremia, did not affect the PK of raxibacumab [82]. Likewise, raxibacumab did not alter the PK of ciprofloxacin.

Raxibacumab is the first biologic product that was developed and approved under the FDA Animal Rule that may be applied when it is not ethical or feasible to conduct controlled clinical trials in humans. The effectiveness of raxibacumab for treatment of inhalational anthrax thus is based on efficacy studies in rabbits and monkeys. Treatment with raxibacumab was initiated when PA was detected in serum (28–42 h) or when body temperature was sustained above baseline for 2 h in animals after challenge with aerosolized *B. anthracis* spores. Significantly improved survival was demonstrated in infected New Zealand White (NZW) rabbits and cynomolgus macaques (44% and 64% survival, respectively), when treated with 40 mg/kg raxibacumab compared to placebo groups (0% survival) [82]. In addition, the combination of raxibacumab and levofloxacin provided significantly enhanced protection (82% survival) compared to the antibiotic alone (65% survival) in *B. anthracis* challenged NZW rabbits [83]. Based on the observed and simulated systemic exposure of raxibacumab in animals versus humans, a single intravenous dose of 40 mg/kg was suggested to provide protection in humans.

5.2. Obiltoxaximab

Obiltoxaximab (Anthim) is also an anti-PA mAb that was approved for the same indication and usage as raxibacumab. However, premedication with diphenhydramine is recommended and close monitoring of individuals who receive obiltoxaximab is also required due to common adverse reactions including hypersensitivity (10.6%, 34/320 healthy subjects) and anaphylaxis (0.9% cases) observed in Phase 1 clinical trials [84]. Obiltoxaximab (K_d = 0.33 nM) protects against anthrax toxin through inhibition of PA binding to cellular receptors on host cells [85]. Obiltoxaximab demonstrated linear PK in dose range of 4–16 mg/kg following single IV administration in healthy humans. Although obiltoxaximab PK has not been studied in infected patients [84], infection of NZW rabbits and cynomolgus monkeys with *B. anthracis* led to significantly faster clearance (17.0 mL/day/kg and 8.6 mL/day/kg) compared to values observed in non-infected animals (8.7 and 4.2 mL/day/kg, respectively) [13]. These data are suggestive of target-mediated elimination upon binding of obiltoxaximab to PA; however, this hypothesis requires further investigation. The estimated half-life and volume of distribution of obiltoxaximab in healthy volunteers was 17–23 days and 6.3–7.5 L, respectively [84]. Low titers (1:20–1:320) of anti-obiltoxaximab antibodies were detected in eight subjects (2.5%) during phase 1 studies, but alterations in PK and toxicity profile were not observed in these individuals [84]. Further, the PK of obiltoxaximab was not affected by concomitant intravenous and oral doses of ciprofloxacin in healthy humans and vice versa [84].

Obiltoxaximab was also approved under the US FDA Animal Rule. Therapeutic efficacy of obiltoxaximab was assessed in animals challenged with aerosolized *B. anthracis* spores. The mAb was administered after animals exhibited clinical signs of systemic anthrax (i.e., presence of PA in serum or sustained elevation of body temperature above baseline), and intravenous obiltoxaximab at 16 mg/kg was able to significantly improve survival in NZW rabbits (62–93%) and cynomolgus macaques (31–47%) compared to 0–6% survival in placebo groups [86]. In prophylaxis studies, a single dose of obiltoxaximab (16 mg/kg) administered 24–72 h prior to *B. anthracis* infection provided full protection (i.e., 100% survival) in cynomolgus macaques versus 10% survival in control animals [13]. Furthermore, obiltoxaximab administered in combination with antibiotics such as levofloxacin, ciprofloxacin, and doxycycline resulted in higher survival rates than the antibiotic alone in *B. anthracis* infected animals [13].

5.3. Bezlotoxumab

Bezlotoxumab (Zinplava) is a human IgG1 that has been approved for use to reduce recurrence of *Clostridium difficile* infection (CDI) in patients ≥18 years of age who are receiving antibacterial drugs for CDI and are at high risk for CDI recurrence. Bezlotoxumab binds with high affinity (K_d < 1 nM) to toxin B, a pivotal virulence factor of *C. difficile*. The mAb inhibits toxin B binding to host cells and hence prevents toxin B-mediated inactivation of Rho GTPases and downstream signaling pathways in cells [87]. The PK of bezlotoxumab was assessed in *C. difficile*-infected patients in Phase 3 clinical trials, with estimated mean clearance, volume of distribution, and half-life of 0.317 L/day, 7.33 L, and 19 days, respectively [88]. Recurrence of CDI (i.e., development of a new episode of *C. difficile*-associated diarrhea following clinical cure of the presenting CDI episode) was significantly lower in patients receiving 10 mg/kg bezlotoxumab with SoC (17.4% and 15.7%) than the subjects receiving placebo with SoC therapy (27.6% and 25.7%) in two Phase 3 studies [89]. However, addition of bezlotoxumab to SoC did not improve clinical cure rate in *C. difficile*-infected patients compared to the SoC group [89]. Thus bezlotoxumab is indicated only for prevention of recurrence of CDI, but not for treatment of CDI.

6. Antibacterial mAbs in Clinical Trials

In addition to the three marketed mAb products, there are nine mAbs that are currently being investigated in clinical trials. Among the nine products listed in Table 2, five mAbs are developed against *Staphylococcus aureus*, three are targeting *Pseudomonas aeruginosa*, and one is for *Escherichia coli*. Released data from preclinical and clinical studies are summarized here to give a broad overview of the products that may be clinically available in the next few years.

6.1. MEDI4893

MEDI4893 is a human IgG1 mAb that specifically binds to and neutralizes alpha-toxin (AT) of *Staphylococcus aureus* and hence inhibits AT-mediated cytotoxic activity toward host cells [90]. AT is a 33-kDa pore-forming toxin that forms heptameric pores in host cells membranes and results in cell lysis [91]. Animal studies using isogenic AT negative mutants demonstrated that AT is a key virulence factor in *S. aureus* infections including sepsis, skin and soft tissue infection, and pneumonia [91–93]. AT was found to be expressed in 83% clinical isolates worldwide, and 91% of the isolates encoded AT subtypes that were neutralized by MEDI4893 [90]. In an acute pneumonia infection model, MEDI4893 was shown to provide both prophylactic and therapeutic effects in immunocompetent and immunocompromised mice. Further, sub-therapeutic MEDI4893 doses administered in combination with sub-therapeutic doses of antibiotics (vancomycin or linezolid) provided significantly improved survival rates compared to monotherapies [94,95]. In a recent phase 1 clinical trial, MEDI4893 exhibited linear PK in the dose range of 225–5000 mg/subject. YTE mutations (amino acid substitutions M252Y/S254T/T256E) in Fc region of the mAb, which increase binding affinity for FcRn, contribute to its favorable clearance of 42–50 mL/day and extended half-life of 80–112 days [96].

6.2. ASN100

ASN100 is a mAb combination of two human IgG1, ASN-1 and ASN-2, which is in development for the prevention of ventilator-associated *S. aureus* pneumonia (VASP). ASN-1 targets alpha-toxin and four leukocidins including gamma hemolysins (HlgAB and HlgCB), Panton-Valentine leukocidin (LukSF or PVL), and LukED. ASN-2 binds another leukocidin LukGH (LukAB) [97,98]. Leukocidins are pore-forming toxins that typically lyse human phagocytic cells and thus play a key role in bacterial evasion of the innate immune response [99–102]. Therefore, ASN100 binds six different toxin molecules to protect against lysis of multiple human cells, including polymorphonuclear leukocytes, monocytes, macrophages, red blood cells, T cells, epithelial, and endothelial cells. Among the five leukocidins, HlgAB, HlgCB, and LukGH are highly conserved in *S. aureus* clinical isolates. LukED is expressed in 50–75% isolates, while LukSF is only present in 5–10% isolates but is correlated with more severe infections [99]. ASN-1 and ASN-2 exhibit linear serum PK over the dose range of 200–4000 mg/subject either when administered alone or simultaneously in healthy human volunteers [103]. Estimated mean clearance, volume of distribution, and half-life of ASN-1 are 0.256 L/day, 7.14 L, and 23.5 days. Values for ASN-2 are 0.186 L/day, 6.45 L, and 26.7 days [103].

6.3. DSTA4637S

DSTA4637S is a THIOMAB™ (Genentech, South San Francisco, CA, USA) antibody antibiotic conjugate (AAC) that is comprised of an anti-*S. aureus* THIOMAB™ (Genentech, South San Francisco, CA, USA) antibody and a potent antibiotic, 4-dimethylamino piperidino-hydroxybenzoxazino rifamycin (dmDNA31), linked through a protease cleavable valine-citrulline linker [35]. It has been known for more than half-century that *S. aureus* can survive inside neutrophils and turn them into "Trojan horses", which assist in systemic bacterial dissemination and contribute to recurrence of infection following antibacterial therapy [104]. DSTA4637A (a preclinical formulation of DSTA4637S) demonstrated potent intracellular bactericidal activity against *S. aureus* both in vitro and in a mouse bacteremia model [35]. The antibody module of the AAC specifically targets the β-O-linked N-acetylglucosamine sugar modifications on cell wall teichoic acid residues of *S. aureus* and is responsible for opsonization of bacteria. Once the opsonized bacteria are taken up into phagolysosomes, proteases such as cathepsins cleave the linker and release the potent dmDNA31 antibiotic, which eradicates intracellular *S. aureus* [35]. Total concentrations of the DSTA4637A antibody (TAb) and antibody-conjugated dmDNA31 (ac-dmDNA31) were consistent with linear plasma PK over the dose range of 5–50 mg/kg in non-infected mice and 25–50 mg/kg in *S. aureus* bacteremia mice [14]. Infection with *S. aureus* had negligible impact on plasma PK of TAb and ac-dmDNA31 over the efficacious dose range of 25–50 mg/kg, with mean clearance of 4.95 vs. 6.08 mL/day/kg, volume of distribution of 94.9 vs. 119 mL/day/kg, and half-life of 14.3 vs. 13.9 days for TAb in non-infected and infected mice, respectively [14]. PK data for DSTA4637S in human subjects have not been published.

6.4. Salvecin

Salvecin (AR-301) is a mAb developed as an adjunctive therapy to SoC antibiotics for ventilator-associated *S. aureus* pneumonia [105]. It binds and neutralizes alpha-toxin and hence prevents AT-mediated lysis of host cells. Phase 1/2a study results met their primary endpoints, and showed that VASP patients who received Salvecin in combination with SoC antibiotics spent shorter time under mechanical ventilation than patients treated with placebo plus antibiotics [106]. In addition, blood bacterial burden was consistently lower in Salvecin-treated patients compared to the control group [106].

6.5. 514.G3

514G3 is a human mAb targeting *Staphylococcus* Protein A (SpA), a key virulence determinant of *S. aureus* that is expressed in all clinical isolates [107]. SpA is present in the *S. aureus* cell wall envelope and is released during bacterial growth [108]. SpA binds the Fc domain of human IgG and protects *S. aureus* from antibody-dependent phagocytic killing [109,110]. Additionally, released SpA triggers B cell superantigen activity through cross-linking of B cell receptors at V_H3 domain [111,112]. 514G3 displaces SpA-bound serum IgG on *S. aureus* surface and enhances opsonophagocytosis or other mechanisms of immune clearance of bacteria [107]. In a pilot Phase 2 study in patients hospitalized with *S. aureus* bacteremia, treatment with 40 mg/kg 514G3 led to 49% reduction in relative risk of overall incidence of serious adverse events (SAEs) and 56% relative risk reduction in *S. aureus* related SAEs compared to the placebo group [113]. More importantly, the duration of hospitalization was reduced by 33% in 514G3 treated patients compared to patients who received placebo (8.6 ± 7 days vs. 12.7 ± 9 days, respectively) [113].

6.6. MEDI3902

MEDI3902 is a bispecific mAb that targets both type III secretion injectisome PcrV anchored on bacterial cell wall and serotype-independent Psl exopolysaccharide of *Pseudomonas aeruginosa* [114]. PcrV is a critical component of the type III secretion system (T3SS) that delivers bacterial toxins and effector molecules into host cells in order to initiate infection. Psl exopolysaccharide is important for *P. aeruginosa* colonization/attachment to mammalian cells and formation of biofilms [115,116]. The majority of *P. aeruginosa* clinical isolates express Psl (89.8–91.2%) and PcrV (87.7–90.2%), and at least one of the targets were identified in 97.3–100% of isolates [114]. While binding of MEDI3902 to PcrV inhibits T3SS-mediated cytotoxicity, targeting Psl prevents *P. aeruginosa* attachment to host cells and enhances opsonophagocytic killing of bacteria. Intravenous administration of MEDI3902 (5 or 15 mg/kg) at 24 h before or 1 h after lethal *P. aeruginosa* challenge conferred 100% survival and significant reductions on tissue bacterial burdens in acute pneumonia and bacteremia animal models including mice, New Zealand rabbits, and pigs [114,117,118].

6.7. Aerumab

Aerumab (AR-101), previously known as panobacumab, is a human IgM mAb directed against the O-antigen of *P. aeruginosa* lipopolysaccharide serotype O11, which accounts for ~20% of clinical isolates. Aerumab is being developed as an adjunctive immunotherapy to SoC antibiotics for ventilator associated pneumonia caused by *P. aeruginosa* [119,120]. Binding of Aerumab to *P. aeruginosa* leads to enhanced bacterial clearance through either phagocytosis or complement-mediated bacterial killing [120]. Aerumab demonstrated linear PK over the dose range of 0.1–4 mg/kg in healthy human volunteers, with mean clearance of 0.039–0.120 L/h, volume of distribution of 4.75–5.47 L, and half-life of 70–95 h [121]. *P. aeruginosa* infection in patients did not affect the PK of Aerumab following IV doses of 1.2 mg/kg, where estimated clearance, volume of distribution, and half-life are 0.0579 L/h, 7.5 L, and 102 h, respectively [122]. Further, all 13 patients who received three doses of 1.2 mg/kg Aerumab as an adjunctive therapy given every 72 h survived, with a mean clinical resolution rate of 85% (11/13) in 8 days compared to a rate of 64% (9/14) in 18.5 days in patients who did not receive the mAb [122,123].

6.8. Aerucin

As indicated above, Aerumab can only recognize ~20% of *P. aeruginosa* clinical isolates. Aerucin is a second generation anti-*P. aeruginosa* mAb that binds to alginate (i.e., exopolysaccharide) in greater than 90% of clinical isolates [124]. Aerucin is also developed as an adjunctive therapy to SoC antibiotics for hospital-acquired and ventilator-associated pneumonia caused by *P. aeruginosa*, and binding of Aerucin is also expected to augment the opsonophagocytic killing and complement-dependent bactericidal activity against *P. aeruginosa* [124]. However, preclinical and clinical study results for Aerucin have not been published.

6.9. Shigamab

Shiga toxin (Stx)-producing *Escherichia coli* (STEC) is the major cause of hemorrhagic colitis by infectious agents in the United States. A serious consequence of STEC infection is hemolytic uremic syndrome (HUS) that can lead to renal failure and death in 5–15% of infected children [125]. Treatments for STEC infections are currently not available, and antibiotics may increase the risk of HUS [126]. Shigamab is a combination of two chimeric mabs, cαStx1 and cαStx2, which were developed to neutralize Stx1 and Stx2, respectively. Stx1 and Stx2 are the two major types of shiga toxin that are the key virulence factors contributing to the pathogenesis of HUS [127]. Treatment with 20 mg/kg of Shigamab conferred 90% survival in mice challenged with lethal doses of Stx1 and Stx2, whereas cαStx1 or cαStx2 alone did not protect mice against infection [128]. In addition, infection with STEC strain B2F1 in mice did not affect the PK of cαStx2 at 15 mg/kg [128]. Shigamab exhibited linear PK over the dose range of 1–3 mg/kg, and cαStx1 was shown to have greater clearance (0.38 ± 0.16 mL/h/kg) and shorter half-life (190 ± 140 h) than cαStx2 (0.20 ± 0.07 mL/h/kg and 261 ± 112 h, respectively) [129].

7. Conclusions

Pathogen-specific antibacterial mAbs have become an appealing therapeutic option due to recent advances in mAb production and engineering technologies. Antibodies kill bacteria or attenuate bacterial pathological activity via various mechanisms, including opsonophagocytosis, complement-mediated bactericidal activity, antibody-dependent cellular cytotoxicity, and neutralization of bacterial toxins. These pharmacodynamic mechanisms are distinct from those of small-molecule antimicrobials and therefore, such mAbs provide an attractive therapeutic option for antimicrobial resistant strains. The high specificity of mAbs may be expected to allow less disturbance to normal flora and less selective pressure for cross-resistance. Extended half-lives of mAbs may allow less frequent dosing and long-term prophylaxis. Antibacterial mAbs may also exhibit pharmacokinetic properties such as target-mediated drug disposition due to opsonophagocytosis or formation of antibody-toxin complexes, and there is some potential for complicated tissue distribution during the course of bacterial infection. These possible complexities require further study. Though there are only three mAbs marketed for prophylaxis or treatment of bacterial infection as of today, there is promise for a more prominent future role for antibacterial mAbs in view of their many advantages over traditional antimicrobials, and in view of the positive findings from clinical investigations of several mAbs in development.

Acknowledgments: This work was supported through funding provided by the Center of Protein Therapeutics (J.P.B).

Author Contributions: S.X.W.-L. performed the literature research. S.X.W.-L. and J.P.B. designed, wrote, and edited the review.

References

1.   Winau, F.; Winau, R. Emil von Behring and serum therapy. *Microbes Infect.* **2002**, *4*, 185–188. [CrossRef]
2.   Casadevall, A. Antibody-based therapies for emerging infectious diseases. *Emerg. Infect. Dis.* **1996**, *2*, 200–208. [CrossRef] [PubMed]
3.   Felton, L.D. The units of protective antibody in antipneumococcus serum and antibody solution. *J. Infect. Dis.* **1928**, *43*, 531–542. [CrossRef]
4.   Weisman, L.E.; Cruess, D.F.; Fischer, G.W. Opsonic activity of commercially available standard intravenous immunoglobulin preparations. *Pediatr. Infect. Dis. J.* **1994**, *13*, 1122–1125. [CrossRef] [PubMed]
5.   Slade, H.B. Human immunoglobulins for intravenous use and hepatitis C viral transmission. *Clin. Diagn. Lab. Immunol.* **1994**, *1*, 613–619. [PubMed]
6.   Davies, J.; Davies, D. Origins and evolution of antibiotic resistance. *Microbiol. Mol. Biol. Rev.* **2010**, *74*, 417–433. [CrossRef] [PubMed]
7.   Ventola, C.L. The antibiotic resistance crisis: Part 1: Causes and threats. *Pharm. Ther.* **2015**, *40*, 277–283.
8.   Kohler, G.; Milstein, C. Continuous cultures of fused cells secreting antibody of predefined specificity. *Nature* **1975**, *256*, 495–497. [CrossRef] [PubMed]
9.   Wright, A.; Shin, S.U.; Morrison, S.L. Genetically engineered antibodies: Progress and prospects. *Crit. Rev. Immunol.* **1992**, *12*, 125–168. [PubMed]
10. Waldmann, T.A.; Strober, W. Metabolism of immunoglobulins. *Prog. Allergy* **1969**, *13*, 1–110. [PubMed]
11. Junghans, R.P. Finally! The brambell receptor (FcRB). Mediator of transmission of immunity and protection from catabolism for IgG. *Immunol. Res.* **1997**, *16*, 29–57. [CrossRef] [PubMed]
12. Levy, G. Pharmacologic target-mediated drug disposition. *Clin. Pharmacol. Ther.* **1994**, *56*, 248–252. [CrossRef] [PubMed]
13. Greig, S.L. Obiltoxaximab: First global approval. *Drugs* **2016**, *76*, 823–830. [CrossRef] [PubMed]
14. Zhou, C.; Lehar, S.; Gutierrez, J.; Rosenberger, C.M.; Ljumanovic, N.; Dinoso, J.; Koppada, N.; Hong, K.; Baruch, A.; Carrasco-Triguero, M.; et al. Pharmacokinetics and pharmacodynamics of DSTA4637A: A novel THIOMAB antibody antibiotic conjugate against *staphylococcus aureus* in mice. *MAbs* **2016**, *8*, 1612–1619. [CrossRef] [PubMed]
15. Wang-Lin, S.X.; Russo, T.A.; Balthasar, J.P. Pharmacokinetics of a monoclonal anti-*acinetobacter baumannii* k2 capsule antibody in mice. Unpublished work. 2018.
16. Baxter, L.T.; Zhu, H.; Mackensen, D.G.; Jain, R.K. Physiologically based pharmacokinetic model for specific and nonspecific monoclonal antibodies and fragments in normal tissues and human tumor xenografts in nude mice. *Cancer Res.* **1994**, *54*, 1517–1528. [PubMed]
17. Flessner, M.F.; Lofthouse, J.; El Zakaria, R. In vivo diffusion of immunoglobulin G in muscle: Effects of binding, solute exclusion, and lymphatic removal. *Am. J. Physiol.* **1997**, *273*, H2783–H2793. [CrossRef] [PubMed]
18. Baxter, L.T.; Jain, R.K. Transport of fluid and macromolecules in tumors. I. Role of interstitial pressure and convection. *Microvasc. Res.* **1989**, *37*, 77–104. [CrossRef]
19. Lobo, E.D.; Hansen, R.J.; Balthasar, J.P. Antibody pharmacokinetics and pharmacodynamics. *J. Pharm. Sci.* **2004**, *93*, 2645–2668. [CrossRef] [PubMed]
20. Wang, W.; Wang, E.Q.; Balthasar, J.P. Monoclonal antibody pharmacokinetics and pharmacodynamics. *Clin. Pharmacol. Ther.* **2008**, *84*, 548–558. [CrossRef] [PubMed]
21. Cerca, N.; Jefferson, K.K.; Oliveira, R.; Pier, G.B.; Azeredo, J. Comparative antibody-mediated phagocytosis of staphylococcus epidermidis cells grown in a biofilm or in the planktonic state. *Infect. Immun.* **2006**, *74*, 4849–4855. [CrossRef] [PubMed]
22. Sawada-Hirai, R.; Jiang, I.; Wang, F.; Sun, S.M.; Nedellec, R.; Ruther, P.; Alvarez, A.; Millis, D.; Morrow, P.R.; Kang, A.S. Human anti-anthrax protective antigen neutralizing monoclonal antibodies derived from donors vaccinated with anthrax vaccine adsorbed. *J. Immune Based Ther. Vaccines* **2004**, *2*, 5. [CrossRef] [PubMed]

23. Abboud, N.; Chow, S.K.; Saylor, C.; Janda, A.; Ravetch, J.V.; Scharff, M.D.; Casadevall, A. A requirement for FcγR in antibody-mediated bacterial toxin neutralization. *J. Exp. Med.* **2010**, *207*, 2395–2405. [CrossRef] [PubMed]

24. Frank, D.W.; Vallis, A.; Wiener-Kronish, J.P.; Roy-Burman, A.; Spack, E.G.; Mullaney, B.P.; Megdoud, M.; Marks, J.D.; Fritz, R.; Sawa, T. Generation and characterization of a protective monoclonal antibody to pseudomonas aeruginosa PcrV. *J. Infect. Dis.* **2002**, *186*, 64–73. [CrossRef] [PubMed]

25. Baer, M.; Sawa, T.; Flynn, P.; Luehrsen, K.; Martinez, D.; Wiener-Kronish, J.P.; Yarranton, G.; Bebbington, C. An engineered human antibody Fab fragment specific for *Pseudomonas aeruginosa* PcrV antigen has potent antibacterial activity. *Infect. Immun.* **2009**, *77*, 1083–1090. [CrossRef] [PubMed]

26. Kuhn, D.A.; Vanhecke, D.; Michen, B.; Blank, F.; Gehr, P.; Petri-Fink, A.; Rothen-Rutishauser, B. Different endocytotic uptake mechanisms for nanoparticles in epithelial cells and macrophages. *Beilstein J. Nanotechnol.* **2014**, *5*, 1625–1636. [CrossRef] [PubMed]

27. Lewis, J.T.; Hafeman, D.G.; McConnell, H.M. Kinetics of antibody-dependent binding of haptenated phospholipid vesicles to a macrophage-related cell line. *Biochemistry* **1980**, *19*, 5376–5386. [CrossRef] [PubMed]

28. Russo, T.A.; Beanan, J.M.; Olson, R.; MacDonald, U.; Cox, A.D.; St Michael, F.; Vinogradov, E.V.; Spellberg, B.; Luke-Marshall, N.R.; Campagnari, A.A. The K1 capsular polysaccharide from *Acinetobacter baumannii* is a potential therapeutic target via passive immunization. *Infect. Immun.* **2013**, *81*, 915–922. [CrossRef] [PubMed]

29. Sompayrac, L. *How the Immune System Works*, 4th ed.; Wiley-Blackwell: Chichester, UK; Hoboken, NJ, USA, 2012; p. 1.

30. Salvador-Morales, C.; Sim, R.B. Complement activation. In *Frontiers in Nanobiomedical Research*; World Scientific Singapore: Singapore, 2012.

31. An, J.; Li, Z.; Dong, Y.; Wu, J.; Ren, J. Complement activation contributes to the anti-methicillin-resistant staphylococcus aureus effect of natural anti-keratin antibody. *Biochem. Biophys. Res. Commun.* **2015**, *461*, 142–147. [CrossRef] [PubMed]

32. LaRocca, T.J.; Holthausen, D.J.; Hsieh, C.; Renken, C.; Mannella, C.A.; Benach, J.L. The bactericidal effect of a complement-independent antibody is osmolytic and specific to *Borrelia*. *Proc. Natl. Acad. Sci. USA* **2009**, *106*, 10752–10757. [CrossRef] [PubMed]

33. LaRocca, T.J.; Crowley, J.T.; Cusack, B.J.; Pathak, P.; Benach, J.; London, E.; Garcia-Monco, J.C.; Benach, J.L. Cholesterol lipids of *Borrelia burgdorferi* form lipid rafts and are required for the bactericidal activity of a complement-independent antibody. *Cell Host Microbe* **2010**, *8*, 331–342. [CrossRef] [PubMed]

34. Beck, A.; Reichert, J.M. Antibody-drug conjugates: Present and future. *MAbs* **2014**, *6*, 15–17. [CrossRef] [PubMed]

35. Lehar, S.M.; Pillow, T.; Xu, M.; Staben, L.; Kajihara, K.K.; Vandlen, R.; DePalatis, L.; Raab, H.; Hazenbos, W.L.; Morisaki, J.H.; et al. Novel antibody-antibiotic conjugate eliminates intracellular *S. Aureus*. *Nature* **2015**, *527*, 323–328. [CrossRef] [PubMed]

36. Gresham, H.D.; Lowrance, J.H.; Caver, T.E.; Wilson, B.S.; Cheung, A.L.; Lindberg, F.P. Survival of *Staphylococcus aureus* inside neutrophils contributes to infection. *J. Immunol.* **2000**, *164*, 3713–3722. [CrossRef] [PubMed]

37. Dadachova, E.; Burns, T.; Bryan, R.A.; Apostolidis, C.; Brechbiel, M.W.; Nosanchuk, J.D.; Casadevall, A.; Pirofski, L. Feasibility of radioimmunotherapy of experimental pneumococcal infection. *Antimicrob. Agents Chemother.* **2004**, *48*, 1624–1629. [CrossRef] [PubMed]

38. Dadachova, E.; Patel, M.C.; Toussi, S.; Apostolidis, C.; Morgenstern, A.; Brechbiel, M.W.; Gorny, M.K.; Zolla-Pazner, S.; Casadevall, A.; Goldstein, H. Targeted killing of virally infected cells by radiolabeled antibodies to viral proteins. *PLoS Med.* **2006**, *3*, e427. [CrossRef] [PubMed]

39. Wherry, E.J.; Kurachi, M. Molecular and cellular insights into T cell exhaustion. *Nat. Rev. Immunol.* **2015**, *15*, 486–499. [CrossRef] [PubMed]

40. Hassan, S.S.; Akram, M.; King, E.C.; Dockrell, H.M.; Cliff, J.M. PD-1, PD-l1 and PD-l2 gene expression on T-cells and natural killer cells declines in conjunction with a reduction in PD-1 protein during the intensive phase of tuberculosis treatment. *PLoS ONE* **2015**, *10*, e0137646. [CrossRef] [PubMed]

41. Bandaru, A.; Devalraju, K.P.; Paidipally, P.; Dhiman, R.; Venkatasubramanian, S.; Barnes, P.F.; Vankayalapati, R.; Valluri, V. Phosphorylated STAT3 and PD-1 regulate IL-17 production and IL-23 receptor expression in mycobacterium tuberculosis infection. *Eur. J. Immunol.* **2014**, *44*, 2013–2024. [CrossRef] [PubMed]

42. Beher, M.G.; Schnaitman, C.A.; Pugsley, A.P. Major heat-modifiable outer membrane protein in gram-negative bacteria: Comparison with the ompa protein of *Escherichia coli*. *J. Bacteriol.* **1980**, *143*, 906–913. [PubMed]

43. Luo, G.; Lin, L.; Ibrahim, A.S.; Baquir, B.; Pantapalangkoor, P.; Bonomo, R.A.; Doi, Y.; Adams, M.D.; Russo, T.A.; Spellberg, B. Active and passive immunization protects against lethal, extreme drug resistant-*Acinetobacter baumannii* infection. *PLoS ONE* **2012**, *7*, e29446. [CrossRef] [PubMed]

44. Hyams, C.; Camberlein, E.; Cohen, J.M.; Bax, K.; Brown, J.S. The *Streptococcus pneumoniae* capsule inhibits complement activity and neutrophil phagocytosis by multiple mechanisms. *Infect. Immun.* **2010**, *78*, 704–715. [CrossRef] [PubMed]

45. Russo, T.A.; Beanan, J.M.; Olson, R.; MacDonald, U.; Cope, J.J. Capsular polysaccharide and the O-specific antigen impede antibody binding: A potential obstacle for the successful development of an extraintestinal pathogenic *Escherichia coli* vaccine. *Vaccine* **2009**, *27*, 388–395. [CrossRef] [PubMed]

46. Pluschke, G.; Mayden, J.; Achtman, M.; Levine, R.P. Role of the capsule and the O antigen in resistance of O18:K1 *Escherichia coli* to complement-mediated killing. *Infect. Immun.* **1983**, *42*, 907–913. [PubMed]

47. Van der Ley, P.; Kuipers, O.; Tommassen, J.; Lugtenberg, B. O-antigenic chains of lipopolysaccharide prevent binding of antibody molecules to an outer membrane pore protein in *Enterobacteriaceae*. *Microb. Pathog.* **1986**, *1*, 43–49. [CrossRef]

48. Wang-Lin, S.X.; Olson, R.; Beanan, J.M.; MacDonald, U.; Balthasar, J.P.; Russo, T.A. The capsular polysaccharide of *Acinetobacter baumannii* is an obstacle for therapeutic passive immunization strategies. *Infect. Immun.* **2017**, *85*, e00591-17. [CrossRef] [PubMed]

49. O'Riordan, K.; Lee, J.C. *Staphylococcus aureus* capsular polysaccharides. *Clin. Microbiol. Rev.* **2004**, *17*, 218–234. [CrossRef] [PubMed]

50. Henrichsen, J. Six newly recognized types of Streptococcus pneumoniae. *J. Clin. Microbiol.* **1995**, *33*, 2759–2762. [PubMed]

51. Llobet, E.; Tomas, J.M.; Bengoechea, J.A. Capsule polysaccharide is a bacterial decoy for antimicrobial peptides. *Microbiology* **2008**, *154*, 3877–3886. [CrossRef] [PubMed]

52. Hawkes, R.A. Enhancement of the infectivity of arboviruses by specific antisera produced in domestic fowls. *Aust. J. Exp. Biol. Med. Sci.* **1964**, *42*, 465–482. [CrossRef] [PubMed]

53. Sasaki, T.; Setthapramote, C.; Kurosu, T.; Nishimura, M.; Asai, A.; Omokoko, M.D.; Pipattanaboon, C.; Pitaksajjakul, P.; Limkittikul, K.; Subchareon, A.; et al. Dengue virus neutralization and antibody-dependent enhancement activities of human monoclonal antibodies derived from dengue patients at acute phase of secondary infection. *Antiviral Res.* **2013**, *98*, 423–431. [CrossRef] [PubMed]

54. Bardina, S.V.; Bunduc, P.; Tripathi, S.; Duehr, J.; Frere, J.J.; Brown, J.A.; Nachbagauer, R.; Foster, G.A.; Krysztof, D.; Tortorella, D.; et al. Enhancement of Zika virus pathogenesis by preexisting antiflavivirus immunity. *Science* **2017**, *356*, 175–180. [CrossRef] [PubMed]

55. Halstead, S.B. Pathogenesis of dengue: Challenges to molecular biology. *Science* **1988**, *239*, 476–481. [CrossRef] [PubMed]

56. Takada, A.; Feldmann, H.; Ksiazek, T.G.; Kawaoka, Y. Antibody-dependent enhancement of Ebola virus infection. *J. Virol.* **2003**, *77*, 7539–7544. [CrossRef] [PubMed]

57. Toth, F.D.; Mosborg-Petersen, P.; Kiss, J.; Aboagye-Mathiesen, G.; Zdravkovic, M.; Hager, H.; Aranyosi, J.; Lampe, L.; Ebbesen, P. Antibody-dependent enhancement of HIV-1 infection in human term syncytiotrophoblast cells cultured in vitro. *Clin. Exp. Immunol.* **1994**, *96*, 389–394. [CrossRef] [PubMed]

58. Tirado, S.M.; Yoon, K.J. Antibody-dependent enhancement of virus infection and disease. *Viral. Immunol.* **2003**, *16*, 69–86. [CrossRef] [PubMed]

59. Takada, A.; Kawaoka, Y. Antibody-dependent enhancement of viral infection: Molecular mechanisms and in vivo implications. *Rev. Med. Virol.* **2003**, *13*, 387–398. [CrossRef] [PubMed]

60. Weiser, J.N.; Bae, D.; Fasching, C.; Scamurra, R.W.; Ratner, A.J.; Janoff, E.N. Antibody-enhanced pneumococcal adherence requires IgA1 protease. *Proc. Natl. Acad. Sci. USA* **2003**, *100*, 4215–4220. [CrossRef] [PubMed]

61. Casadevall, A. Antibodies to mycobacterium tuberculosis. *N. Engl. J. Med.* **2017**, *376*, 283–285. [CrossRef] [PubMed]

62. Lu, L.L.; Chung, A.W.; Rosebrock, T.R.; Ghebremichael, M.; Yu, W.H.; Grace, P.S.; Schoen, M.K.; Tafesse, F.; Martin, C.; Leung, V.; et al. A functional role for antibodies in tuberculosis. *Cell* **2016**, *167*, 433–443. [CrossRef] [PubMed]

63. Zimmermann, N.; Thormann, V.; Hu, B.; Kohler, A.B.; Imai-Matsushima, A.; Locht, C.; Arnett, E.; Schlesinger, L.S.; Zoller, T.; Schurmann, M.; et al. Human isotype-dependent inhibitory antibody responses against *Mycobacterium tuberculosis*. *EMBO Mol. Med.* **2016**, *8*, 1325–1339. [CrossRef] [PubMed]

64. Wang-Lin, S.X.; Olson, R.; Beanan, J.M.; MacDonald, U.; Russo, T.A.; Balthasar, J.P. Antibody dependent enhancement of *acinetobacter baumannii* infection through immunoglobulin g engagement of fc gamma receptors. *J. Immunol.* **2017**. submitted.

65. Bjorck, L.; Kronvall, G. Purification and some properties of streptococcal protein G, a novel IgG-binding reagent. *J. Immunol.* **1984**, *133*, 969–974. [PubMed]

66. Akerstrom, B.; Brodin, T.; Reis, K.; Bjorck, L. Protein G: A powerful tool for binding and detection of monoclonal and polyclonal antibodies. *J. Immunol.* **1985**, *135*, 2589–2592. [PubMed]

67. Falugi, F.; Kim, H.K.; Missiakas, D.M.; Schneewind, O. Role of protein A in the evasion of host adaptive immune responses by *Staphylococcus aureus*. *MBio* **2013**, *4*, e00575-13. [CrossRef] [PubMed]

68. Von Pawel-Rammingen, U.; Johansson, B.P.; Bjorck, L. Ides, a novel streptococcal cysteine proteinase with unique specificity for immunoglobulin G. *EMBO J.* **2002**, *21*, 1607–1615. [CrossRef] [PubMed]

69. Collin, M.; Olsen, A. Effect of SpeB and EndoS from *Streptococcus pyogenes* on human immunoglobulins. *Infect. Immun.* **2001**, *69*, 7187–7189. [CrossRef] [PubMed]

70. Fick, R.B., Jr.; Naegel, G.P.; Squier, S.U.; Wood, R.E.; Gee, J.B.; Reynolds, H.Y. Proteins of the cystic fibrosis respiratory tract. Fragmented immunoglobulin g opsonic antibody causing defective opsonophagocytosis. *J. Clin. Investig.* **1984**, *74*, 236–248. [CrossRef] [PubMed]

71. Karlsson, A.; Arvidson, S. Variation in extracellular protease production among clinical isolates of *Staphylococcus aureus* due to different levels of expression of the protease repressor sarA. *Infect. Immun.* **2002**, *70*, 4239–4246. [CrossRef] [PubMed]

72. Rooijakkers, S.H.; van Wamel, W.J.; Ruyken, M.; van Kessel, K.P.; van Strijp, J.A. Anti-opsonic properties of staphylokinase. *Microbes Infect.* **2005**, *7*, 476–484. [CrossRef] [PubMed]

73. Fick, R.B., Jr.; Baltimore, R.S.; Squier, S.U.; Reynolds, H.Y. IgG proteolytic activity of *Pseudomonas aeruginosa* in cystic fibrosis. *J. Infect. Dis.* **1985**, *151*, 589–598. [CrossRef] [PubMed]

74. Mulks, M.H.; Kornfeld, S.J.; Plaut, A.G. Specific proteolysis of human IgA by *Streptococcus pneumoniae* and *Haemophilus influenzae*. *J. Infect. Dis.* **1980**, *141*, 450–456. [CrossRef] [PubMed]

75. Hart, P.D.; Young, M.R.; Gordon, A.H.; Sullivan, K.H. Inhibition of phagosome-lysosome fusion in macrophages by certain mycobacteria can be explained by inhibition of lysosomal movements observed after phagocytosis. *J. Exp. Med.* **1987**, *166*, 933–946. [CrossRef] [PubMed]

76. Whitworth, T.; Popov, V.L.; Yu, X.J.; Walker, D.H.; Bouyer, D.H. Expression of the *Rickettsia prowazekii* pld or tlyC gene in *Salmonella enterica* serovar typhimurium mediates phagosomal escape. *Infect. Immun.* **2005**, *73*, 6668–6673. [CrossRef] [PubMed]

77. Flannagan, R.S.; Heit, B.; Heinrichs, D.E. Intracellular replication of staphylococcus aureus in mature phagolysosomes in macrophages precedes host cell death, and bacterial escape and dissemination. *Cell. Microbiol.* **2016**, *18*, 514–535. [CrossRef] [PubMed]

78. Voyich, J.M.; Braughton, K.R.; Sturdevant, D.E.; Whitney, A.R.; Said-Salim, B.; Porcella, S.F.; Long, R.D.; Dorward, D.W.; Gardner, D.J.; Kreiswirth, B.N.; et al. Insights into mechanisms used by staphylococcus aureus to avoid destruction by human neutrophils. *J. Immunol.* **2005**, *175*, 3907–3919. [CrossRef] [PubMed]

79. Chen, Z.; Moayeri, M.; Purcell, R. Monoclonal antibody therapies against anthrax. *Toxins (Basel)* **2011**, *3*, 1004–1019. [CrossRef] [PubMed]

80. Mazumdar, S. Raxibacumab. *MAbs* **2009**, *1*, 531–538. [CrossRef] [PubMed]

81. Subramanian, G.M.; Cronin, P.W.; Poley, G.; Weinstein, A.; Stoughton, S.M.; Zhong, J.; Ou, Y.; Zmuda, J.F.; Osborn, B.L.; Freimuth, W.W. A phase 1 study of Pamab, a fully human monoclonal antibody against *Bacillus anthracis* protective antigen, in healthy volunteers. *Clin. Infect. Dis.* **2005**, *41*, 12–20. [CrossRef] [PubMed]

82. Migone, T.S.; Subramanian, G.M.; Zhong, J.; Healey, L.M.; Corey, A.; Devalaraja, M.; Lo, L.; Ullrich, S.; Zimmerman, J.; Chen, A.; et al. Raxibacumab for the treatment of inhalational anthrax. *N. Engl. J. Med.* **2009**, *361*, 135–144. [CrossRef] [PubMed]

83. Corey, A.; Migone, T.S.; Bolmer, S.; Fiscella, M.; Ward, C.; Chen, C.; Meister, G. *Bacillus anthracis* protective antigen kinetics in inhalation spore-challenged untreated or levofloxacin/raxibacumab-treated New Zealand white rabbits. *Toxins (Basel)* **2013**, *5*, 120–138. [CrossRef] [PubMed]

84. Nagy, C.F.; Leach, T.S.; Hoffman, J.H.; Czech, A.; Carpenter, S.E.; Guttendorf, R. Pharmacokinetics and tolerability of obiltoxaximab: A report of 5 healthy volunteer studies. *Clin. Ther.* **2016**, *38*, 2083–2097. [CrossRef] [PubMed]

85. Nagy, C.F.; Mondick, J.; Serbina, N.; Casey, L.S.; Carpenter, S.E.; French, J.; Guttendorf, R. Animal-to-Human Dose Translation of Obiltoxaximab for Treatment of Inhalational Anthrax Under the US FDA Animal Rule. *Clin. Transl. Sci.* **2017**, *10*, 12–19. [CrossRef] [PubMed]

86. Yamamoto, B.J.; Shadiack, A.M.; Carpenter, S.; Sanford, D.; Henning, L.N.; O'Connor, E.; Gonzales, N.; Mondick, J.; French, J.; Stark, G.V.; et al. Efficacy projection of obiltoxaximab for treatment of inhalational anthrax across a range of disease severity. *Antimicrob. Agents Chemother.* **2016**, *60*, 5787–5795. [CrossRef] [PubMed]

87. Orth, P.; Xiao, L.; Hernandez, L.D.; Reichert, P.; Sheth, P.R.; Beaumont, M.; Yang, X.; Murgolo, N.; Ermakov, G.; DiNunzio, E.; et al. Mechanism of action and epitopes of *Clostridium difficile* toxin B-neutralizing antibody bezlotoxumab revealed by X-ray crystallography. *J. Biol. Chem.* **2014**, *289*, 18008–18021. [CrossRef] [PubMed]

88. Markham, A. Bezlotoxumab: First global approval. *Drugs* **2016**, *76*, 1793–1798. [CrossRef] [PubMed]

89. Wilcox, M.H.; Gerding, D.N.; Poxton, I.R.; Kelly, C.; Nathan, R.; Birch, T.; Cornely, O.A.; Rahav, G.; Bouza, E.; Lee, C.; et al. Bezlotoxumab for prevention of recurrent clostridium difficile infection. *N. Engl. J. Med.* **2017**, *376*, 305–317. [CrossRef] [PubMed]

90. Tabor, D.E.; Yu, L.; Mok, H.; Tkaczyk, C.; Sellman, B.R.; Wu, Y.; Oganesyan, V.; Slidel, T.; Jafri, H.; McCarthy, M.; et al. *Staphylococcus aureus* alpha-toxin is conserved among diverse hospital respiratory isolates collected from a global surveillance study and is neutralized by monoclonal antibody MEDI4893. *Antimicrob. Agents Chemother.* **2016**, *60*, 5312–5321. [CrossRef] [PubMed]

91. Bubeck Wardenburg, J.; Bae, T.; Otto, M.; Deleo, F.R.; Schneewind, O. Poring over pores: Alpha-hemolysin and panton-valentine leukocidin in *Staphylococcus aureus* pneumonia. *Nat. Med.* **2007**, *13*, 1405–1406. [CrossRef] [PubMed]

92. Powers, M.E.; Kim, H.K.; Wang, Y.; Bubeck Wardenburg, J. Adam10 mediates vascular injury induced by *Staphylococcus aureus* alpha-hemolysin. *J. Infect. Dis.* **2012**, *206*, 352–356. [CrossRef] [PubMed]

93. Tkaczyk, C.; Hamilton, M.M.; Datta, V.; Yang, X.P.; Hilliard, J.J.; Stephens, G.L.; Sadowska, A.; Hua, L.; O'Day, T.; Suzich, J.; et al. *Staphylococcus aureus* alpha toxin suppresses effective innate and adaptive immune responses in a murine dermonecrosis model. *PLoS ONE* **2013**, *8*, e75103. [CrossRef] [PubMed]

94. Hua, L.; Hilliard, J.J.; Shi, Y.; Tkaczyk, C.; Cheng, L.I.; Yu, X.; Datta, V.; Ren, S.; Feng, H.; Zinsou, R.; et al. Assessment of an anti-alpha-toxin monoclonal antibody for prevention and treatment of *Staphylococcus aureus*-induced pneumonia. *Antimicrob. Agents Chemother.* **2014**, *58*, 1108–1117. [CrossRef] [PubMed]

95. Hua, L.; Cohen, T.S.; Shi, Y.; Datta, V.; Hilliard, J.J.; Tkaczyk, C.; Suzich, J.; Stover, C.K.; Sellman, B.R. MEDI4893* promotes survival and extends the antibiotic treatment window in a *Staphylococcus aureus* immunocompromised pneumonia model. *Antimicrob. Agents Chemother.* **2015**, *59*, 4526–4532. [CrossRef] [PubMed]

96. Yu, X.Q.; Robbie, G.J.; Wu, Y.; Esser, M.T.; Jensen, K.; Schwartz, H.I.; Bellamy, T.; Hernandez-Illas, M.; Jafri, H.S. Safety, tolerability, and pharmacokinetics of MEDI4893, an investigational, extended-half-life, anti-*Staphylococcus aureus* alpha-toxin human monoclonal antibody, in healthy adults. *Antimicrob. Agents Chemother.* **2017**, *61*, e01020-16. [CrossRef] [PubMed]

97. Badarau, A.; Rouha, H.; Malafa, S.; Battles, M.B.; Walker, L.; Nielson, N.; Dolezilkova, I.; Teubenbacher, A.; Banerjee, S.; Maierhofer, B.; et al. Context matters: The importance of dimerization-induced conformation of the lukgh leukocidin of *Staphylococcus aureus* for the generation of neutralizing antibodies. *MAbs* **2016**, *8*, 1347–1360. [CrossRef] [PubMed]

98.   Rouha, H.; Badarau, A.; Visram, Z.C.; Battles, M.B.; Prinz, B.; Magyarics, Z.; Nagy, G.; Mirkina, I.; Stulik, L.; Zerbs, M.; et al. Five birds, one stone: Neutralization of alpha-hemolysin and 4 bi-component leukocidins of *Staphylococcus aureus* with a single human monoclonal antibody. *MAbs* **2015**, *7*, 243–254. [CrossRef] [PubMed]

99.   Vandenesch, F.; Lina, G.; Henry, T. *Staphylococcus aureus* hemolysins, bi-component leukocidins, and cytolytic peptides: A redundant arsenal of membrane-damaging virulence factors? *Front. Cell. Infect. Microbiol.* **2012**, *2*, 12. [CrossRef] [PubMed]

100. Alonzo, F., III; Torres, V.J. The bicomponent pore-forming leucocidins of *Staphylococcus aureus*. *Microbiol. Mol. Biol. Rev.* **2014**, *78*, 199–230. [CrossRef] [PubMed]

101. DuMont, A.L.; Torres, V.J. Cell targeting by the *Staphylococcus aureus* pore-forming toxins: It's not just about lipids. *Trends Microbiol.* **2014**, *22*, 21–27. [CrossRef] [PubMed]

102. DeLeo, F.R.; Diep, B.A.; Otto, M. Host defense and pathogenesis in *Staphylococcus aureus* infections. *Infect. Dis. Clin. North Am.* **2009**, *23*, 17–34. [CrossRef] [PubMed]

103. Magyarics, Z.; Leslie, F.; Luperchio, S.; Bartko, J.; Schorgenhofer, C.; Schwameis, M.; Derhaschnig, U.; Lagler, H.; Stiebellehner, L.; Jilma, B.; et al. Safety and pharmacokinetics of ASN100, a monoclonal antibody combination for the prevention and treatment of *Staphylococcus aureus* infections, from a single ascending dose phase 1 clinical study in healthy adult volunteers. In Proceedings of the European Congress of Clinical Microbiology and Infectious Diseases, Vienna, Austria, 22–25 April 2017.

104. Rogers, D.E. Studies on bacteriemia. I. Mechanisms relating to the persistence of bacteriemia in rabbits following the intravenous injection of staphylococci. *J. Exp. Med.* **1956**, *103*, 713–742. [CrossRef] [PubMed]

105. Health, N.I.O. Safety, Pharmacokinetics and Efficacy of KBSA301 in Severe Pneumonia (*S. Aureus*). Available online: https://clinicaltrials.gov/ct2/show/NCT01589185?recrs=abdefghim&cond=Staphylococcus+Aureus&intr=Antibodies%2C+Monoclonal&rank=2 (accessed on 22 July 2017).

106. Aridis Pharmaceuticals. Ar-301: Fully Human mAb against *Straphylococcus aureus*. Available online: http://www.aridispharma.com/ar-301/ (accessed on 22 July 2017).

107. Huynh, T.; Stecher, M.; McKinnon, J.; Jung, N.; Rupp, M. Safety and tolerability of 514G3, a ture human anti-protein a monoclonal antibody for the treatment of *S. Aureus* bacteremia. In *Open Forum Infectious Diseases*; Oxford University Press: Oxford, UK, 2016.

108. Ton-That, H.; Liu, G.; Mazmanian, S.K.; Faull, K.F.; Schneewind, O. Purification and characterization of sortase, the transpeptidase that cleaves surface proteins of *Staphylococcus aureus* at the LPXTG motif. *Proc. Natl. Acad. Sci. USA* **1999**, *96*, 12424–12429. [CrossRef] [PubMed]

109. Sjodahl, J. Repetitive sequences in protein a from *Staphylococcus aureus*. Arrangement of five regions within the protein, four being highly homologous and Fc-binding. *Eur. J. Biochem.* **1977**, *73*, 343–351. [CrossRef] [PubMed]

110. Forsgren, A.; Quie, P.G. Effects of staphylococcal protein A on heat labile opsonins. *J. Immunol.* **1974**, *112*, 1177–1180. [PubMed]

111. Cary, S.; Krishnan, M.; Marion, T.N.; Silverman, G.J. The murine clan V$_h$ III related 7183, J606 and S107 and DNA4 families commonly encode for binding to a bacterial B cell superantigen. *Mol. Immunol.* **1999**, *36*, 769–776. [CrossRef]

112. Goodyear, C.S.; Silverman, G.J. Death by a B cell superantigen: In vivo VH-targeted apoptotic supraclonal B cell deletion by a staphylococcal toxin. *J. Exp. Med.* **2003**, *197*, 1125–1139. [CrossRef] [PubMed]

113. Otero, A. Patients Receiving 514G3 Therapy Had Reduced Hospitalization and Fewer Infection-Related Serious Adverse Events. Available online: http://investors.xbiotech.com/phoenix.zhtml?c=253990&p=irol-newsArticle&ID=2259222 (accessed on 22 July 2017).

114. DiGiandomenico, A.; Keller, A.E.; Gao, C.; Rainey, G.J.; Warrener, P.; Camara, M.M.; Bonnell, J.; Fleming, R.; Bezabeh, B.; Dimasi, N.; et al. A multifunctional bispecific antibody protects against *Pseudomonas aeruginosa*. *Sci. Transl. Med.* **2014**, *6*, 262ra155. [CrossRef] [PubMed]

115. DiGiandomenico, A.; Warrener, P.; Hamilton, M.; Guillard, S.; Ravn, P.; Minter, R.; Camara, M.M.; Venkatraman, V.; Macgill, R.S.; Lin, J.; et al. Identification of broadly protective human antibodies to *Pseudomonas aeruginosa* exopolysaccharide Psl by phenotypic screening. *J. Exp. Med.* **2012**, *209*, 1273–1287. [CrossRef] [PubMed]

116. Warrener, P.; Varkey, R.; Bonnell, J.C.; DiGiandomenico, A.; Camara, M.; Cook, K.; Peng, L.; Zha, J.; Chowdury, P.; Sellman, B.; et al. A novel anti-PcrV antibody providing enhanced protection against *Pseudomonas aeruginosa* in multiple animal infection models. *Antimicrob. Agents Chemother.* **2014**, *58*, 4384–4391. [CrossRef] [PubMed]

117. Li Bassi, G.; Aguilera, E.; Senussi, T.; Iodone, F.A.; Motos, A.; Chiurazzi, C.; Travierso, C.; Amaro, R.; Hua, Y.; Bobi, J.; et al. MEDI3902 targeting *P. Aeruginosa* virulence factors PcrV and Psl for the prevention of pulmonary colonization during mechanical ventilation. In Proceedings of the American Thoracic Society 2017 International Conference, Washington, DC, USA, 19–24 May 2017.

118. DiGiandomenico, A.; Le, H.; Pinheiro, M.G.; Le, V.T.M.; Aguiar-Alves, F.; Quetz, J.; Tran, V.G.; Stover, C.K.; Diep, B.A. Protective activity of MEDI3902 for the prevention or treatment of lethal pneumonia and bloodstream infection caused by *pseudomonas aeruginosa* in rabbits. In Proceedings of the American Thoracic Society 2017 International Conference, Washington, DC, USA, 19–24 May 2017.

119. Secher, T.; Fas, S.; Fauconnier, L.; Mathieu, M.; Rutschi, O.; Ryffel, B.; Rudolf, M. The anti-*Pseudomonas aeruginosa* antibody panobacumab is efficacious on acute pneumonia in neutropenic mice and has additive effects with meropenem. *PLoS ONE* **2013**, *8*, e73396. [CrossRef] [PubMed]

120. Secher, T.; Fauconnier, L.; Szade, A.; Rutschi, O.; Fas, S.C.; Ryffel, B.; Rudolf, M.P. Anti-*Pseudomonas aeruginosa* serotype O11 LPS immunoglobulin M monoclonal antibody panobacumab (KBPA101) confers protection in a murine model of acute lung infection. *J. Antimicrob. Chemother.* **2011**, *66*, 1100–1109. [CrossRef] [PubMed]

121. Lazar, H.; Horn, M.P.; Zuercher, A.W.; Imboden, M.A.; Durrer, P.; Seiberling, M.; Pokorny, R.; Hammer, C.; Lang, A.B. Pharmacokinetics and safety profile of the human anti-*Pseudomonas aeruginosa* serotype O11 immunoglobulin M monoclonal antibody KBPA-101 in healthy volunteers. *Antimicrob. Agents Chemother.* **2009**, *53*, 3442–3446. [CrossRef] [PubMed]

122. Lu, Q.; Rouby, J.J.; Laterre, P.F.; Eggimann, P.; Dugard, A.; Giamarellos-Bourboulis, E.J.; Mercier, E.; Garbino, J.; Luyt, C.E.; Chastre, J.; et al. Pharmacokinetics and safety of panobacumab: Specific adjunctive immunotherapy in critical patients with nosocomial *Pseudomonas aeruginosa* O11 pneumonia. *J. Antimicrob. Chemother.* **2011**, *66*, 1110–1116. [CrossRef] [PubMed]

123. Que, Y.A.; Lazar, H.; Wolff, M.; Francois, B.; Laterre, P.F.; Mercier, E.; Garbino, J.; Pagani, J.L.; Revelly, J.P.; Mus, E.; et al. Assessment of panobacumab as adjunctive immunotherapy for the treatment of nosocomial *Pseudomonas aeruginosa* pneumonia. *Eur. J. Clin. Microbiol. Infect. Dis.* **2014**, *33*, 1861–1867. [CrossRef] [PubMed]

124. Aridis Pharmaceuticals. Aerucin: Broadly Active Human IgG Mab against *P. Aeruginosa*. Available online: http://www.aridispharma.com/aerucin/ (accessed on 23 July 2017).

125. Tarr, P.I.; Gordon, C.A.; Chandler, W.L. Shiga-toxin-producing *Escherichia coli* and haemolytic uraemic syndrome. *Lancet* **2005**, *365*, 1073–1086. [CrossRef]

126. Ahn, C.K.; Holt, N.J.; Tarr, P.I. Shiga-toxin producing *Escherichia coli* and the hemolytic uremic syndrome: What have we learned in the past 25 years? *Adv. Exp. Med. Biol.* **2009**, *634*, 1–17. [PubMed]

127. Melton-Celsa, A.R.; Smith, M.J.; O'Brien, A.D. Shiga toxins: Potent poisons, pathogenicity determinants, and pharmacological agents. *EcoSal Plus* **2005**, *1*. [CrossRef] [PubMed]

128. Melton-Celsa, A.R.; Carvalho, H.M.; Thuning-Roberson, C.; O'Brien, A.D. Protective efficacy and pharmacokinetics of human/mouse chimeric anti-stx1 and anti-stx2 antibodies in mice. *Clin. Vaccine Immunol.* **2015**, *22*, 448–455. [CrossRef] [PubMed]

129. Bitzan, M.; Poole, R.; Mehran, M.; Sicard, E.; Brockus, C.; Thuning-Roberson, C.; Riviere, M. Safety and pharmacokinetics of chimeric anti-shiga toxin 1 and anti-shiga toxin 2 monoclonal antibodies in healthy volunteers. *Antimicrob. Agents Chemother.* **2009**, *53*, 3081–3087. [CrossRef] [PubMed]

4

Antibody Conjugates - Recent Advances and Future Innovations

Donmienne Leung [1,*], Jacqueline M. Wurst [2], Tao Liu [2], Ruben M. Martinez [2], Amita Datta-Mannan [3] and Yiqing Feng [4]

[1] Biotechnology Discovery Research, Lilly Research Laboratories, Lilly Biotechnology Center, Eli Lilly and Company, San Diego, CA 92121, USA
[2] Discovery Chemistry and Research Technology, Lilly Research Laboratories, Lilly Biotechnology Center, Eli Lilly and Company, San Diego, CA 92121, USA; jwurst@lilly.com (J.M.W.); liu_tao2@lilly.com (T.L.); Martinez_ruben_martin@lilly.com (R.M.M.)
[3] Exploratory Medicine & Pharmacology, Lilly Research Laboratories, Lilly Corporate Center, Eli Lilly and Company, Indianapolis, IN 46225, USA; datta_amita@lilly.com
[4] Biotechnology Discovery Research, Lilly Research Laboratories, Lilly Technology Center North, Eli Lilly and Company, Indianapolis, IN 46221, USA; feng_yiqing@lilly.com
* Correspondence: leung_donmienne@lilly.com

Abstract: Monoclonal antibodies have evolved from research tools to powerful therapeutics in the past 30 years. Clinical success rates of antibodies have exceeded expectations, resulting in heavy investment in biologics discovery and development in addition to traditional small molecules across the industry. However, protein therapeutics cannot drug targets intracellularly and are limited to soluble and cell-surface antigens. Tremendous strides have been made in antibody discovery, protein engineering, formulation, and delivery devices. These advances continue to push the boundaries of biologics to enable antibody conjugates to take advantage of the target specificity and long half-life from an antibody, while delivering highly potent small molecule drugs. While the "magic bullet" concept produced the first wave of antibody conjugates, these entities were met with limited clinical success. This review summarizes the advances and challenges in the field to date with emphasis on antibody conjugation, linker-payload chemistry, novel payload classes, absorption, distribution, metabolism, and excretion (ADME), and product developability. We discuss lessons learned in the development of oncology antibody conjugates and look towards future innovations enabling other therapeutic indications.

Keywords: antibodies; site-specific conjugation; bioconjugates; ADC; antibody-drug conjugates; payloads; linkers; nucleic acids; ADME; developability; formulation

1. Introduction

Since the first monoclonal antibody drug approval (OKT3) in 1986, over 60 antibody therapeutics have become marketed drugs to date [1]. The number of protein therapeutics entering clinical development, including antibodies, antibody fragments, bispecifics, Fc-fusion proteins, and antibody-drug conjugates is expected to grow due to robust pipelines and high success rates for treating various diseases [2,3]. With the advances and extensive experience in antibody engineering over the past decades [4], antibody therapeutics have evolved from murine (e.g., OKT3) to chimeric (e.g., Rituxan®) to fully human (e.g., Humira®) as depicted in Figure 1. Monoclonal antibody-based therapeutics have been built to deliver specific effector functions or as bispecifics and conjugates to achieve the desired pharmacological effects [5,6]. Antibody discovery was enabled by murine hybridoma technology [7] followed by humanization [8] to deliver therapeutic antibodies with lower risk of immunogenicity [9]. Display technologies and transgenic animals have pushed the boundaries to produce antibodies with fully human sequences [10]. Antibody conjugates have similarly taken advantage of the progress made in monoclonal antibody development and improvements in conjugation chemistries [11–13] to expand the druggable target space for antibody-based therapies. These advances in antibody development are crucial to the success of antibody conjugates.

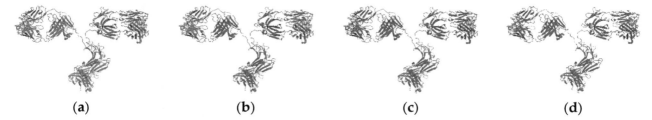

(a) (b) (c) (d)

Figure 1. The evolution of (**a**) murine, (**b**) chimeric, (**c**) humanized, and (**d**) fully human monoclonal antibodies through protein engineering. Red and blue represents mouse and human antibody sequence respectively. The antigen binding complementarity determining regions (CDRs) are shown as sticks. The new generation of antibody-drug-conjugates (ADCs) utilized humanized (**c**) and fully human antibodies (**d**).

While chemotherapy and radiation have been the dominant treatments of cancer for decades, their lack of ability to distinguish between healthy and tumor cells has fueled the desire to create tumor specific delivery of cytotoxic payloads and radionuclides via antibody conjugates. Oncology antibody conjugates have successfully delivered potent chemotherapeutic and radioactive agents to kill tumor cells [12]. Currently, all of the FDA approved antibody-drug-conjugates (ADCs) are targeted cancer therapies (Table 1) [14], including the latest approval in June 2019 for Polivy® [15]. Herein, we review the progress made in oncology ADCs in terms of conjugate design and development, linker payload conjugation chemistries and highlight novel non-oncology conjugate innovations.

2. Critical Considerations for Antibody Conjugates

First generation oncology ADCs in the 1990s were based on murine or chimeric antibodies which were plagued with immunogenicity issues [16] and linker instability [17]. Immunogenicity of protein therapeutics has a critical impact on the pharmacokinetics and drug disposition and ultimately clinical success [18,19]. These molecules were designed to deliver a variety of protein toxins [20] and microtubule binding drugs [21] as the cytotoxic payloads. Limited antigen density on tumors, low potency of the payloads, and the low average drug-antibody-ratio (DAR ~3–4) prevented efficacious quantity of drug delivered, which was proposed to be one of the reasons for initial ADC failures, while higher DAR conjugates suffered from toxicity and low therapeutic index. Second generation ADCs from the last 10+ years approved by the FDA were armed humanized antibodies coupled to stabilized linkers and more potent payloads, such as auristatins, calicheamicins, and maytansinoids (Table 1).

In an ideal situation, ADC payloads should be inactive in circulation when conjugated to an antibody via a linker and remain stably conjugated until the conjugate reaches the target of interest. Upon internalization of the conjugate-target complex, active payload is released inside target cells after lysosomal degradation of the linker or the antibody itself. In addition to reducing target-independent uptake, conjugate stability remains crucial for specific delivery and distribution of payload to the target tissue from systemic circulation. Conjugation sites, chemistries and linker designs coupled with DAR load greatly affect plasma stability, biophysical properties, and consequently pharmacokinetics of the conjugate. Next generation ADCs will likely incorporate fully human antibodies with site-specific conjugation and novel linkers to reduce immunogenicity and optimize biodistribution and payload delivery. These topics will be discussed in this review.

Table 1. FDA approved antibody-drug-conjugates (ADCs).

ADC Product	Indications	Approval Date	Target Antigen	Antibody Conjugation	Average Drug Antibody Ratio (DAR)	Linker	Payload
Mylotarg® (Gemtuzumab ozogamicin)	Relapsed AML	2001, withdrawn 2010; (reapproved 2017)	CD33	Humanized IgG4—lysine	2–3	Hydrazone	Calicheamicin
Adcetris® (Brentuximab vedotin)	Relapsed HL and sALCL	2011	CD30	Chimeric IgG1—cysteine	~4	Dipeptide cleavable (Val-Cit)	Monomethyl auristatin E (MMAE)
Kadcyla® (Trastuzumab emtansine)	HER2 + metastatic breast cancer	2013	HER2	Humanized IgG1—lysine	3.5	Thioether Non-cleavable	Emtansine (DM1)
Besponsa® (Inotuzumab ozogamicin)	Relapsed or refractory CD22 + B-ALL	2017	CD22	Humanized IgG4—lysine	~4	Hydrazone	Calicheamicin
Polivy® (Polatuzumab vedotin)	Relapsed or refractory DLBCL	2019	CD79b	Humanized IgG1—cysteine	3.5	Dipeptide cleavable (Val-Cit)	Monomethyl auristatin E (MMAE)

2.1. Target and Antibody Selection

One of the key contributing factors to clinical failures has been the bio-distribution of an ADC, which is critically dependent on the relative target expression as well as target-independent uptake. Other aspects such as conjugate and linker stability and payload properties are described in other sections. Preferably for an oncology treatment with a biologic, antigen targets should have high expression levels on tumor cells and little to no expression on normal tissues. Internalization of the target-antibody complex is crucial for specific intracellular release of payloads. Antibodies are ideal delivery vehicles due to their high specificity to targets and long half-life, which is the result of pinocytosis and subsequent neonatal Fc receptor (FcRn)-mediated recycling [22]. Prolonged systemic circulation enables conjugate accumulation at the target sites.

The antibody Fc choice is an important consideration for both monoclonal antibody therapeutics and ADC therapeutics [23]. Fc-mediated effector functions such as antibody-dependent cellular cytotoxicity (ADCC) or complement-dependent cytotoxicity (CDC) are part of the mechanism of action for depleting antibodies [24]. However, with ADCs, the contribution of effector functions to efficacy and toxicity are not well understood. It is noted that two out of the five currently FDA approved ADCs (Mylotarg® and Besponsa®) employed IgG4 antibodies which lack effector functions. Although the effector functions have the potential to augment the anti-tumor activities of the ADCs, engaging Fcγ receptors is also a possible cause for off-target and dose-limiting toxicity (reviewed in [25].) Emerging literature suggests that the antibody internalization and delivery of the toxic drug to the target cells serves as the primary mechanism of action for ADCs that is far more efficient than ADCC and Antibody-Dependent Cellular Phagocytosis (ADCP). For example, trastuzumab-DM1, SYD985, and DS-8201a all target HER2 and have shown similar ADCC activity as trastuzumab but they have demonstrated dramatically more anti-tumor activity than trastuzumab [26–31]. The anti-Trop-2 ADC IMMU-132 represents a more striking case as this ADC lost 60%–70% of the ADCC activity compared with the unconjugated mAb upon the conjugation of SN38 [32]. Nevertheless, this ADC demonstrated significant antitumor effects in mice bearing human pancreatic or gastric cancer xenografts [32] and is showing promise in clinical trials [33,34]. On the other hand, it is well established that afucosylated IgG1 increased binding to FcγRIIIa on effector cell such as natural killer cells and led to enhanced ADCC activity [35]. An example is GSK2857916, an afucosylated IgG1 antibody as a non-cleavable MMAF conjugate targeting B-cell maturation antigen (BCMA), in the clinic for multiple myeloma and demonstrated potent anti-tumor activity while it harnessed multiple cytotoxic mechanisms [36,37].

Due to the large size of an antibody conjugate, the stromal barrier [38] and tumor tissue penetration is an obvious obstacle for oncology ADCs to overcome for the treatment of solid tumors. Nonetheless, the successful targeting and delivery of payload to liquid tumor in circulation pushed the concept and led to a new frontier in ADCs to deliver small molecules for non-oncology indications [39,40]. Novel non-cytotoxic payloads have been conjugated to antibodies in the hopes of extending the pharmacokinetic properties and increasing therapeutic index of the drugs. Genentech has pioneered antibody-antibiotic conjugates [41,42] to target intracellular *Staphylococcus aureus* within host cells. Others have leveraged the internalization mechanism of antibodies to deliver immunosuppressive, cardiovascular or metabolic disorder small molecule drugs to specific cells using cell surface targets such as E-selectin [43], CD11a [44,45], CD25 [46], a3(IV)NC1 [47], CXCR4 [40,48], CD45 [49], CD70 [50], CD74 [51], and CD163 [52,53]. Examples of linker payloads as well as formulation and delivery challenges for non-oncology indications are discussed below. Additionally, genes of interest have been targeted in specific cell types to produce durable response using antibody-oligonucleotide conjugates [54,55]. Delivery of oligonucleotides have traditionally been challenging and various modifications have been employed to facilitate better cell penetration. This is explored in a later section.

2.2. Conjugation Methods

Antibody conjugation methods (Figure 2) have been extensively reviewed [11,56–58]. To date, all the FDA approved ADCs have relied on coupling reactions using either the nucleophilic primary amino group of surface-exposed lysines or the thiol group of reduced structural disulfides. The resulting product is a controlled heterogeneous mixture of antibodies with average drug load. High DAR species leads to aggregate formation, lower tolerated dose, and faster systemic clearance while low DAR species suffer from low efficacy [59]. Although DAR profile can be controlled by conjugation process development and specific DAR can be purified, site-specific methods to produce more homogeneous drug products would improve yield and biophysical properties, which will be critical for the next generation of ADCs. Towards these ends, extensive experience in protein engineering has allowed strategic placements of residues at specific locations enabling chemo-selective conjugation reactions. Researchers at Genentech first demonstrated that conjugation stability is location dependent and specific engineered cysteine sites were able to improve therapeutic index [60–62]. Cysteine insertions at specific sites can also efficiently produce stable conjugations [63]. Others have shown similarly that location of the conjugation sites can impact the stability and pharmacokinetics of the ADCs using alternative residues and chemistries [64,65].

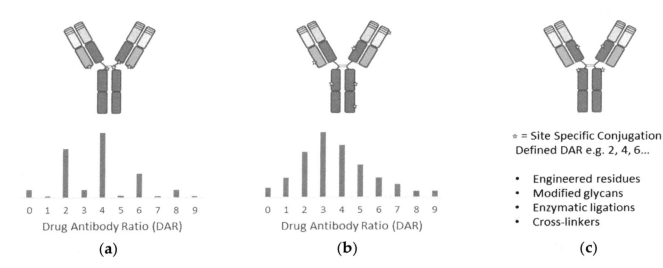

Drug Antibody Ratio (DAR)   Drug Antibody Ratio (DAR)

(a)   (b)   (c)

☆ = Site Specific Conjugation
Defined DAR e.g. 2, 4, 6...

- Engineered residues
- Modified glycans
- Enzymatic ligations
- Cross-linkers

Figure 2. Antibody conjugation methods include (**a**) cysteine-reactive, and (**b**) lysine-reactive chemistries which generate heterogeneous mixtures of drug-antibody-ratio (DAR), while (**c**) site specific conjugation methods deliver more homogeneous product with defined DAR using engineered residues, modified glycans, enzymatic ligations, and chemical cross-linkers. Schematic representation of antibody heavy chains and light chains are colored blue and green respectively. complementarity determining regions (CDRs) and conjugation sites are depicted as red bars and stars respectively. Approximate DAR distribution for stochastic cysteine and lysine conjugations are presented as bar charts.

Enzymatic methods have also been explored (reviewed in [66]) where recognition sequences have been engineered into the antibody to facilitate site-specific conjugation. Most well-exemplified in this category are enzymes such as transglutaminase [65,67–69], sortase [70–72] and formylglycine-generating enzyme (FGE) [73,74]. Transglutaminases (TG) catalyze a stable isopeptide bond between an amine of a lysine and the γ-carbonyl amide of a glutamine. Deglycosylation of N-linked glycan on a native antibody exposes glutamine at position 295 for site-specific conjugation with TG either through direct coupling with an amine-functionalized linker payload or via a two-step coupling by installing bio-orthogonal azide or thiol for strain-promoted azide-alkyne cycloaddition and maleimide chemistry respectively [67]. Alternatively, glutamine residues can be engineered and short glutamine (LLQG) tags were introduced into different regions to yield highly stable site-specific conjugates with good pharmacokinetic profiles [65,68,69]. Sortase catalyzes a transpeptidation reaction between a N-terminal glycine of GGG peptide or linker payload with the threonine-glycine bond in a LPXTG motif to produce a peptide fusion or site-specific ADC with high in vitro and in vivo potency [70–72]. Lastly, SMARTag® [75] is an example where formylglycine-generating enzyme (FGE) converts an engineered cysteine residue in a specific peptide sequence to produce an aldehyde tag in cell culture [73,74] to enable conjugation with linkers via oxime formation or a Pictet–Spengler reaction [76,77].

Other conjugation chemistries involved the engineering of unnatural amino acids [78–82] to install reactive groups in the antibody for bio-orthogonal chemistry [77]. Companies such as Ambrx [81] and Sutro Biopharma [83] have utilized these elegant approaches to generate site-specific ADCs. An orthogonal amber suppressor tRNA/aminoacyl-tRNA synthetase pair is used to incorporate the unnatural amino acids such as para-acetylphenylalanine (pAF), para-azidophenylalanine (pAZ), and para-azidomethylphenylalanine (pAMF) into recombinantly expressed antibodies in cell-based or cell-free systems. Reactive ketone in pAF forms a stable oxime linkage with alkoxyamine containing linkers, while the azido group in pAZ and pAMF undergoes click chemistry with alkynes to produce homogenous ADCs.

Alternatively, native antibodies can be conjugated site-specifically [84] after enzymatic modification of natural amino acids such as tyrosines [85] and glutamines [67], and carbohydrates can be oxidized chemically or modified with enzymes to produce reactive groups for conjugation [86–88]. For instance, sodium periodate oxidation of fucose at the native N-linked glycan of an antibody installed an aldehyde for conjugation with hydrazides [86]. Glyco-remodeling methods include enzymatic transfer of galactose and sialic acid with a mixture of transferases yielded glycans which can be oxidized with periodate to form oxime conjugates with aminooxy linker payloads [87], while sialytransferase can also incorporate an azide modified sialic acid derivative into the antibody for click chemistry [89]. Similarly, SynAffix BV utilized a 2-steps GlycoConnect™ process to trim a mixture of glycoforms with endoglycosidase, followed by enzymatic transfer of azido sialic acid for copper-free click chemistry [88]. Lastly, site-specific conjugation approach to retain the structural stability of a native antibody is to cross-link the reduced interchain disulfides with re-bridging chemical reagents [90–94].

Taken together, the various novel site-specific conjugation methods often require additional investments in manufacturing processes to produce the clinically viable products at large scale. Many development advances have been made in site-specific conjugations enabled a new generation of ADCs to enter the clinic in recent years, but this topic is outside the scope of this review.

3. Current Small Molecule Payloads and Beyond

ADC payloads have been mostly anti-mitotic small molecules for oncology indications [13,39]. The clear advantage of conjugates in this space is targeted delivery at efficacious doses that are below what could be given systemically due to the toxicity of the payload. Current approved ADCs such as Adcetris®, Kadcyla®, and Polivy® carry cytotoxic payloads that rely on the anti-mitotic mechanism of action (MOA) such as monomethyl auristatin E and emtansine (Table 1; Figure 3a,b, respectively). This class of payloads still predominates in clinical stage research, including novel derivates of these small molecules, despite efforts to use payloads with alternative MOAs [13,39,95].

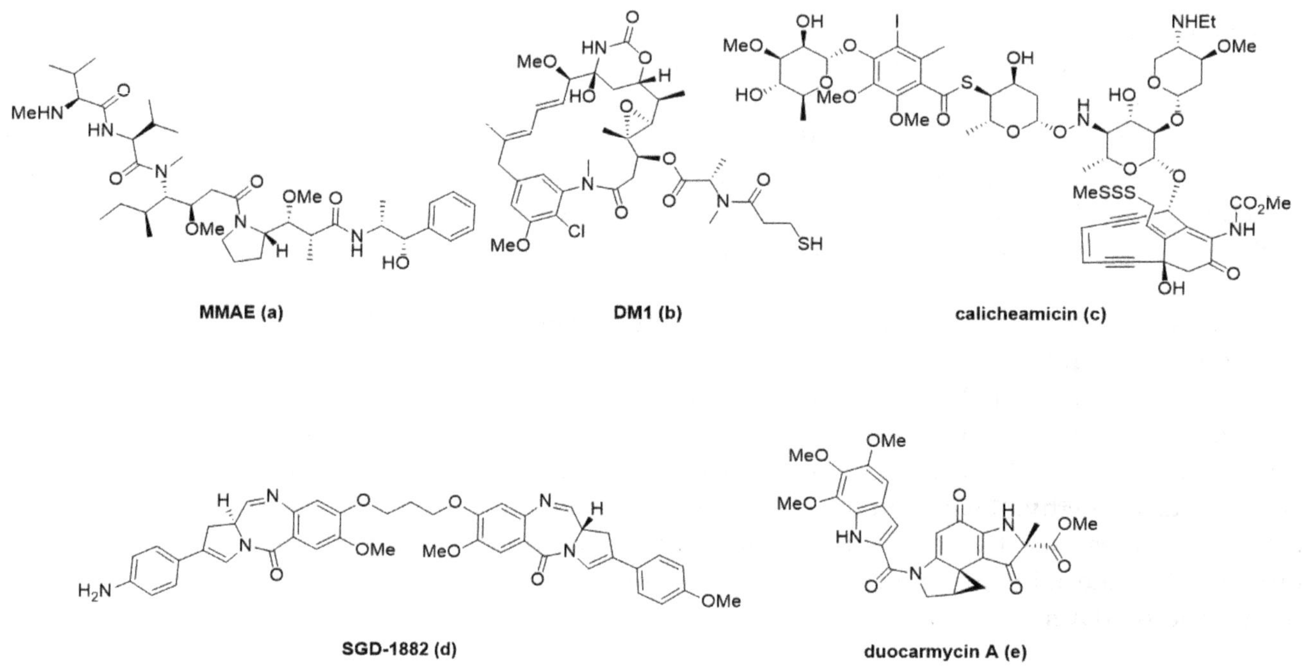

Figure 3. Examples of ADC payloads used clinically include, monomethyl auristatin E (MMAE, **a**, emtansine (DM1, **b**), calicheamicin (**c**), pyrrolobenzodiazepine dimer (PBD, SGD-1882, **d**), and duocarmycin A (**e**).

DNA damaging agents are another class of well-studied payloads [96–98]. Enediynes, such as calicheamicin **c**, are the warhead in Mylotarg® and Besponsa® (Table 1, Figure 3). They act through DNA-binding and induction of DNA-double strand breaking to produce a cytotoxic response in target cells. Other important DNA damaging agents currently used as payloads in clinical trials are duocarmycins **e** and pyrrolobenzodiazepines (PBD, **d**); they have unique, well-understood minor groove binding mechanisms that disrupt normal DNA function leading to cell death. Novel payloads have been explored recently in this space such as bis-intercalator depsipeptides with nanomolar affinity to DNA [99]. Pfizer demonstrated that this ultra-potent payload **a** (Figure 4) can overcome the previous limits of efficacy in animal models, therefore, expanding their relevance to indications beyond liquid tumors.

Further, highly-potent payloads described in the conjugate space (Figure 4) are pyrrole-based KSP (kinesin spindle protein) inhibitors **b** [100], which are traditional in the sense of their antimitotic mechanism-of-action, but newly incorporated pyrrole functionality provided an increase in efficacy against a wide-range of cancers previously untouched by this class. Continuing the push beyond the limits of first-generation payloads, Daiichi Sankyo® has incorporated a topoisomerase I inhibitor, exatecan derivative (DXd, **c**) into an ADC (DS-8201a). With superior pharmacodynamic and safety properties, in large part from the payload, DS-8201a has shown promising response in trastuzumab emtansine-insensitive cancers [31].

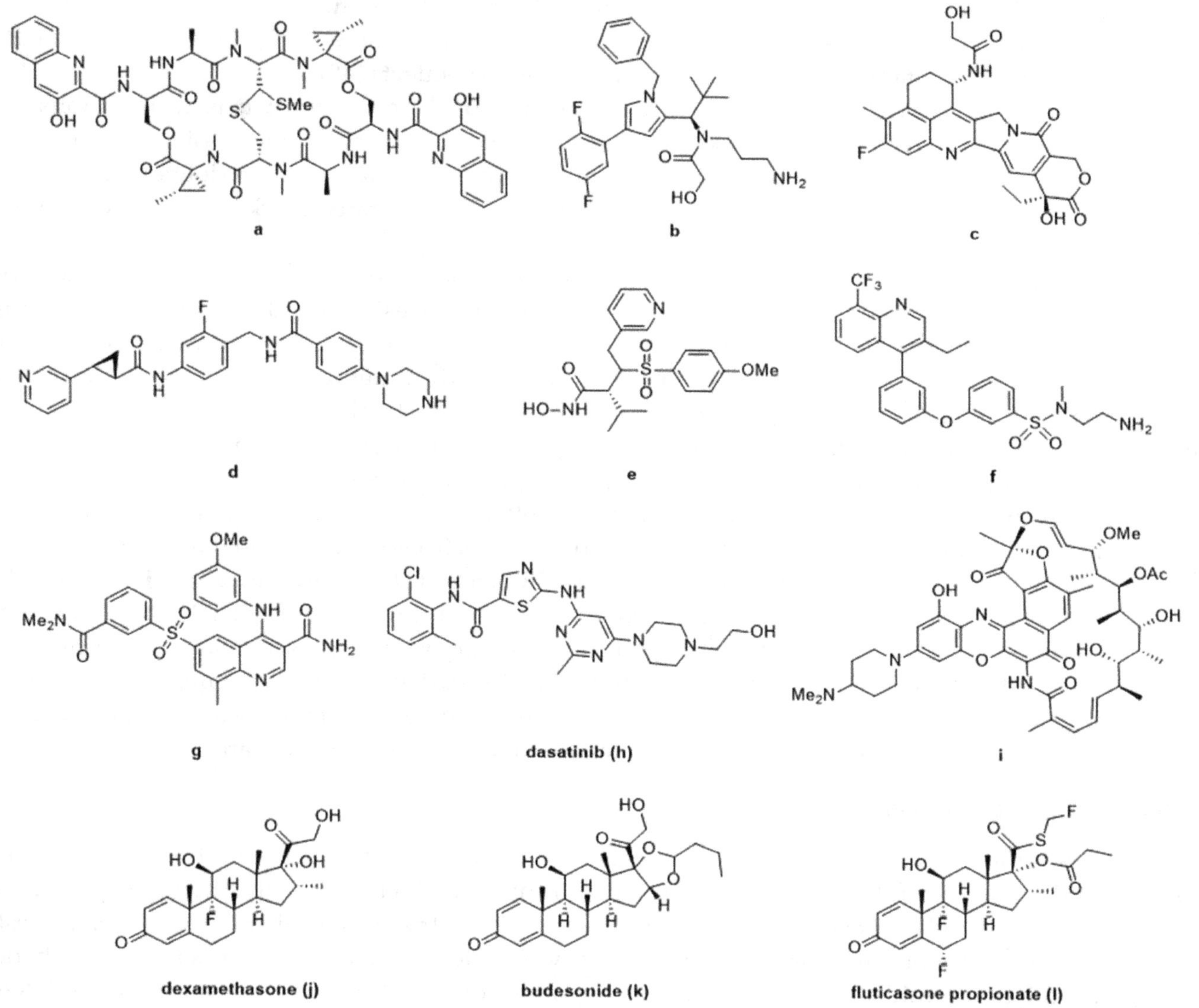

Figure 4. Expanding payload space in oncology with DNA disrupting bis-intercalator depsipeptide (SW-163D, **a**), pyrrole-based kinesin spindle protein (KSP) inhibitor (**b**), topoisomerase I inhibitor (DXd, **c**), nicotinamide phosphoribosyltransferase (NAMPT) inhibitor (**d**), and MMP9 inhibitor (CGS27023A, **e**). Examples of non-oncology payloads include LXR agonist (**f**), PDE4 inhibitor (GSK256066, **g**), kinase inhibitor dasatinib (**h**), antimicrobial rifamycin analog (**i**), GR agonists dexamethasone (**j**), budesonide (**k**), and fluticasone propionate (**l**).

As with other oncology examples, nicotinamide phosphoribosyltransferase (NAMPT) inhibitors **d** have not succeeded in the clinic due to low therapeutic index with limiting toxicities, but exploitation of ADC targeted delivery of NAMPT inhibitors provides an outlet for these potent payloads [101] in preclinical studies. Similarly, an anti-MMP9 antibody was conjugated to a non-selective MMP inhibitor (CGS27023A, **e**), showing remarkable selectivity for MMP9 alone, due to the antibody targeting in vitro [102].

Beyond oncology, ADCs are just beginning to show promise as a novel modality, offering a potential solution to the pitfalls of traditional drug discovery. Using an anti-CD11a antibody conjugated to an LXR (Liver X Receptor) agonist **f**, researchers were able to target macrophages to reverse cholesterol transport and reduce inflammation without negatively affecting hepatocytes, which have previously shown on-target toxicity with LXR agonists [44]. Antibody targeting CD11a was also used to selectively deliver a known PDE4 (Phosphodiesterase 4) inhibitor (GSK256066, **g**) and reduce inflammatory cytokine production, showing promise for the treatment of chronic inflammatory conditions with a more optimal therapeutic index [45]. In a similar fashion, dasatinib **h**, a known Src-family kinase inhibitor against leukemia was re-purposed as an immunosuppressive ADC using an anti-CXCR4 antibody to specifically target T-cells without undesirable side-effects [48].

Antimicrobial research is another area demanding novel approaches; it is well established that our current arsenal against microbes is failing and the discovery of new molecules has been limited [103]. Genentech pioneered the antibody-antibiotic conjugate (AAC) to deliver a rifamycin analog **i** intracellularly via an anti-*S. aureus* antibody which demonstrated marked clearance of latent bacteria reservoirs thought to be the cause of recurring infection [41].

Other known classes of molecules, namely, glucocorticoids are used as a standard of care for many immunological indications. They come with less-than-desirable side-effects at efficacious doses [104,105] with chronic use. One of the first examples of targeted glucocorticoid delivery via antibody used an anti-E-selectin conjugate to deliver dexamethasone to TNFα stimulated endothelial cells [43]. These early proof-of-concept experiments tracked conjugate internalization, intracellular release of steroid, and reduction of the pro-inflammatory IL-8 expression. Expanding on these preliminary experiments, an anti-CD163 conjugate was used to deliver dexamethasone to macrophages showing a synergistic anti-inflammatory effect of the conjugate versus its components alone, and a significant reduction in the systemic steroidal side-effects of orally dosed dexamethasone at the same efficacy [52]. Known glucocorticoid receptor (GR) agonists (i.e., dexamethasone **j**, budesonide **k**, and fluticasone propionate **l**) have also been attached to anti-CD74, anti-CD70, and anti-CD25 antibodies showing an immune cell targeted anti-inflammatory response, as well as highlighting the complexities of developing ADCs in this therapeutic area [46,50,51,106]. This novel modality promises treatment to larger populations of patients with autoimmune disorders, in a disease specific fashion that could potentially replace traditional steroid treatments as the standard of care.

4. Nucleic Acid Conjugates

For traditional oncolytic ADCs, the challenge of delivery manifests in the form of systemic toxicity of the potent cytotoxic payloads. However, similar molecular calculus may be applied to extensively cleared molecular entities which may otherwise have trouble reaching the tissues of interest. A rapidly-advancing molecular space which is typically impeded by delivery issues is that of synthetic therapeutic oligonucleotides including antisense oligonucleotides (ASOs) and short interfering RNA (siRNA) [107–109].

While traditional ADC payloads are small molecules which act on cellular machinery to elicit their desired phenotype via action on a molecular target, the current generation of synthetic oligonucleotide therapeutics instead act on information molecules upstream of their targets such as endogenous mRNA, achieving specificity through base-pair complementarity. Several different mechanisms of action have been clinically validated. Examples include intronic splice modulation (i.e., nusinersen, an ASO for treating spinal muscular atrophy) and formation of a catalytic mRNA silencing complex (i.e., patisiran, a lipid-nanoparticle formulated siRNA for treating ATTR amyloidosis). The details of these mechanisms, along with others, have been recently reviewed [110] and are beyond the scope of this discussion. The chemical structures and properties of oligonucleotides that make this therapeutic space challenging, however, are central to this discussion; their poor tissue penetration and circulation half-life are often attributed to the polyanionic backbone characteristics [111,112].

A number of advances in both oligonucleotide chemistry as well as conjugate chemistry have been enabling oligonucleotide clinical candidates as a class and will likely impact oligonucleotide bioconjugates [113]. For example, it has been demonstrated that appending of N-acetylgalactosamine (GalNAc, Figure 5b) residues to the end of siRNA strands allows for efficacious loading of hepatocytes in vivo with sustained target knockdown [114]. Along with GalNAc, number of other common modifications in oligonucleotide chemistry have been utilized, such as 2'-modification (i.e., 2'-F and 2'-OMe nucleosides, Figure 5a) and sulfurized phosphate analogs (i.e., phosphorothiolates, Figure 5a). Similar themes of heavy chemical modification have been utilized in ASOs. For example, one report principally noted that GalNAc conjugation ameliorated some nephrotoxicity signals in PCSK9-targeting ASOs, with data suggesting such conjugation could be a path towards addressing oligo-induced nephrotoxicity concerns more generally [115]. Beyond GalNAc, other oligonucleotide conjugation strategies have been found effective pre-clinically in targeting specific cellular populations or promoting systemic availability, as with conjugation of a GLP1R agonist [116] or conjugation to various lipids such as cholesterol or docosahexaenoic acid (DHA, Figure 5b) [117], respectively.

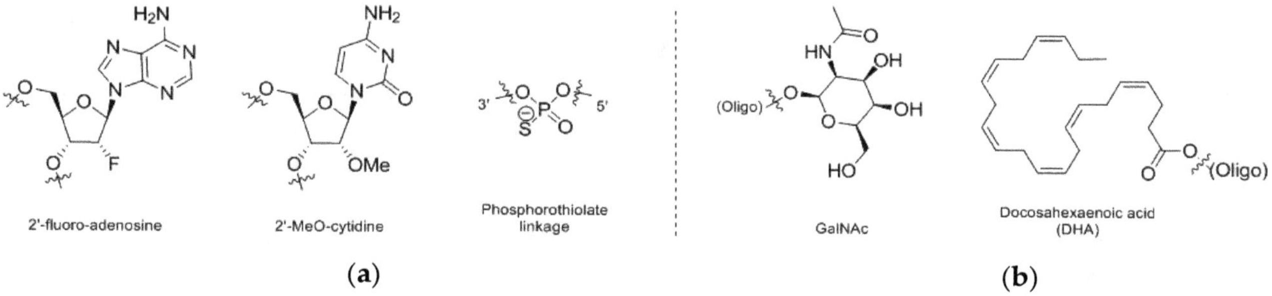

Figure 5. (a) stabilizing chemical modifications for siRNA, (b) oligo delivery conjugate moieties.

Although there are limited examples of discreet therapeutically-oriented antibody-oligonucleotide conjugates in the literature, the current studies have made significant headway and put to use many of the strategies discussed herein. In an early example reported, hu3S193, an internalizing humanized Lewis-Y mAb was conjugated to a largely unmodified STAT3 siRNA [118]. This conjugation by utilizing non-specific amino residue labeling of hu3S193 with activated hydrazonal nicotinamide (HyNic) reagent which was covalently coupled with STAT3 siRNA using an aldehyde linker. Cellular specificity was confirmed through flow cytometry and internalization by confocal microscopy, the construct could only effect STAT3 knockdown when high doses (100 µM) of chloroquine as an endosomal disrupting agent was added.

The disconnect between specific internalization and siRNA target knockdown was further demonstrated in a systematic study which applied a number of important antibody-drug conjugate parameters [119], which included variations of linker chemistry, cell surface receptor identity, receptor internalization types and count, antibody linkage positions, and antibody formats. This study utilized several sophisticated methods, including the application of site-specific engineered cysteine conjugation (Genentech's THIOMAB™ platform) to deliver reproducible and largely homogeneous conjugates, as well as highly modified chemically-stabilized housekeeping gene (PPIB) siRNA constructs to enable in vivo studies. While seven different internalizing antigens were profiled, only three showed any knockdown of the target gene and of those only TENB2 on cell lines with high surface receptor density was able to achieve knockdown levels of greater than 50% in vitro. It was inconclusive what properties of the different active conjugates enabled effective knockdown, but importantly, conjugates were able to demonstrate 33% transcript knockdown with cellular specificity to tumor cells near the vasculature in a mouse xenograft model.

At this time, there have yet to be any clinical studies on antibody-oligonucleotide conjugates, but several of the requisite preclinical proof-of-concept studies have been reported. One notable example has demonstrated application of a myostatin-silencing siRNA-antibody conjugate in a mouse model of muscular regeneration [120]. In this study, the well-profiled CD71 receptor (transferrin receptor) was chosen for muscular target engagement utilizing anti-CD71 Fab'-siRNA conjugates. In profiling methods of administration, principal findings were that equivalent target engagement was achievable through different perfused systemic administration routes. PCR-based detection methods were used to verify conjugate was detectable 24 h post-dose, but notably durable silencing up to a month out was observed. Additionally, intramuscular injection enabled superior levels of target engagement in a model of peripheral artery disease, with muscular regeneration due to myostatin knockdown observed with microgram-scale injections. While this Fab'-based study utilized structural cystines for conjugation, other therapeutic antibody-oligonucleotide conjugation systems not yet described in this section have been reported, including two oncology examples which applied two-step conjugations for azide-labeling the antibody which were then treated with cyclooctyne-appended ASOs to generate the conjugates [121,122]. Other antibody-oligonucleotide conjugation methods beyond the scope of this review (i.e., for immuno PCR applications, pre-targeted radiotherapy, or those which utilize non-covalent heterogeneous complexes) have been recently reviewed [109].

While these results are promising, further analytical work must demonstrate pharmacokinetic profiling of these conjugates to enable clinical study. In this vein, a report describing a triplex forming oligonucleotide ELISA assay utilized locked nucleic acid-containing probes [123] for conjugate quantification. This assay is distinguished from PCR-based methods as a direct, quantitative readout of intact oligonucleotide-antibody conjugate. The authors demonstrated that this assay is capable of accurately detecting conjugate doped into cellular matrices such as serum or tissue homogenate down to a limit of detection of 120 pg/mL. These early developments in antibody-oligonucleotide conjugates can help propel the next wave of novel conjugates to leverage the cellular specificity of antibodies and target-gene specificity of oligonucleotide therapies.

5. Linkers

While a simple concept at first glance, a linker is far more complex than a mundane spanning element between the small molecule payload and the antibody which make up the ADC. It ensures the fundamental principles of targeted drug delivery of ADCs-minimizing premature drug release in plasma and promoting selective release of payload to the target cell. Additionally, it can modulate the physiochemical property of the overall conjugate. This requires the linker design to be stable in circulation and upon antibody-mediated internalization, the payload is efficiently released.

To meet the desired therapeutic effect, cytotoxic payloads can be designed to be released either intracellularly or extracellularly [10,13,124–126]. For instance, intracellular hydrolytic enzymes can recognize specific linker motifs (Figure 6a) and catalyze the cleavage reactions to release payloads inside endosomes or lysosomes. Cathepsin family enzymes and other proteolytic enzymes are responsible for the digestion of peptide linkers in lysosomes [69]. Selection of the linker peptide sequence affects the plasma stability of ADCs and the efficiency of proteolytic cleavage of linkers in target cells [127,128]. Phosphatases [106] and glycosidases [129,130] are other examples of hydrolytic enzymes that are present in lysosomes at high concentrations and break down respective linkers of internalized ADCs. Alternatively, through exploitation of the relatively acidic and reductive tumor microenvironment, payloads may also be released extracellularly through non-enzymatic cleavable linkers (Figure 6b) at a tumor site. For example, hydrazine and acyl hydrazine (approved products in Table 1) [25,131], ketal and acetal [132], as well as carbonate [133] are acid-labile linkages that are designed to degrade at low pH in cell chambers (pH 5.5 in endosome, pH 4.5 in lysosome) and remain intact in circulation (pH 7.4). Disulfide linkages are subjected to glutathione attack in cytosol, thus offering a chance of selective releasing toxic payloads in tumor cell. How the conjugation site and steric hindrance around disulfide linkage modulates its stability in plasma is a subject that has attracted extensive studies [134,135].

Both enzymatic cleavable linkers and non-enzymatic cleavable linkers have been conjugated onto antibodies through naturally occurring cysteine and lysine residues (Figure 6c). Nucleophilic thiol groups can react with maleimide and alkyl-halide to produce stable conjugates. In cases of maleimide-based ADCs where stability is a concern, semi-hydrolysis of maleimide has been reported as an effective strategy to minimize the retro-Michael reaction of thiomaleimide and preventing premature payload loss [136]. Amino groups on surface exposed lysines can form stable amide via alkylation of an activated ester on the linker. Side chains of natural amino acids can be modified or engineered to produce ketones to form imines or hydrazones. Notably, recent site-specific ADCs utilize novel linker conjugation chemistries with unnatural amino acids that are incorporated on engineered antibodies through imine/hydrazine formation, copper-catalyzed azide alkyne cycloaddition (CuAAC), and strain promoted azide alkyne cycloaddition (SPAAC) [44,78,80].

(a) Enzymatic cleavable linkers

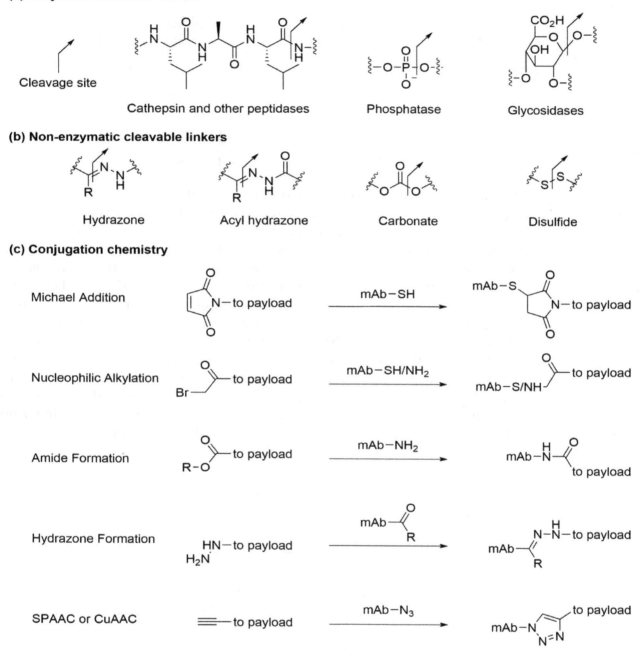

Cleavage site

Cathepsin and other peptidases   Phosphatase   Glycosidases

(b) Non-enzymatic cleavable linkers

Hydrazone   Acyl hydrazone   Carbonate   Disulfide

(c) Conjugation chemistry

Michael Addition

Nucleophilic Alkylation

Amide Formation

Hydrazone Formation

SPAAC or CuAAC

Figure 6. (**a**) Enzymatic cleavable linkers; (**b**) non-enzymatic cleavable linkers; (**c**) conjugation chemistry.

In sharp contrast to approved cytotoxic ADCs for oncological indications, the goal of ADCs for non-oncological applications is the selective modulation of target cells without on-target adverse bystander effects. Besides selection of non-toxin-based payloads, this new direction also demands new concepts in linker-payload design. Linker-payload design is critical in modulating bystander effect of payloads. A diphosphatase-cleavable linker has been reported for the selective delivery of immune suppressing payloads to immune cells following ADC internalization and diphosphate cleavage (Figure 7) [51]. In this study, the fluticasone propionate derived payload has a high intrinsic binding affinity to target, but also bears a charged phosphate moiety. Due to antibody-driven delivery and limited free payload permeability, the target exposure of payload to cell is increased, and a superior in vitro potency is observed. Further in vivo testing may require additional linker development.

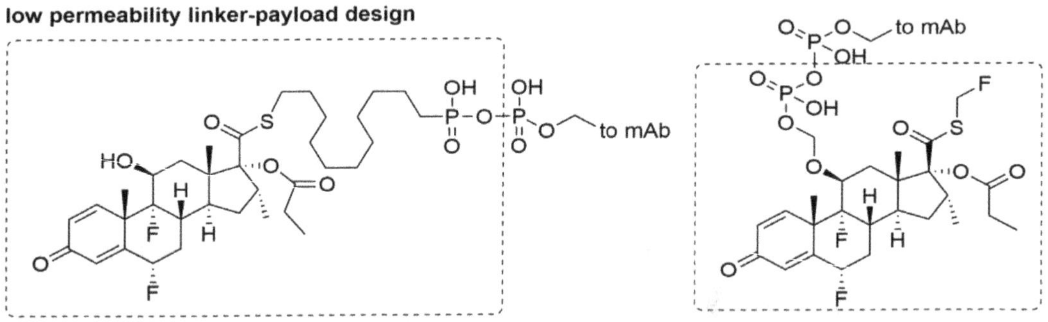

low permeability linker-payload design

Figure 7. Low permeability linker-payload design.

Linker-payload design is also critical to the successful implementation of high-DAR ADCs, via reduced aggregation and improved overall pharmacokinetics profiles. Even though increasing DAR instinctively increases in vitro potency of ADCs, it may not translate to an improvement of in vivo potency since the plasma clearance of ADCs rises along with DAR [129]. The aggregation and fast clearance problem may be largely mitigated without extensive linker optimization for water-soluble payloads such as the topoisomerase I inhibitor DXd in DS8201a, which is an ADC with DAR 8 that has shown remarkable in vivo stability both pre-clinically and clinically [31]. For highly hydrophobic payloads, the paradoxical effect of higher DAR resulting in lower exposure can be corrected by novel linker design. Several linker modifications to enhance hydrophilicity have been reported that allowed ADC to be produced with DAR as high as 8 (reviewed in [124]). These modifications include addition of a polyethylene glycol (PEG) moiety [127,128], a glucuronic acid unit [129], or a combination of branched PEG moiety and glucuronic acid unit [130]. For instance, hydrophilic linker construct in Figure 8 [129] minimizes the detrimental hydrophobicity associated with increasing DAR, imparting an optimal pharmacokinetic profile to the high DAR ADC, thereby reduces non-specific clearance and improves in vivo potency.

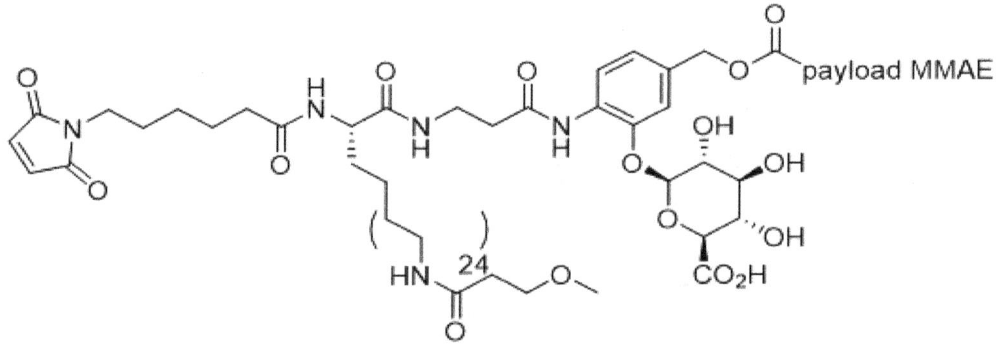

Figure 8. Hydrophilic linker-payload design.

6. Absorption, Distribution, Metabolism, and Excretion (ADME) of ADCs

As discussed in the sections above, considerable advancements in next generation ADCs are anticipated to further explore both the chemical and biological design elements for ADCs. This includes, but is not limited to, antibody engineering to facilitate direct site-specific conjugation, modification of conjugation chemistry and introduction of novel linker compositions to confer enhanced stability, as well as, the exploration of additional existing and novel chemical entities/modalities as conjugates to increase the pharmacological applications of ADCs. Many of these advancements to design better molecules are intricately interdependent with optimizing or improving the ADME drug-ability properties of ADCs, such as linker-payload stability, distribution, and pharmacokinetics (PK). This is because defining the exposure-response relationship for both safety and efficacy has been intimately tied with ADC peripheral PK, target tissue or site of action concentration and the disposition of the payload at the intended site. The criticality of understanding the exposure-response relationship and therapeutic index (TI) for ADCs is exemplified by Mylotarg® (gemtuzumab ozogamicin) which is composed of a CD33 mAb linked to the cytotoxic drug calicheamicin via an acid-liable hydrazine linker. While initially approved for the treatment of acute myeloid leukemia (AML) in 2000, it was pulled from the market at the request of regulatory agencies in 2010 due to safety concerns and the failure to reproduce the clinical benefit connected to linker stability in AML patients. Following additional interrogation of exposure-response relationships, examining alternative lower dosing and scheduling, Mylotarg found a path back to the market and received a new FDA approval for newly diagnosed CD-33 positive acute AML patients in 2017.

Dissecting the ADME properties of ADCs is a complex endeavor given the unique properties of each component within the molecules. ADC ADME involves delineating the intertwined properties of linker-payload stability, pharmacokinetics, clearance, metabolism, and disposition of mAb, conjugate (i.e., small molecule chemical entity for traditional ADCs), as well as, the ADC entity itself. The ADME properties of ADCs are influenced by the mAb, target antigen, linker, site of conjugation, DAR number, and the conjugated species (i.e., payload). Table 2 summarizes the various types of in vitro and in vivo studies to characterize ADC ADME.

Table 2. ADME Characterization approaches for ADCs and their constituents.

Species	ADME Information
Antibody	• Determine PK-dose relationship in vivo • Characterize target affinity/specificity in vitro, target expression/turnover in vivo, unintended or off-target binding in vitro and in vivo
ADC	• Linker Component (1) Characterize linker stability and kinetics of catabolism in vitro and in vivo across species (2) Evaluate nature of the released species (active payload and its catabolites) • Conjugation Site (1) Evaluate influence of conjugation site on linker stability in vitro and in vivo (2) Determine the effect of conjugation site on PK • DAR (1) Determine in vivo PK and disposition with heterogenous and homogenous DAR species
Payload	• Metabolite identification, characterize DDI potential (CYP inhibition, induction and reaction phenotypes) • P-gp substrate or inhibitor • Characterize non-P-gp transporters • Plasma protein binding

The antibody component of ADCs is the primary driver of the slow clearance, long systemic half-life and restricted tissue distribution of these modalities compared to their payload counterparts. Similar to mAbs, the properties related to target (expression pattern, density and turnover), as well as, antibody structure (including physiochemical properties, FcRn binding, Fcγ receptor interactions and isotype) that affect antibody PK and disposition also impact ADCs. An anti-drug antibody (ADA) or neutralizing antibody (Nab) response against the therapeutic antibody component can affect the PK profile and shorten the half-life of the ADCs in the body [9,19]. Nevertheless, idiotype networks have an important biological role in avoiding the expansion of autoreactive B or T-cells [137,138]. Uniquely, ADC PK is also impacted by linker composition, chemical nature of the payload and DAR. These are both speculated to affect the physiochemical properties of the ADC which are linked to the PK and clearance of the molecules. For example, ADCs with high DAR values have been shown to aggregate and have higher clearance rates than their unconjugated mAb counterparts or lower DAR species [59,129,139]. Similarly, decreasing the hydrophobicity and improving the hydrophilicity of the linker component within an anti-CD70 and anti-HER2 mAbs improved the exposure and changed the disposition of the ADCs [129,140].

In addition to the antibody, the linker and payload components of ADCs are also subject to their own clearance mechanisms. The stability of the linker to premature release of the payload in the systemic circulation has been demonstrated to be a critical ADC ADME component for determining the exposure-response and exposure-toxicity relationships [141]. From a stability perspective, well-behaved ADCs should only release the payload in the intended target tissue to minimize payload toxicity to unintended tissue and maximize efficacy in target tissues/organs, especially with payloads with cytotoxic properties. The ADC linker stability is noted to be a challenge due to the long circulating half-life (days to weeks) imparted by the mAb component resulting in the continuous assault of the linker to endogenous proteases. Mechanistically, linker stability can be evaluated both in vitro using plasma/serum incubations and in vivo following administration to multiple species by following the formation of the released payload and DAR changes over time. As covered above, linker composition continues to be an intense area of focus in the development of ADCs. In terms of the payload, initial reports with limited chemical entities suggested that type of payloads did not impact the PK of ADCs; however, more recent studies of conjugation sites and of site-specific conjugations have demonstrated the connectivity of the site of conjugation with various payloads to impact ADC PK and disposition [142,143]. Engineering ADCs for site-specific conjugation to control the DAR and PK has shown some evidence of improving the TI in non-clinical oncology studies [144]. Approaches such as engineered cysteines, unnatural amino acids, and the inclusion of tags (i.e., selenocysteine, aldehyde, or glutamine) continue to be intense areas of research for the application of site-specific payload conjugation to optimize ADC ADME.

Like mAbs, ADCs are likely trafficked via the vascular and lymphatic systems. The biodistribution of ADCs follows that of the antibody component. ADC are removed from the systemic circulation by target-mediated drug disposition (TMDD); thus, highly vascularized organs or tissues that express the target antigen are involved in the clearance of ADCs from the periphery. The TMDD is believed to be followed by intracellular trafficking of the target: ADC complex to lysosomes where degradation of the ADC occurs, and the payload is released from the mAb to elicit its activity. In addition, nonspecific uptake of ADCs by pinocytosis also facilitates their systemic depletion. This form of uptake could lead to degradation and/or recycling of the ADC by the neonatal Fc receptor (FcRn). Indeed, in terms of tissue distribution the preponderance of ADCs are observed in four organs including the liver, kidneys, lungs, and skin [145,146]; however, the amount in each tissue differs between ADCs based on their target binding and physiochemical properties [147]. Importantly, irrespective of the mode of ADC degradation, the payload or chemical moiety can be released into the blood. The unconjugated payload is expected to follow the biodistribution pattern of a typical small molecule drug which is widely distributed throughout the tissues.

The elimination of ADCs involves two processes. First, intracellular catabolism through proteolysis in the tissues (i.e., TMDD- or pinocytosis-mediated). Second, complete deconjugation of the payload which can result in both mAb or mAb with a partial linker along with free drug [148]. While the mAb based species are expected to follow catabolism through the same mechanisms as the ADC, there is increased attention in the elimination of the unconjugated payload under conditions of impairment of renal and hepatic processes. For example, a study of brentuximab vedotin showed that the major route of MMAE excretion was through the feces (~72%) and the remaining MMAE was recovered in urine in humans [149]. Given these data, the relationship of hepatic and renal insufficiency to ADC exposure is an important aspect of clinical development.

Another area of intense research is dissecting the noted phenomenon of resistance against ADCs. A few mechanisms of resistance have been noted including to the antibody portion of the ADCs by mutation and/or down-regulation of the target antigen, as well as, to the payload via drug efflux transporters that remove the payload from cells [150]. Changes in the intracellular processing of ADCs through alterations of the linker cleavage caused by lysosomal or endosomal abnormalities can also significantly affect the PK profiles. These changes impair the release of payloads in the cytosol and consequently affect the therapeutic indexes of the ADCs [150].

7. Conjugate Developability, Formulations, and Characteristics

An antibody conjugate combines an inherently complex antibody with a small synthetic molecule drug to create an even more complex large molecule. Despite the relatively small addition in molecular weight, the small molecule drug has a profound impact on the characteristics and properties of the conjugate.

Over the last decade, significant advancements in analytical methods have been made to characterize ADCs and have been extensively reviewed [151–154]. These methods have focused on the major ADC attributes such as DAR, drug load distribution, residual linker-payload and related impurity levels, in addition to typical attributes for antibodies such as aggregation level, charge variants, and host cell protein level. The DAR number has a strong influence on the properties of ADCs. Currently, many of the ADCs in the clinic have DAR numbers in the range of 2–4, although ADCs with higher DAR numbers have also been reported [31,155–158]. For stochastically conjugated ADCs, the small molecule drug is covalently linked to either the lysine or the interchain cysteine residues of the antibody, resulting in a heterogeneous mixture with various DAR species which are more difficult to characterize and control. For example, as many as 40 lysines were found to be partially modified in a lysine conjugated ADC molecule using LC-MS and peptide mapping methods [159]. The aforementioned site-specific conjugation approaches have drastically improved the DAR homogeneity albeit process development is required to further control the remaining heterogeneity during the production process [160]. At present, nearly all the antibody conjugate characterization literature has focused on antibody-small organic molecule conjugates. Based on the molecular nature of each payload, chromatographic and electrophoretic methods as well as spectroscopic methods have been commonly employed in DAR determination along with mass spectrometer method which provides more detail. The analytical methods will continue to evolve as the payload expands to nucleic acids which possess very different properties compared with small organic molecules [120,161].

It is well-documented that the addition of a small molecule drug to an otherwise soluble and stable antibody can cause aggregation and other physicochemical instability in the ADC [162,163]. This is not only because many of the small molecule drugs are bulky and hydrophobic in nature leading to a significant increase in the hydrophobicity of the ADC, but also because the conjugation can induce perturbations to secondary and tertiary structures of the antibody resulting in reduced conformational stabilities. To this point, a systematic study of trastuzumab, trastuzumab-MCC conjugate intermediate, and trastuzumab-DM1 found that both conjugates suffered decreased thermal stability and increased aggregation compared with trastuzumab [164]. Recently, the impact of drug conjugation on intra- and intermolecular interactions of trastuzumab-DM1 compared with trastuzumab was studied and the results confirmed that the lower colloidal stability and higher aggregation propensity for trastuzumab-DM1 are attributed to both reduced repulsive charge interaction and increased hydrophobicity [165]. Multiple publications have reported a more pronounced conjugation destabilizing effect on interchain cysteine conjugated ADCs and an inverse correlation between the drug load and stability [166–170]. Consistent with the findings on the interchain cysteine conjugated ADCs, the high DAR species in trastuzumab-DM1, a lysine conjugate, have also been found to be less stable and more prone to aggregation than the low DAR species [171]. Site-specific conjugation approaches with carefully chosen conjugation sites are expected to have less negative impact on stability and aggregation propensity of ADCs [64,65,172]. Most site-specific conjugates in the clinical pipeline have homogeneous DAR of 2 resulting in reduced hydrophobicity and aggregation compared to stochastic conjugates of average DAR of 3.5–4 where DAR species range from 0 to 8 or higher. In order to achieve sufficient efficacy with a relatively low DAR number, potent payloads such as PBD, a MDR1-resistant maytansine payload, and an auristatin payload Aur0101 have been developed. However, the DAR 2 site-specific conjugates with PBD and Aur0101 have shown limited therapeutic index in clinic thus far [173–176], while the clinical data for the DAR 2 maytansine ADC is pending [177]. While extensive characterization studies have been reported for antibody conjugated to cytotoxic payloads, there is a scarcity of literature on the molecular properties of conjugates with non-toxic small organic molecule payloads and nucleic acids. The optimal DAR number and solution property of conjugates with oligonucleotides, which are highly charged and significantly larger than small organic molecules, remains to be determined.

In addition to all the issues encountered during antibody formulation development, the formulation development of ADC drugs must find suitable pH and excipient conditions to simultaneously maintain the stability of the antibody, the linker, and the small molecule drug (reviewed in [162,163]). Even if there is an in-depth understanding of the stability of the parental antibody in aqueous solution, its physical stability may change upon conjugation in the presence of organic solvent or through possible cross-linking mechanism, and its chemical stability may depend on the conjugation method [178]. An example is the light-sensitivity in a model ADC using trastuzumab whereas trastuzumab itself does not show such sensitivity [179]. While much is known in the literature regarding the chemical stability of monoclonal antibodies [180] and the data on commonly used cytotoxic linker-payloads is accumulating [153,181,182], novel and non-toxic linker-payloads including siRNA will require a clear understanding of their degradation pathways in order to form control strategies during drug development process, similar to what has been demonstrated on payload metabolism [183]. Therefore, a comprehensive evaluation of the combined system will always be necessary for novel ADCs.

All the current ADC drugs on the market are lyophilized products suitable for intravenous administration. Such a freeze-dried state protects the ADCs from chemical degradation and aggregation which occur under long-term solution storage conditions. Although interest has been growing for liquid formulation based on the increased experience with ADCs and the improved solubility and stability of the new generation of ADCs, few such feasibility studies have been reported in the literature to date. It can be particularly challenging to prevent payloads from falling off the antibody over a long period of time in solution. In addition, the currently approved ADC drugs are reconstituted to 0.25–20 mg/mL in solution, significantly below the concentrations for most therapeutic antibody products. While the above is a viable approach for intravenous administration commonly used for oncology therapies, the emerging non-oncology application of the ADCs will likely demand stable liquid formulation and subcutaneous administration as commonly expected for many antibody drugs to increase convenience for patients. This growing trend exerts pressure on linker-payload design and conjugation methods in addition to the properties of the parental antibodies, as well as on formulation and device development. The current pre-clinical data for non-oncology ADCs suggest that the ADC doses might not be significantly lower than those for antibodies [41,45,47,52]. The clinical efficacy and therapeutic index of the non-oncology ADCs will ultimately determine the dose requirement and the appropriate drug product concentration.

8. Conclusions

Antibody conjugates in oncology have thus far delivered several successfully approved therapeutics. Extensive research into novel payloads, more developable linkers and conjugation chemistries further enable the field of oncology conjugates to cross the finish line. These learnings and advances also help propel the next generation of conjugates for non-oncology indications. Additional challenges such as in vivo stability, formulation and delivery will drive the field to seek solutions to broaden the therapeutic horizon to include payloads like nucleic acids. Overall, the rise of non-oncology ADC therapeutics offers a huge opportunity for innovation at multiple fronts of drug discovery and development for years to come.

Author Contributions: Writing—Original Draft Preparation, Review & Editing, D.L., J.M.W., T.L., R.M.M., A.D.-M. and Y.F. All authors have read and agreed to the published version of the manuscript.

References

1. Singh, S.; Kumar, N.K.; Dwiwedi, P.; Charan, J.; Kaur, R.; Sidhu, P.; Chugh, V.K. Monoclonal antibodies: A review. *Curr. Clin. Pharmacol.* **2018**, *13*, 85–99. [CrossRef]
2. Grilo, A.L.; Mantalaris, A. The increasingly human and profitable monoclonal antibody market. *Trends Biotechnol.* **2019**, *37*, 9–16. [CrossRef]
3. Kaplon, H.; Reichert, J.M. Antibodies to watch in 2019. *mAbs* **2019**, *11*, 219–238. [CrossRef]
4. Sifniotis, V.; Cruz, E.; Eroglu, B.; Kayser, V. Current advancements in addressing key challenges of therapeutic antibody design, manufacture, and formulation. *Antibodies* **2019**, *8*, 36. [CrossRef]
5. Weiner, G.J. Building better monoclonal antibody-based therapeutics. *Nat. Rev. Cancer* **2015**, *15*, 361–370. [CrossRef] [PubMed]
6. Saeed, A.F.U.H.; Wang, R.; Ling, S.; Wang, S. Antibody engineering for pursuing a healthier future. *Front. Microbiol.* **2017**, *8*, 495. [CrossRef] [PubMed]
7. Kohler, G.; Milstein, C. Continuous cultures of fused cells secreting antibody of predefined specificity. *Nature* **1975**, *256*, 495–497. [CrossRef] [PubMed]
8. Riechmann, L.; Clark, M.; Waldmann, H.; Winter, G. Reshaping human antibodies for therapy. *Nature* **1988**, *332*, 323–327. [CrossRef]
9. Harding, F.A.; Stickler, M.M.; Razo, J.; DuBridge, R.B. The immunogenicity of humanized and fully human antibodies: Residual immunogenicity resides in the CDR regions. *mAbs* **2010**, *2*, 256–265. [CrossRef]
10. Strohl, W.R. Human antibody discovery platforms. In *Protein Therapeutics*; Wiley-VCH Verlag GmbH & Co. KgaA: Weinheim, Germany, 2017; pp. 113–159. [CrossRef]
11. Tsuchikama, K.; An, Z. Antibody-drug conjugates: Recent advances in conjugation and linker chemistries. *Protein Cell* **2018**, *9*, 33–46. [CrossRef]
12. Mukherjee, A.; Waters, A.K.; Babic, I.; Nurmemmedov, E.; Glassy, M.C.; Kesari, S.; Yenugonda, V.M. Antibody drug conjugates: Progress, pitfalls, and promises. *Hum. Antibodies* **2019**, *27*, 53–62. [CrossRef]
13. Beck, A.; Goetsch, L.; Dumontet, C.; Corvaia, N. Strategies and challenges for the next generation of antibody-drug conjugates. *Nat. Rev. Drug Discov.* **2017**, *16*, 315–337. [CrossRef] [PubMed]
14. Chau, C.H.; Steeg, P.S.; Figg, W.D. Antibody–drug conjugates for cancer. *Lancet* **2019**, *394*, 793–804. [CrossRef]
15. FDA Approves First Chemoimmunotherapy Regimen for Patients with Relapsed or Refractory Diffuse Large B-Cell Lymphoma. Available online: https://www.fda.gov/news-events/press-announcements/fda-approves-first-chemoimmunotherapy-regimen-patients-relapsed-or-refractory-diffuse-large-b-cell (accessed on 25 June 2019).
16. Petersen, B.H.; DeHerdt, S.V.; Schneck, D.W.; Bumol, T.F. The human immune response to KS1/4-desacetylvinblastine (LY256787) and KS1/4-desacetylvinblastine hydrazide (LY203728) in single and multiple dose clinical studies. *Cancer Res.* **1991**, *51*, 2286–2290. [PubMed]
17. Abdollahpour-Alitappeh, M.; Lotfinia, M.; Gharibi, T.; Mardaneh, J.; Farhadihosseinabadi, B.; Larki, P.; Faghfourian, B.; Sepehr, K.S.; Abbaszadeh-Goudarzi, K.; Abbaszadeh-Goudarzi, G.; et al. Antibody-drug conjugates (ADCs) for cancer therapy: Strategies, challenges, and successes. *J. Cell. Physiol.* **2019**, *234*, 5628–5642. [CrossRef] [PubMed]
18. Boehncke, W.H.; Brembilla, N.C. Immunogenicity of biologic therapies: Causes and consequences. *Expert Rev. Clin. Immunol.* **2018**, *14*, 513–523. [CrossRef] [PubMed]
19. Pineda, C.; Castaneda Hernandez, G.; Jacobs, I.A.; Alvarez, D.F.; Carini, C. Assessing the immunogenicity of biopharmaceuticals. *BioDrugs* **2016**, *30*, 195–206. [CrossRef]
20. Ghetie, V.; Vitetta, E. Immunotoxins in the therapy of cancer: From bench to clinic. *Pharmacol. Ther.* **1994**, *63*, 209–234. [CrossRef]

19. Pineda, C.; Castaneda Hernandez, G.; Jacobs, I.A.; Alvarez, D.F.; Carini, C. Assessing the immunogenicity of biopharmaceuticals. *BioDrugs* **2016**, *30*, 195–206. [CrossRef]
20. Ghetie, V.; Vitetta, E. Immunotoxins in the therapy of cancer: From bench to clinic. *Pharmacol. Ther.* **1994**, *63*, 209–234. [CrossRef]
21. Dumontet, C.; Jordan, M.A. Microtubule-binding agents: A dynamic field of cancer therapeutics. *Nat. Rev. Drug Discov.* **2010**, *9*, 790–803. [CrossRef]
22. Pyzik, M.; Sand, K.M.K.; Hubbard, J.J.; Andersen, J.T.; Sandlie, I.; Blumberg, R.S. The neonatal Fc Receptor (FcRn): A misnomer? *Front. Immunol.* **2019**, *10*, 1540. [CrossRef]
23. Datta-Mannan, A.; Choi, H.; Stokell, D.; Tang, J.; Murphy, A.; Wrobleski, A.; Feng, Y. The properties of cysteine-conjugated antibody-drug conjugates are impacted by the IgG subclass. *AAPS J.* **2018**, *20*, 103. [CrossRef]
24. Mohammed, R.; Milne, A.; Kayani, K.; Ojha, U. How the discovery of rituximab impacted the treatment of B-cell non-Hodgkin's lymphomas. *J. Blood Med.* **2019**, *10*, 71–84. [CrossRef] [PubMed]
25. Hoffmann, R.M.; Coumbe, B.G.T.; Josephs, D.H.; Mele, S.; Ilieva, K.M.; Cheung, A.; Tutt, A.N.; Spicer, J.F.; Thurston, D.E.; Crescioli, S.; et al. Antibody structure and engineering considerations for the design and function of Antibody Drug Conjugates (ADCs). *Oncoimmunology* **2018**, *7*, e1395127. [CrossRef] [PubMed]
26. Junttila, T.T.; Li, G.; Parsons, K.; Phillips, G.L.; Sliwkowski, M.X. Trastuzumab-DM1 (T-DM1) retains all the mechanisms of action of trastuzumab and efficiently inhibits growth of lapatinib insensitive breast cancer. *Breast Cancer Res. Treat.* **2011**, *128*, 347–356. [CrossRef] [PubMed]
27. English, D.P.; Bellone, S.; Schwab, C.L.; Bortolomai, I.; Bonazzoli, E.; Cocco, E.; Buza, N.; Hui, P.; Lopez, S.; Ratner, E.; et al. T-DM1, a novel antibody-drug conjugate, is highly effective against primary HER2 overexpressing uterine serous carcinoma in vitro and in vivo. *Cancer Med.* **2014**, *3*, 1256–1265. [CrossRef] [PubMed]
28. Nicoletti, R.; Lopez, S.; Bellone, S.; Cocco, E.; Schwab, C.L.; Black, J.D.; Centritto, F.; Zhu, L.; Bonazzoli, E.; Buza, N.; et al. T-DM1, a novel antibody-drug conjugate, is highly effective against uterine and ovarian carcinosarcomas overexpressing HER2. *Clin. Exp. Metastasis* **2015**, *32*, 29–38. [CrossRef] [PubMed]
29. Black, J.; Menderes, G.; Bellone, S.; Schwab, C.L.; Bonazzoli, E.; Ferrari, F.; Predolini, F.; De Haydu, C.; Cocco, E.; Buza, N.; et al. SYD985, a novel duocarmycin-based HER2-targeting antibody-drug conjugate, shows antitumor activity in uterine serous carcinoma with HER2/Neu expression. *Mol. Cancer Ther.* **2016**, *15*, 1900–1909. [CrossRef]
30. Menderes, G.; Bonazzoli, E.; Bellone, S.; Black, J.; Altwerger, G.; Masserdotti, A.; Pettinella, F.; Zammataro, L.; Buza, N.; Hui, P.; et al. SYD985, a novel duocarmycin-based HER2-targeting antibody-drug conjugate, shows promising antitumor activity in epithelial ovarian carcinoma with HER2/Neu expression. *Gynecol. Oncol.* **2017**, *146*, 179–186. [CrossRef]
31. Ogitani, Y.; Aida, T.; Hagihara, K.; Yamaguchi, J.; Ishii, C.; Harada, N.; Soma, M.; Okamoto, H.; Oitate, M.; Arakawa, S.; et al. DS-8201a, a novel HER2-targeting ADC with a novel DNA topoisomerase i inhibitor, demonstrates a promising antitumor efficacy with differentiation from T-DM1. *Clin. Cancer Res.* **2016**, *22*, 5097–5108. [CrossRef]
32. Cardillo, T.M.; Govindan, S.V.; Sharkey, R.M.; Trisal, P.; Arrojo, R.; Liu, D.; Rossi, E.A.; Chang, C.H.; Goldenberg, D.M. Sacituzumab govitecan (IMMU-132), an Anti-Trop-2/SN-38 antibody-drug conjugate: Characterization and efficacy in pancreatic, gastric, and other cancers. *Bioconjug. Chem.* **2015**, *26*, 919–931. [CrossRef]
33. Bardia, A.; Mayer, I.A.; Vahdat, L.T.; Tolaney, S.M.; Isakoff, S.J.; Diamond, J.R.; O'Shaughnessy, J.; Moroose, R.L.; Santin, A.D.; Abramson, V.G.; et al. Sacituzumab govitecan-hziy in refractory metastatic triple-negative breast cancer. *N. Engl. J. Med.* **2019**, *380*, 741–751. [CrossRef] [PubMed]
34. Heist, R.S.; Guarino, M.J.; Masters, G.; Purcell, W.T.; Starodub, A.N.; Horn, L.; Scheff, R.J.; Bardia, A.; Messersmith, W.A.; Berlin, J.; et al. Therapy of advanced non-small-cell lung cancer with an SN-38-Anti-Trop-2 drug conjugate, sacituzumab govitecan. *J. Clin. Oncol.* **2017**, *35*, 2790–2797. [CrossRef] [PubMed]
35. Pereira, N.A.; Chan, K.F.; Lin, P.C.; Song, Z. The "less-is-more" in therapeutic antibodies: Afucosylated anti-cancer antibodies with enhanced antibody-dependent cellular cytotoxicity. *mAbs* **2018**, *10*, 693–711. [CrossRef] [PubMed]

36. Tai, Y.-T.; Mayes, P.A.; Acharya, C.; Zhong, M.Y.; Cea, M.; Cagnetta, A.; Craigen, J.; Yates, J.; Gliddon, L.; Fieles, W.; et al. Novel anti-B-cell maturation antigen antibody-drug conjugate (GSK2857916) selectively induces killing of multiple myeloma. *Blood* **2014**, *123*, 3128–3138. [CrossRef] [PubMed]

37. Trudel, S.; Lendvai, N.; Popat, R.; Voorhees, P.M.; Reeves, B.; Libby, E.N.; Richardson, P.G.; Hoos, A.; Gupta, I.; Bragulat, V.; et al. Antibody–drug conjugate, GSK2857916, in relapsed/refractory multiple myeloma: An update on safety and efficacy from dose expansion phase I study. *Blood Cancer J.* **2019**, *9*, 37. [CrossRef]

38. Szot, C.; Saha, S.; Zhang, X.M.; Zhu, Z.; Hilton, M.B.; Morris, K.; Seaman, S.; Dunleavey, J.M.; Hsu, K.-S.; Yu, G.-J.; et al. Tumor stroma–targeted antibody-drug conjugate triggers localized anticancer drug release. *J. Clin. Investig.* **2018**, *128*, 2927–2943. [CrossRef]

39. Liu, R.; Wang, R.E.; Wang, F. Antibody-drug conjugates for non-oncological indications. *Expert Opin. Biol. Ther.* **2016**, *16*, 591–593. [CrossRef]

40. Yu, S.; Lim, A.; Tremblay, M.S. Next horizons: ADCs beyond oncology. In *Innovations for Next-Generation Antibody-Drug Conjugates*; Humana Press: Totowa, NJ, USA, 2018; pp. 321–347. [CrossRef]

41. Lehar, S.M.; Pillow, T.; Xu, M.; Staben, L.; Kajihara, K.K.; Vandlen, R.; DePalatis, L.; Raab, H.; Hazenbos, W.L.; Morisaki, J.H.; et al. Novel antibody-antibiotic conjugate eliminates intracellular S. aureus. *Nature* **2015**, *527*, 323–328. [CrossRef]

42. Mariathasan, S.; Tan, M.-W. Antibody–antibiotic conjugates: A novel therapeutic platform against bacterial infections. *Trends Mol. Med.* **2017**, *23*, 135–149. [CrossRef]

43. Everts, M.; Kok, R.J.; Ásgeirsdóttir, S.A.; Melgert, B.N.; Moolenaar, T.J.M.; Koning, G.A.; van Luyn, M.J.A.; Meijer, D.K.F.; Molema, G. Selective intracellular delivery of dexamethasone into activated endothelial cells using an e-selectin-directed immunoconjugate. *J. Immunol.* **2002**, *168*, 883–889. [CrossRef]

44. Lim, R.K.; Yu, S.; Cheng, B.; Li, S.; Kim, N.J.; Cao, Y.; Chi, V.; Kim, J.Y.; Chatterjee, A.K.; Schultz, P.G.; et al. Targeted delivery of LXR agonist using a site-specific antibody-drug conjugate. *Bioconjug. Chem.* **2015**, *26*, 2216–2222. [CrossRef] [PubMed]

45. Yu, S.; Pearson, A.D.; Lim, R.K.; Rodgers, D.T.; Li, S.; Parker, H.B.; Weglarz, M.; Hampton, E.N.; Bollong, M.J.; Shen, J.; et al. Targeted delivery of an anti-inflammatory PDE4 inhibitor to immune cells via an antibody-drug conjugate. *Mol. Ther.* **2016**, *24*, 2078–2089. [CrossRef]

46. Beaumont, M.; Tomazela, D.; Hodges, D.; Ermakov, G.; Hsieh, E.; Figueroa, I.; So, O.-Y.; Song, Y.; Ma, H.; Antonenko, S.; et al. Antibody-drug conjugates: Integrated bioanalytical and biodisposition assessments in lead optimization and selection. *AAPS Open* **2018**, *4*, 6. [CrossRef]

47. Kvirkvelia, N.; McMenamin, M.; Gutierrez, V.I.; Lasareishvili, B.; Madaio, M.P. Human anti-alpha3(IV)NC1 antibody drug conjugates target glomeruli to resolve nephritis. *Am. J. Physiol. Ren. Physiol.* **2015**, *309*, F680–F684. [CrossRef] [PubMed]

48. Wang, R.E.; Liu, T.; Wang, Y.; Cao, Y.; Du, J.; Luo, X.; Deshmukh, V.; Kim, C.H.; Lawson, B.R.; Tremblay, M.S.; et al. An immunosuppressive antibody-drug conjugate. *J. Am. Chem. Soc.* **2015**, *137*, 3229–3232. [CrossRef] [PubMed]

49. Palchaudhuri, R.; Saez, B.; Hoggatt, J.; Schajnovitz, A.; Sykes, D.B.; Tate, T.A.; Czechowicz, A.; Kfoury, Y.; Ruchika, F.; Rossi, D.J.; et al. Non-genotoxic conditioning for hematopoietic stem cell transplantation using a hematopoietic-cell-specific internalizing immunotoxin. *Nat. Biotechnol.* **2016**, *34*, 738–745. [CrossRef]

50. Kern, J.C.; Dooney, D.; Zhang, R.; Liang, L.; Brandish, P.E.; Cheng, M.; Feng, G.; Beck, A.; Bresson, D.; Firdos, J.; et al. Novel phosphate modified cathepsin B linkers: Improving aqueous solubility and enhancing payload scope of ADCs. *Bioconjug. Chem.* **2016**, *27*, 2081–2088. [CrossRef]

51. Brandish, P.E.; Palmieri, A.; Antonenko, S.; Beaumont, M.; Benso, L.; Cancilla, M.; Cheng, M.; Fayadat-Dilman, L.; Feng, G.; Figueroa, I.; et al. Development of Anti-CD74 antibody-drug conjugates to target glucocorticoids to immune cells. *Bioconjug. Chem.* **2018**, *29*, 2357–2369. [CrossRef]

52. Graversen, J.H.; Svendsen, P.; Dagnaes-Hansen, F.; Dal, J.; Anton, G.; Etzerodt, A.; Petersen, M.D.; Christensen, P.A.; Moller, H.J.; Moestrup, S.K. Targeting the hemoglobin scavenger receptor CD163 in macrophages highly increases the anti-inflammatory potency of dexamethasone. *Mol. Ther.* **2012**, *20*, 1550–1558. [CrossRef]

53. Thomsen, K.L.; Møller, H.J.; Graversen, J.H.; Magnusson, N.E.; Moestrup, S.K.; Vilstrup, H.; Grønbæk, H. Anti-CD163-dexamethasone conjugate inhibits the acute phase response to lipopolysaccharide in rats. *World J. Hepatol.* **2016**, *8*, 726–730. [CrossRef]

54. Yarian, F.; Alibakhshi, A.; Eyvazi, S.; Arezumand, R.; Ahangarzadeh, S. Antibody-drug therapeutic conjugates: Potential of antibody-siRNAs in cancer therapy. *J. Cell. Physiol.* **2019.** [CrossRef] [PubMed]

55. Lu, H.; Wang, D.; Kazane, S.; Javahishvili, T.; Tian, F.; Song, F.; Sellers, A.; Barnett, B.; Schultz, P.G. Site-specific antibody–polymer conjugates for siRNA delivery. *J. Am. Chem. Soc.* **2013**, *135*, 13885–13891. [CrossRef] [PubMed]

56. Zhou, Q. Site-specific antibody conjugation for ADC and beyond. *Biomedicines* **2017**, *5*, 64. [CrossRef] [PubMed]

57. Behrens, C.R.; Liu, B. Methods for site-specific drug conjugation to antibodies. *mAbs* **2014**, *6*, 46–53. [CrossRef] [PubMed]

58. Schumacher, D.; Hackenberger, C.P.; Leonhardt, H.; Helma, J. Current status: Site-specific antibody drug conjugates. *J. Clin. Immunol.* **2016**, *36* (Suppl. S1), 100–107. [CrossRef] [PubMed]

59. Hamblett, K.J.; Senter, P.D.; Chace, D.F.; Sun, M.M.; Lenox, J.; Cerveny, C.G.; Kissler, K.M.; Bernhardt, S.X.; Kopcha, A.K.; Zabinski, R.F.; et al. Effects of drug loading on the antitumor activity of a monoclonal antibody drug conjugate. *Clin. Cancer Res.* **2004**, *10*, 7063–7070. [CrossRef]

60. Junutula, J.R.; Flagella, K.M.; Graham, R.A.; Parsons, K.L.; Ha, E.; Raab, H.; Bhakta, S.; Nguyen, T.; Dugger, D.L.; Li, G.; et al. Engineered thio-trastuzumab-DM1 conjugate with an improved therapeutic index to target human epidermal growth factor receptor 2-positive breast cancer. *Clin. Cancer Res.* **2010**, *16*, 4769–4778. [CrossRef]

61. Junutula, J.R.; Raab, H.; Clark, S.; Bhakta, S.; Leipold, D.D.; Weir, S.; Chen, Y.; Simpson, M.; Tsai, S.P.; Dennis, M.S.; et al. Site-specific conjugation of a cytotoxic drug to an antibody improves the therapeutic index. *Nat. Biotechnol.* **2008**, *26*, 925–932. [CrossRef]

62. Shen, B.Q.; Xu, K.; Liu, L.; Raab, H.; Bhakta, S.; Kenrick, M.; Parsons-Reponte, K.L.; Tien, J.; Yu, S.F.; Mai, E.; et al. Conjugation site modulates the in vivo stability and therapeutic activity of antibody-drug conjugates. *Nat. Biotechnol.* **2012**, *30*, 184–189. [CrossRef]

63. Dimasi, N.; Fleming, R.; Zhong, H.; Bezabeh, B.; Kinneer, K.; Christie, R.J.; Fazenbaker, C.; Wu, H.; Gao, C. Efficient preparation of site-specific antibody-drug conjugates using cysteine insertion. *Mol. Pharm.* **2017**, *14*, 1501–1516. [CrossRef]

64. Sussman, D.; Westendorf, L.; Meyer, D.W.; Leiske, C.I.; Anderson, M.; Okeley, N.M.; Alley, S.C.; Lyon, R.; Sanderson, R.J.; Carter, P.J.; et al. Engineered cysteine antibodies: An improved antibody-drug conjugate platform with a novel mechanism of drug-linker stability. *Protein Eng. Des. Sel.* **2018**, *31*, 47–54. [CrossRef] [PubMed]

65. Strop, P.; Liu, S.H.; Dorywalska, M.; Delaria, K.; Dushin, R.G.; Tran, T.T.; Ho, W.H.; Farias, S.; Casas, M.G.; Abdiche, Y.; et al. Location matters: Site of conjugation modulates stability and pharmacokinetics of antibody drug conjugates. *Chem. Biol.* **2013**, *20*, 161–167. [CrossRef] [PubMed]

66. Falck, G.; Müller, K.M. Enzyme-based labeling strategies for antibody–drug conjugates and antibody mimetics. *Antibodies* **2018**, *7*, 4. [CrossRef] [PubMed]

67. Dennler, P.; Chiotellis, A.; Fischer, E.; Bregeon, D.; Belmant, C.; Gauthier, L.; Lhospice, F.; Romagne, F.; Schibli, R. Transglutaminase-based chemo-enzymatic conjugation approach yields homogeneous antibody-drug conjugates. *Bioconjug. Chem.* **2014**, *25*, 569–578. [CrossRef] [PubMed]

68. Jeger, S.; Zimmermann, K.; Blanc, A.; Grunberg, J.; Honer, M.; Hunziker, P.; Struthers, H.; Schibli, R. Site-specific and stoichiometric modification of antibodies by bacterial transglutaminase. *Angew. Chem. Int. Ed. Engl.* **2010**, *49*, 9995–9997. [CrossRef] [PubMed]

69. Dorywalska, M.; Strop, P.; Melton-Witt, J.A.; Hasa-Moreno, A.; Farias, S.E.; Galindo Casas, M.; Delaria, K.; Lui, V.; Poulsen, K.; Loo, C.; et al. Effect of attachment site on stability of cleavable antibody drug conjugates. *Bioconjug. Chem.* **2015**, *26*, 650–659. [CrossRef]

70. Ritzefeld, M. Sortagging: A robust and efficient chemoenzymatic ligation strategy. *Chemistry* **2014**, *20*, 8516–8529. [CrossRef]

71. Beerli, R.R.; Hell, T.; Merkel, A.S.; Grawunder, U. Sortase enzyme-mediated generation of site-specifically conjugated antibody drug conjugates with high in vitro and in vivo potency. *PLoS ONE* **2015**, *10*, e0131177. [CrossRef]

72. Pishesha, N.; Ingram, J.R.; Ploegh, H.L. Sortase A: A model for transpeptidation and its biological applications. *Annu. Rev. Cell Dev. Biol.* **2018**, *34*, 163–188. [CrossRef]

73. Carrico, I.S.; Carlson, B.L.; Bertozzi, C.R. Introducing genetically encoded aldehydes into proteins. *Nat. Chem. Biol.* **2007**, *3*, 321. [CrossRef]

74. Rabuka, D.; Rush, J.S.; deHart, G.W.; Wu, P.; Bertozzi, C.R. Site-specific chemical protein conjugation using genetically encoded aldehyde tags. *Nat. Protoc.* **2012**, *7*, 1052–1067. [CrossRef] [PubMed]

75. Liu, J.; Barfield, R.M.; Rabuka, D. Site-specific bioconjugation using SMARTag((R)) Technology: A practical and effective chemoenzymatic approach to generate antibody-drug conjugates. *Methods Mol. Biol.* **2019**, *2033*, 131–147. [CrossRef] [PubMed]

76. Agarwal, P.; van der Weijden, J.; Sletten, E.M.; Rabuka, D.; Bertozzi, C.R. A Pictet-Spengler ligation for protein chemical modification. *Proc. Natl. Acad. Sci. USA* **2013**, *110*, 46–51. [CrossRef] [PubMed]

77. Agarwal, P.; Bertozzi, C.R. Site-specific antibody–drug conjugates: The nexus of bioorthogonal chemistry, protein engineering, and drug development. *Bioconjug. Chem.* **2015**, *26*, 176–192. [CrossRef] [PubMed]

78. Hallam, T.J.; Smider, V.V. Unnatural amino acids in novel antibody conjugates. *Future Med. Chem.* **2014**, *6*, 1309–1324. [CrossRef] [PubMed]

79. Kim, C.H.; Axup, J.Y.; Schultz, P.G. Protein conjugation with genetically encoded unnatural amino acids. *Curr. Opin. Chem. Biol.* **2013**, *17*, 412–419. [CrossRef]

80. Axup, J.Y.; Bajjuri, K.M.; Ritland, M.; Hutchins, B.M.; Kim, C.H.; Kazane, S.A.; Halder, R.; Forsyth, J.S.; Santidrian, A.F.; Stafin, K.; et al. Synthesis of site-specific antibody-drug conjugates using unnatural amino acids. *Proc. Natl. Acad. Sci. USA* **2012**, *109*, 16101–16106. [CrossRef]

81. Tian, F.; Lu, Y.; Manibusan, A.; Sellers, A.; Tran, H.; Sun, Y.; Phuong, T.; Barnett, R.; Hehli, B.; Song, F.; et al. A general approach to site-specific antibody drug conjugates. *Proc. Natl. Acad. Sci. USA* **2014**, *111*, 1766–1771. [CrossRef]

82. Hofer, T.; Skeffington, L.R.; Chapman, C.M.; Rader, C. Molecularly defined antibody conjugation through a selenocysteine interface. *Biochemistry* **2009**, *48*, 12047–12057. [CrossRef]

83. Zimmerman, E.S.; Heibeck, T.H.; Gill, A.; Li, X.; Murray, C.J.; Madlansacay, M.R.; Tran, C.; Uter, N.T.; Yin, G.; Rivers, P.J.; et al. Production of site-specific antibody–drug conjugates using optimized non-natural amino acids in a cell-free expression system. *Bioconjug. Chem.* **2014**, *25*, 351–361. [CrossRef]

84. Yamada, K.; Ito, Y. Recent chemical approaches for site-specific conjugation of native antibodies: Technologies toward next generation antibody-drug conjugates. *ChemBioChem* **2019**, *20*, 2729–2737. [CrossRef] [PubMed]

85. Ban, H.; Nagano, M.; Gavrilyuk, J.; Hakamata, W.; Inokuma, T.; Barbas, C.F., 3rd. Facile and stabile linkages through tyrosine: Bioconjugation strategies with the tyrosine-click reaction. *Bioconjug. Chem.* **2013**, *24*, 520–532. [CrossRef] [PubMed]

86. Zuberbuhler, K.; Casi, G.; Bernardes, G.J.; Neri, D. Fucose-specific conjugation of hydrazide derivatives to a vascular-targeting monoclonal antibody in IgG format. *Chem. Commun.* **2012**, *48*, 7100–7102. [CrossRef] [PubMed]

87. Zhou, Q.; Stefano, J.E.; Manning, C.; Kyazike, J.; Chen, B.; Gianolio, D.A.; Park, A.; Busch, M.; Bird, J.; Zheng, X.; et al. Site-specific antibody–drug conjugation through glycoengineering. *Bioconjug. Chem.* **2014**, *25*, 510–520. [CrossRef] [PubMed]

88. van Geel, R.; Wijdeven, M.A.; Heesbeen, R.; Verkade, J.M.; Wasiel, A.A.; van Berkel, S.S.; van Delft, F.L. Chemoenzymatic conjugation of toxic payloads to the globally conserved N-Glycan of native mAbs provides homogeneous and highly efficacious antibody-drug conjugates. *Bioconjug. Chem.* **2015**, *26*, 2233–2242. [CrossRef] [PubMed]

89. Li, X.; Fang, T.; Boons, G.J. Preparation of well-defined antibody-drug conjugates through glycan remodeling and strain-promoted azide-alkyne cycloadditions. *Angew. Chem. Int. Ed. Engl.* **2014**, *53*, 7179–7182. [CrossRef]

90. Badescu, G.; Bryant, P.; Bird, M.; Henseleit, K.; Swierkosz, J.; Parekh, V.; Tommasi, R.; Pawlisz, E.; Jurlewicz, K.; Farys, M.; et al. Bridging disulfides for stable and defined antibody drug conjugates. *Bioconjug. Chem.* **2014**, *25*, 1124–1136. [CrossRef]

91. Behrens, C.R.; Ha, E.H.; Chinn, L.L.; Bowers, S.; Probst, G.; Fitch-Bruhns, M.; Monteon, J.; Valdiosera, A.; Bermudez, A.; Liao-Chan, S.; et al. Antibody-Drug Conjugates (ADCs) derived from interchain cysteine cross-linking demonstrate improved homogeneity and other pharmacological properties over conventional heterogeneous ADCs. *Mol. Pharm.* **2015**, *12*, 3986–3998. [CrossRef]

92. Bryant, P.; Pabst, M.; Badescu, G.; Bird, M.; McDowell, W.; Jamieson, E.; Swierkosz, J.; Jurlewicz, K.; Tommasi, R.; Henseleit, K.; et al. In vitro and in vivo evaluation of cysteine rebridged trastuzumab-MMAE antibody drug conjugates with defined drug-to-antibody ratios. *Mol. Pharm.* **2015**, *12*, 1872–1879. [CrossRef]

93. Forte, N.; Chudasama, V.; Baker, J.R. Homogeneous antibody-drug conjugates via site-selective disulfide bridging. *Drug Discov. Today Technol.* **2018**, *30*, 11–20. [CrossRef]

94. Schumacher, F.F.; Nunes, J.P.M.; Maruani, A.; Chudasama, V.; Smith, M.E.B.; Chester, K.A.; Baker, J.R.; Caddick, S. Next generation maleimides enable the controlled assembly of antibody-drug conjugates via native disulfide bond bridging. *Org. Biomol. Chem.* **2014**, *12*, 7261–7269. [CrossRef] [PubMed]

95. Altwerger, G.; Bonazzoli, E.; Bellone, S.; Egawa-Takata, T.; Menderes, G.; Pettinella, F.; Bianchi, A.; Riccio, F.; Feinberg, J.; Zammataro, L.; et al. In vitro and in vivo activity of IMGN853, an antibody-drug conjugate targeting folate receptor alpha linked to DM4, in biologically aggressive endometrial cancers. *Mol. Cancer Ther.* **2018**, *17*, 1003–1011. [CrossRef] [PubMed]

96. Pei, Z.; Chen, C.; Chen, J.; Cruz-Chuh, J.D.; Delarosa, R.; Deng, Y.; Fourie-O'Donohue, A.; Figueroa, I.; Guo, J.; Jin, W.; et al. Exploration of pyrrolobenzodiazepine (PBD)-dimers containing disulfide-based prodrugs as payloads for antibody-drug conjugates. *Mol. Pharm.* **2018**, *15*, 3979–3996. [CrossRef] [PubMed]

97. Mantaj, J.; Jackson, P.J.M.; Rahman, K.M.; Thurston, D.E. From anthramycin to pyrrolobenzodiazepine (PBD)-containing antibody-drug conjugates (ADCs). *Angew. Chem. Int. Ed. Engl.* **2017**, *56*, 462–488. [CrossRef]

98. Dan, N.; Setua, S.; Kashyap, V.K.; Khan, S.; Jaggi, M.; Yallapu, M.M.; Chauhan, S.C. Antibody-drug conjugates for cancer therapy: Chemistry to clinical implications. *Pharmaceuticals* **2018**, *11*, 32. [CrossRef]

99. Ratnayake, A.S.; Chang, L.P.; Tumey, L.N.; Loganzo, F.; Chemler, J.A.; Wagenaar, M.; Musto, S.; Li, F.; Janso, J.E.; Ballard, T.E.; et al. Natural product bis-intercalator depsipeptides as a new class of payloads for antibody-drug conjugates. *Bioconjug. Chem.* **2019**, *30*, 200–209. [CrossRef]

100. Lerchen, H.G.; Wittrock, S.; Stelte-Ludwig, B.; Sommer, A.; Berndt, S.; Griebenow, N.; Rebstock, A.S.; Johannes, S.; Cancho-Grande, Y.; Mahlert, C.; et al. Antibody-drug conjugates with pyrrole-based KSP inhibitors as the payload class. *Angew. Chem. Int. Ed. Engl.* **2018**, *57*, 15243–15247. [CrossRef]

101. Karpov, A.S.; Abrams, T.; Clark, S.; Raikar, A.; D'Alessio, J.A.; Dillon, M.P.; Gesner, T.G.; Jones, D.; Lacaud, M.; Mallet, W.; et al. Nicotinamide phosphoribosyltransferase inhibitor as a novel payload for antibody-drug conjugates. *ACS Med. Chem. Lett.* **2018**, *9*, 838–842. [CrossRef]

102. Love, E.A.; Sattikar, A.; Cook, H.; Gillen, K.; Large, J.M.; Patel, S.; Matthews, D.; Merritt, A. Developing an antibody–drug conjugate approach to selective inhibition of an extracellular protein. *ChemBioChem* **2019**, *20*, 754–758. [CrossRef]

103. Brown, E.D.; Wright, G.D. Antibacterial drug discovery in the resistance era. *Nature* **2016**, *529*, 336–343. [CrossRef]

104. van der Goes, M.C.; Jacobs, J.W.; Bijlsma, J.W. The value of glucocorticoid co-therapy in different rheumatic diseases-positive and adverse effects. *Arthritis Res. Ther.* **2014**, *16*, S2. [CrossRef] [PubMed]

105. Schäcke, H.; Döcke, W.-D.; Asadullah, K. Mechanisms involved in the side effects of glucocorticoids. *Pharmacol. Ther.* **2002**, *96*, 23–43. [CrossRef]

106. Kern, J.C.; Cancilla, M.; Dooney, D.; Kwasnjuk, K.; Zhang, R.; Beaumont, M.; Figueroa, I.; Hsieh, S.; Liang, L.; Tomazela, D.; et al. Discovery of pyrophosphate diesters as tunable, soluble, and bioorthogonal linkers for site-specific antibody-drug conjugates. *J. Am. Chem. Soc.* **2016**, *138*, 1430–1445. [CrossRef] [PubMed]

107. Peters, C.; Brown, S. Antibody–drug conjugates as novel anti-cancer chemotherapeutics. *Biosci. Rep.* **2015**, *35*, e00225. [CrossRef] [PubMed]

108. Juliano, R.L. The delivery of therapeutic oligonucleotides. *Nucleic Acids Res.* **2016**, *44*, 6518–6548. [CrossRef]

109. Dovgan, I.; Koniev, O.; Kolodych, S.; Wagner, A. Antibody–oligonucleotide conjugates as therapeutic, imaging, and detection agents. *Bioconjug. Chem.* **2019**, *30*, 2483–2501. [CrossRef]

110. Levin, A.A. Treating disease at the RNA level with oligonucleotides. *N. Engl. J. Med.* **2019**, *380*, 57–70. [CrossRef]

111. Geary, R.S.; Norris, D.; Yu, R.; Bennett, C.F. Pharmacokinetics, biodistribution and cell uptake of antisense oligonucleotides. *Adv. Drug Deliv. Rev.* **2015**, *87*, 46–51. [CrossRef]

112. Park, J.; Park, J.; Pei, Y.; Xu, J.; Yeo, Y. Pharmacokinetics and biodistribution of recently-developed siRNA nanomedicines. *Adv. Drug Deliv. Rev.* **2016**, *104*, 93–109. [CrossRef]

113.	Benizri, S.; Gissot, A.; Martin, A.; Vialet, B.; Grinstaff, M.W.; Barthélémy, P. Bioconjugated oligonucleotides: Recent developments and therapeutic applications. *Bioconjug. Chem.* **2019**, *30*, 366–383. [CrossRef]

114.	Nair, J.K.; Willoughby, J.L.S.; Chan, A.; Charisse, K.; Alam, M.R.; Wang, Q.; Hoekstra, M.; Kandasamy, P.; Kel'in, A.V.; Milstein, S.; et al. Multivalent N-acetylgalactosamine-conjugated siRNA localizes in hepatocytes and elicits robust RNAi-mediated gene silencing. *J. Am. Chem. Soc.* **2014**, *136*, 16958–16961. [CrossRef]

115.	Sewing, S.; Gubler, M.; Gérard, R.; Avignon, B.; Mueller, Y.; Braendli-Baiocco, A.; Odin, M.; Moisan, A. GalNAc conjugation attenuates the cytotoxicity of antisense oligonucleotide drugs in renal tubular cells. *Mol. Ther. Nucleic Acids* **2019**, *14*, 67–79. [CrossRef] [PubMed]

116.	Ämmälä, C.; Drury, W.J.; Knerr, L.; Ahlstedt, I.; Stillemark-Billton, P.; Wennberg-Huldt, C.; Andersson, E.-M.; Valeur, E.; Jansson-Löfmark, R.; Janzén, D.; et al. Targeted delivery of antisense oligonucleotides to pancreatic β-cells. *Sci. Adv.* **2018**, *4*, eaat3386. [CrossRef]

117.	Osborn, M.F.; Coles, A.H.; Biscans, A.; Haraszti, R.A.; Roux, L.; Davis, S.; Ly, S.; Echeverria, D.; Hassler, M.R.; Godinho, B.M.D.C.; et al. Hydrophobicity drives the systemic distribution of lipid-conjugated siRNAs via lipid transport pathways. *Nucleic Acids Res.* **2018**, *47*, 1070–1081. [CrossRef] [PubMed]

118.	Ma, Y.; Kowolik, C.M.; Swiderski, P.M.; Kortylewski, M.; Yu, H.; Horne, D.A.; Jove, R.; Caballero, O.L.; Simpson, A.J.G.; Lee, F.-T.; et al. Humanized lewis-y specific antibody based delivery of STAT3 siRNA. *ACS Chem. Biol.* **2011**, *6*, 962–970. [CrossRef] [PubMed]

119.	Cuellar, T.L.; Barnes, D.; Nelson, C.; Tanguay, J.; Yu, S.-F.; Wen, X.; Scales, S.J.; Gesch, J.; Davis, D.; van Brabant Smith, A.; et al. Systematic evaluation of antibody-mediated siRNA delivery using an industrial platform of THIOMAB–siRNA conjugates. *Nucleic Acids Res.* **2014**, *43*, 1189–1203. [CrossRef]

120.	Sugo, T.; Terada, M.; Oikawa, T.; Miyata, K.; Nishimura, S.; Kenjo, E.; Ogasawara-Shimizu, M.; Makita, Y.; Imaichi, S.; Murata, S.; et al. Development of antibody-siRNA conjugate targeted to cardiac and skeletal muscles. *J. Control. Release* **2016**, *237*, 1–13. [CrossRef]

121.	Satake, N.; Duong, C.; Yoshida, S.; Oestergaard, M.; Chen, C.; Peralta, R.; Guo, S.; Seth, P.P.; Li, Y.; Beckett, L.; et al. Novel targeted therapy for precursor B cell acute lymphoblastic leukemia: Anti-CD22 antibody-MXD3 antisense oligonucleotide conjugate. *Mol. Med.* **2016**, *22*, 632–642. [CrossRef]

122.	Arnold, A.E.; Malek-Adamian, E.; Le, P.U.; Meng, A.; Martinez-Montero, S.; Petrecca, K.; Damha, M.J.; Shoichet, M.S. Antibody-antisense oligonucleotide conjugate downregulates a key gene in glioblastoma stem cells. *Mol. Ther. Nucleic Acids* **2018**, *11*, 518–527. [CrossRef]

123.	Humphreys, S.C.; Thayer, M.B.; Campuzano, I.D.G.; Netirojjanakul, C.; Rock, B.M. Quantification of siRNA-antibody conjugates in biological matrices by triplex-forming oligonucleotide ELISA. *Nucleic Acid Ther.* **2019**, *29*, 161–166. [CrossRef]

124.	Bargh, J.D.; Isidro-Llobet, A.; Parker, J.S.; Spring, D.R. Cleavable linkers in antibody–drug conjugates. *Chem. Soc. Rev.* **2019**, *48*, 4361–4374. [CrossRef] [PubMed]

125.	Dubowchik, G.M.; Walker, M.A. Receptor-mediated and enzyme-dependent targeting of cytotoxic anticancer drugs. *Pharmacol. Ther.* **1999**, *83*, 67–123. [CrossRef]

126.	Kratz, F.; Müller, I.A.; Ryppa, C.; Warnecke, A. Prodrug strategies in anticancer chemotherapy. *ChemMedChem* **2008**, *3*, 20–53. [CrossRef] [PubMed]

127.	Anami, Y.; Yamazaki, C.M.; Xiong, W.; Gui, X.; Zhang, N.; An, Z.; Tsuchikama, K. Glutamic acid–valine–citrulline linkers ensure stability and efficacy of antibody–drug conjugates in mice. *Nat. Commun.* **2018**, *9*, 2512. [CrossRef]

128.	Wei, B.; Gunzner-Toste, J.; Yao, H.; Wang, T.; Wang, J.; Xu, Z.; Chen, J.; Wai, J.; Nonomiya, J.; Tsai, S.P.; et al. Discovery of peptidomimetic antibody–drug conjugate linkers with enhanced protease specificity. *J. Med. Chem.* **2018**, *61*, 989–1000. [CrossRef]

129.	Lyon, R.P.; Bovee, T.D.; Doronina, S.O.; Burke, P.J.; Hunter, J.H.; Neff-LaFord, H.D.; Jonas, M.; Anderson, M.E.; Setter, J.R.; Senter, P.D. Reducing hydrophobicity of homogeneous antibody-drug conjugates improves pharmacokinetics and therapeutic index. *Nat. Biotechnol.* **2015**, *33*, 733–735. [CrossRef]

130.	Kolodych, S.; Michel, C.; Delacroix, S.; Koniev, O.; Ehkirch, A.; Eberova, J.; Cianferani, S.; Renoux, B.; Krezel, W.; Poinot, P.; et al. Development and evaluation of beta-galactosidase-sensitive antibody-drug conjugates. *Eur. J. Med. Chem.* **2017**, *142*, 376–382. [CrossRef]

131. DiJoseph, J.F.; Dougher, M.M.; Kalyandrug, L.B.; Armellino, D.C.; Boghaert, E.R.; Hamann, P.R.; Moran, J.K.; Damle, N.K. Antitumor efficacy of a combination of CMC-544 (Inotuzumab Ozogamicin), a CD22-targeted cytotoxic immunoconjugate of calicheamicin, and rituximab against Non-Hodgkin's B-Cell lymphoma. *Clin. Cancer Res.* **2006**, *12*, 242–249. [CrossRef]

132. Zhou, D.; Casavant, J.; Graziani, E.I.; He, H.; Janso, J.; Loganzo, F.; Musto, S.; Tumey, N.; O'Donnell, C.J.; Dushin, R. Novel PIKK inhibitor antibody-drug conjugates: Synthesis and anti-tumor activity. *Bioorg. Med. Chem. Lett.* **2019**, *29*, 943–947. [CrossRef]

133. Govindan, S.V.; Cardillo, T.M.; Sharkey, R.M.; Tat, F.; Gold, D.V.; Goldenberg, D.M. Milatuzumab-SN-38 conjugates for the treatment of CD74+ cancers. *Mol. Cancer Ther.* **2013**, *12*, 968–978. [CrossRef]

134. Kellogg, B.A.; Garrett, L.; Kovtun, Y.; Lai, K.C.; Leece, B.; Miller, M.; Payne, G.; Steeves, R.; Whiteman, K.R.; Widdison, W.; et al. Disulfide-linked antibody–maytansinoid conjugates: Optimization of in vivo activity by varying the steric hindrance at carbon atoms adjacent to the disulfide linkage. *Bioconjug. Chem.* **2011**, *22*, 717–727. [CrossRef] [PubMed]

135. Bernardes, G.J.L.; Casi, G.; Trüssel, S.; Hartmann, I.; Schwager, K.; Scheuermann, J.; Neri, D. A traceless vascular-targeting antibody–drug conjugate for cancer therapy. *Angew. Chem. Int. Ed.* **2012**, *51*, 941–944. [CrossRef] [PubMed]

136. Baldwin, A.D.; Kiick, K.L. Tunable degradation of maleimide—Thiol adducts in reducing environments. *Bioconjug. Chem.* **2011**, *22*, 1946–1953. [CrossRef] [PubMed]

137. Yasunaga, M.; Manabe, S.; Matsumura, Y. Immunoregulation by IL-7R-targeting antibody-drug conjugates: Overcoming steroid-resistance in cancer and autoimmune disease. *Sci. Rep.* **2017**, *7*, 10735. [CrossRef]

138. Hampe, C.S. Protective role of anti-idiotypic antibodies in autoimmunity—Lessons for type 1 diabetes. *Autoimmunity* **2012**, *45*, 320–331. [CrossRef] [PubMed]

139. Senter, P.D. Potent antibody drug conjugates for cancer therapy. *Curr. Opin. Chem. Biol.* **2009**, *13*, 235–244. [CrossRef]

140. Lewis Phillips, G.D.; Li, G.; Dugger, D.L.; Crocker, L.M.; Parsons, K.L.; Mai, E.; Blättler, W.A.; Lambert, J.M.; Chari, R.V.J.; Lutz, R.J.; et al. Targeting HER2-positive breast cancer with trastuzumab-DM1, an antibody–cytotoxic drug conjugate. *Cancer Res.* **2008**, *68*, 9280–9290. [CrossRef]

141. Kraynov, E.; Kamath, A.V.; Walles, M.; Tarcsa, E.; Deslandes, A.; Iyer, R.A.; Datta-Mannan, A.; Sriraman, P.; Bairlein, M.; Yang, J.J.; et al. Current approaches for absorption, distribution, metabolism, and excretion characterization of antibody-drug conjugates: An industry white paper. *Drug Metab. Dispos.* **2016**, *44*, 617–623. [CrossRef]

142. Drake, P.M.; Rabuka, D. Recent developments in ADC technology: Preclinical studies signal future clinical trends. *BioDrugs* **2017**, *31*, 521–531. [CrossRef]

143. Donaghy, H. Effects of antibody, drug and linker on the preclinical and clinical toxicities of antibody-drug conjugates. *mAbs* **2016**, *8*, 659–671. [CrossRef]

144. Panowski, S.; Bhakta, S.; Raab, H.; Polakis, P.; Junutula, J.R. Site-specific antibody drug conjugates for cancer therapy. *mAbs* **2014**, *6*, 34–45. [CrossRef] [PubMed]

145. Shah, D.K.; Betts, A.M. Antibody biodistribution coefficients. *mAbs* **2013**, *5*, 297–305. [CrossRef] [PubMed]

146. Yip, V.; Palma, E.; Tesar, D.B.; Mundo, E.E.; Bumbaca, D.; Torres, E.K.; Reyes, N.A.; Shen, B.Q.; Fielder, P.J.; Prabhu, S.; et al. Quantitative cumulative biodistribution of antibodies in mice. *mAbs* **2014**, *6*, 689–696. [CrossRef] [PubMed]

147. Herbertson, R.A.; Tebbutt, N.C.; Lee, F.T.; MacFarlane, D.J.; Chappell, B.; Micallef, N.; Lee, S.T.; Saunder, T.; Hopkins, W.; Smyth, F.E.; et al. Phase I biodistribution and pharmacokinetic study of Lewis Y-targeting immunoconjugate CMD-193 in patients with advanced epithelial cancers. *Clin. Cancer Res.* **2009**, *15*, 6709–6715. [CrossRef]

148. Lu, D.; Joshi, A.; Wang, B.; Olsen, S.; Yi, J.H.; Krop, I.E.; Burris, H.A.; Girish, S. An integrated multiple-analyte pharmacokinetic model to characterize trastuzumab emtansine (T-DM1) clearance pathways and to evaluate reduced pharmacokinetic sampling in patients with HER2-positive metastatic breast cancer. *Clin. Pharm.* **2013**, *52*, 657–672. [CrossRef]

149. Han, T.H.; Gopal, A.K.; Ramchandren, R.; Goy, A.; Chen, R.; Matous, J.V.; Cooper, M.; Grove, L.E.; Alley, S.C.; Lynch, C.M.; et al. CYP3A-mediated drug-drug interaction potential and excretion of brentuximab vedotin, an antibody-drug conjugate, in patients with CD30-positive hematologic malignancies. *J. Clin. Pharmacol.* **2013**, *53*, 866–877. [CrossRef]

150. Collins, D.M.; Bossenmaier, B.; Kollmorgen, G.; Niederfellner, G. Acquired resistance to antibody-drug conjugates. *Cancers* **2019**, *11*, 394. [CrossRef]

151. Bobaly, B.; Fleury-Souverain, S.; Beck, A.; Veuthey, J.L.; Guillarme, D.; Fekete, S. Current possibilities of liquid chromatography for the characterization of antibody-drug conjugates. *J. Pharm. Biomed. Anal.* **2018**, *147*, 493–505. [CrossRef]

152. Lechner, A.; Giorgetti, J.; Gahoual, R.; Beck, A.; Leize-Wagner, E.; Francois, Y.N. Insights from capillary electrophoresis approaches for characterization of monoclonal antibodies and antibody drug conjugates in the period 2016–2018. *J. Chromatogr. B* **2019**, *1122*, 1–17. [CrossRef]

153. Wagh, A.; Song, H.; Zeng, M.; Tao, L.; Das, T.K. Challenges and new frontiers in analytical characterization of antibody-drug conjugates. *mAbs* **2018**, *10*, 222–243. [CrossRef]

154. Beck, A.; D'Atri, V.; Ehkirch, A.; Fekete, S.; Hernandez-Alba, O.; Gahoual, R.; Leize-Wagner, E.; Francois, Y.; Guillarme, D.; Cianferani, S. Cutting-edge multi-level analytical and structural characterization of antibody-drug conjugates: Present and future. *Expert Rev. Proteom.* **2019**, *16*, 337–362. [CrossRef] [PubMed]

155. Yurkovetskiy, A.V.; Yin, M.; Bodyak, N.; Stevenson, C.A.; Thomas, J.D.; Hammond, C.E.; Qin, L.; Zhu, B.; Gumerov, D.R.; Ter-Ovanesyan, E.; et al. A polymer-based antibody-vinca drug conjugate platform: Characterization and preclinical efficacy. *Cancer Res.* **2015**, *75*, 3365–3372. [CrossRef] [PubMed]

156. Goldenberg, D.M.; Cardillo, T.M.; Govindan, S.V.; Rossi, E.A.; Sharkey, R.M. Trop-2 is a novel target for solid cancer therapy with sacituzumab govitecan (IMMU-132), an antibody-drug conjugate (ADC). *Oncotarget* **2015**, *6*, 22496–22512. [CrossRef] [PubMed]

157. Viricel, W.; Fournet, G.; Beaumel, S.; Perrial, E.; Papot, S.; Dumontet, C.; Joseph, B. Monodisperse polysarcosine-based highly-loaded antibody-drug conjugates. *Chem. Sci.* **2019**, *10*, 4048–4053. [CrossRef] [PubMed]

158. Schneider, H.; Deweid, L.; Pirzer, T.; Yanakieva, D.; Englert, S.; Becker, B.; Avrutina, O.; Kolmar, H. Dextramabs: A novel format of antibody-drug conjugates featuring a multivalent polysaccharide scaffold. *ChemistryOpen* **2019**, *8*, 354–357. [CrossRef]

159. Wang, L.; Amphlett, G.; Blattler, W.A.; Lambert, J.M.; Zhang, W. Structural characterization of the maytansinoid-monoclonal antibody immunoconjugate, huN901-DM1, by mass spectrometry. *Protein Sci.* **2005**, *14*, 2436–2446. [CrossRef]

160. Cao, M.; De Mel, N.; Jiao, Y.; Howard, J.; Parthemore, C.; Korman, S.; Thompson, C.; Wendeler, M.; Liu, D. Site-specific antibody-drug conjugate heterogeneity characterization and heterogeneity root cause analysis. *mAbs* **2019**, *11*, 1–13. [CrossRef]

161. Mehta, G.; Scheinman, R.I.; Holers, V.M.; Banda, N.K. A new approach for the treatment of arthritis in mice with a novel conjugate of an Anti-C5aR1 antibody and C5 small interfering RNA. *J. Immunol.* **2015**, *194*, 5446–5454. [CrossRef]

162. Ross, P.L.; Wolfe, J.L. Physical and chemical stability of antibody drug conjugates: Current status. *J. Pharm. Sci.* **2016**, *105*, 391–397. [CrossRef]

163. Duerr, C.; Friess, W. Antibody-drug conjugates-stability and formulation. *Eur. J. Pharm. Biopharm.* **2019**, *139*, 168–176. [CrossRef]

164. Wakankar, A.A.; Feeney, M.B.; Rivera, J.; Chen, Y.; Kim, M.; Sharma, V.K.; Wang, Y.J. Physicochemical stability of the antibody-drug conjugate Trastuzumab-DM1: Changes due to modification and conjugation processes. *Bioconjug. Chem.* **2010**, *21*, 1588–1595. [CrossRef] [PubMed]

165. Gandhi, A.V.; Randolph, T.W.; Carpenter, J.F. Conjugation of emtansine onto trastuzumab promotes aggregation of the antibody-drug conjugate by reducing repulsive electrostatic interactions and increasing hydrophobic interactions. *J. Pharm. Sci.* **2019**, *108*, 1973–1983. [CrossRef] [PubMed]

166. Beckley, N.S.; Lazzareschi, K.P.; Chih, H.W.; Sharma, V.K.; Flores, H.L. Investigation into temperature-induced aggregation of an antibody drug conjugate. *Bioconjug. Chem.* **2013**, *24*, 1674–1683. [CrossRef]

167. Adem, Y.T.; Schwarz, K.A.; Duenas, E.; Patapoff, T.W.; Galush, W.J.; Esue, O. Auristatin antibody drug conjugate physical instability and the role of drug payload. *Bioconjug. Chem.* **2014**, *25*, 656–664. [CrossRef] [PubMed]

168. Guo, J.; Kumar, S.; Prashad, A.; Starkey, J.; Singh, S.K. Assessment of physical stability of an antibody drug conjugate by higher order structure analysis: Impact of thiol- maleimide chemistry. *Pharm. Res.* **2014**, *31*, 1710–1723. [CrossRef] [PubMed]

169. Guo, J.; Kumar, S.; Chipley, M.; Marcq, O.; Gupta, D.; Jin, Z.; Tomar, D.S.; Swabowski, C.; Smith, J.; Starkey, J.A.; et al. Characterization and higher-order structure assessment of an interchain cysteine-based ADC: Impact of drug loading and distribution on the mechanism of aggregation. *Bioconjug. Chem.* **2016**, *27*, 604–615. [CrossRef]

170. Buecheler, J.W.; Winzer, M.; Tonillo, J.; Weber, C.; Gieseler, H. Impact of payload hydrophobicity on the stability of antibody-drug conjugates. *Mol. Pharm.* **2018**, *15*, 2656–2664. [CrossRef]

171. Gandhi, A.V.; Arlotta, K.J.; Chen, H.N.; Owen, S.C.; Carpenter, J.F. Biophysical properties and heating-induced aggregation of lysine-conjugated antibody-drug conjugates. *J. Pharm. Sci.* **2018**, *107*, 1858–1869. [CrossRef]

172. Ohri, R.; Bhakta, S.; Fourie-O'Donohue, A.; Dela Cruz-Chuh, J.; Tsai, S.P.; Cook, R.; Wei, B.; Ng, C.; Wong, A.W.; Bos, A.B.; et al. High-throughput cysteine scanning to identify stable antibody conjugation sites for maleimide- and disulfide-based linkers. *Bioconjug. Chem.* **2018**, *29*, 473–485. [CrossRef]

173. Fathi, A.T.; Erba, H.P.; Lancet, J.E.; Stein, E.M.; Ravandi, F.; Faderl, S.; Walter, R.B.; Advani, A.S.; DeAngelo, D.J.; Kovacsovics, T.J.; et al. A phase 1 trial of vadastuximab talirine combined with hypomethylating agents in patients with CD33-positive AML. *Blood* **2018**, *132*, 1125–1133. [CrossRef]

174. King, G.T.; Eaton, K.D.; Beagle, B.R.; Zopf, C.J.; Wong, G.Y.; Krupka, H.I.; Hua, S.Y.; Messersmith, W.A.; El-Khoueiry, A.B. A phase 1, dose-escalation study of PF-06664178, an anti-Trop-2/Aur0101 antibody-drug conjugate in patients with advanced or metastatic solid tumors. *Investig. New Drugs* **2018**, *36*, 836–847. [CrossRef] [PubMed]

175. Phillips, T.; Barr, P.M.; Park, S.I.; Kolibaba, K.; Caimi, P.F.; Chhabra, S.; Kingsley, E.C.; Boyd, T.; Chen, R.; Carret, A.-S.; et al. A phase 1 trial of SGN-CD70A in patients with CD70-positive diffuse large B cell lymphoma and mantle cell lymphoma. *Investig. New Drugs* **2019**, *37*, 297–306. [CrossRef] [PubMed]

176. Saber, H.; Simpson, N.; Ricks, T.K.; Leighton, J.K. An FDA oncology analysis of toxicities associated with PBD-containing antibody-drug conjugates. *Regul. Toxicol. Pharmacol.* **2019**, *107*, 104429. [CrossRef] [PubMed]

177. Drake, P.M.; Carlson, A.; McFarland, J.M.; Banas, S.; Barfield, R.M.; Zmolek, W.; Kim, Y.C.; Huang, B.C.B.; Kudirka, R.; Rabuka, D. CAT-02-106, a site-specifically conjugated Anti-CD22 antibody bearing an MDR1-resistant maytansine payload yields excellent efficacy and safety in preclinical models. *Mol. Cancer Ther.* **2018**, *17*, 161–168. [CrossRef] [PubMed]

178. Buecheler, J.W.; Winzer, M.; Weber, C.; Gieseler, H. Oxidation-induced destabilization of model antibody-drug conjugates. *J. Pharm. Sci.* **2019**, *108*, 1236–1245. [CrossRef]

179. Cockrell, G.M.; Wolfe, M.S.; Wolfe, J.L.; Schoneich, C. Photoinduced aggregation of a model antibody-drug conjugate. *Mol. Pharm.* **2015**, *12*, 1784–1797. [CrossRef]

180. Liu, H.; Gaza-Bulseco, G.; Faldu, D.; Chumsae, C.; Sun, J. Heterogeneity of monoclonal antibodies. *J. Pharm. Sci.* **2008**, *97*, 2426–2447. [CrossRef]

181. Chen, T.; Su, D.; Gruenhagen, J.; Gu, C.; Li, Y.; Yehl, P.; Chetwyn, N.P.; Medley, C.D. Chemical de-conjugation for investigating the stability of small molecule drugs in antibody-drug conjugates. *J. Pharm. Biomed. Anal.* **2016**, *117*, 304–310. [CrossRef]

182. Wakankar, A.; Chen, Y.; Gokarn, Y.; Jacobson, F.S. Analytical methods for physicochemical characterization of antibody drug conjugates. *mAbs* **2011**, *3*, 161–172. [CrossRef]

183. Su, D.; Kozak, K.R.; Sadowsky, J.; Yu, S.-F.; Fourie-O'Donohue, A.; Nelson, C.; Vandlen, R.; Ohri, R.; Liu, L.; Ng, C.; et al. Modulating antibody–drug conjugate payload metabolism by conjugation site and linker modification. *Bioconjug. Chem.* **2018**, *29*, 1155–1167. [CrossRef]

5

Process Analytical Approach towards Quality Controlled Process Automation for the Downstream of Protein Mixtures by Inline Concentration Measurements Based on Ultraviolet/Visible Light (UV/VIS) Spectral Analysis

Steffen Zobel-Roos [1], Mourad Mouellef [1], Christian Siemers [2] and Jochen Strube [1,*]

[1]   Institute for Separation and Process Technology, Clausthal University of Technology, Leibnizstraße 15,
       38678 Clausthal-Zellerfeld, Germany; zobel-roos@itv.tu-clausthal.de (S.Z.-R.);
       mourad.mouellef@tu-clausthal.de (M.M.)

[2]   Institute for Process Control, Clausthal University of Technology, Arnold-Sommerfeld-Straße 1,
       38678 Clausthal-Zellerfeld, Germany; Christian.siemers@tu-clausthal.de

*   Correspondence: strube@itv.tu-clausthal.de

Abstract: Downstream of pharmaceutical proteins, such as monoclonal antibodies, is mainly done by chromatography, where concentration determination of coeluting components presents a major problem. Inline concentration measurements (ICM) by Ultraviolet/Visible light (UV/VIS)-spectral data analysis provide a label-free and noninvasive approach to significantly speed up the analysis and process time. Here, two different approaches are presented. For a test mixture of three proteins, a fast and easily calibrated method based on the non-negative least-squares algorithm is shown, which reduces the calibration effort compared to a partial least-squares approach. The accuracy of ICM for analytical separations of three proteins on an ion exchange column is over 99%, compared to less than 85% for classical peak area evaluation. The power of the partial least squares algorithm (PLS) is shown by measuring the concentrations of Immunoglobulin G (IgG) monomer and dimer under a worst-case scenario of completely overlapping peaks. Here, the faster SIMPLS algorithm is used in comparison to the nonlinear iterative partial least squares (NIPALS) algorithm. Both approaches provide concentrations as well as purities in real-time, enabling live-pooling decisions based on product quality. This is one important step towards advanced process automation of chromatographic processes. Analysis time is less than 100 ms and only one program is used for all the necessary communications and calculations.

Keywords: inline concentration measurements; UV/VIS spectral analysis; PAT for monoclonal antibodies; live pooling; peak deconvolution

---

1. Introduction

Inline concentration measurements (ICM) of individual components in a mixture are critical for almost every unit operation in the field of chemical and biotechnological processes. Although most processes are designed to match specific concentration and purity criteria, the actual values still have to be monitored inline or offline [1].

This becomes even more important for batch operations, like chromatography, where concentration and purity vary over time. For such processes, the inline measurement of concentrations and purities become a game winning objective, but often also a major challenge.

In the field of analytical chromatography, concentration or purity quantifications are usually based on peak areas. Therefore, great effort is put into the chromatographic separation to achieve a baseline separation, if possible. Nevertheless, this is not always achieved. Very closely related components are often especially difficult to separate. The deconvolution of overlapping peaks allows for better results as well as shorter and less expensive separations.

For preparative chromatography, complete baseline separation is not desirable; on the contrary, it conflicts with process efficiency and economy. The separation process is optimized for a maximum resin utilization and productivity. The product fractionation is often controlled via timed cut points, where the exact moment for the fraction start and end points are derived from earlier experiments and are therefore not directly related to the current chromatographic run. In this case, critical product attributes like the concentration and purity have to be measured offline after the run. Anomalies in elution behavior often result in shifts of the chromatogram leading to large variations from the expected design chromatogram. Thus, the time-based cut points do not match the purity criteria and might lead to a batch failure or require reprocessing. This problem becomes even worse for continuous chromatography processes. Start- and end-pooling criteria based on real-time, online detection of volume and Ultraviolet/Visible light (UV/VIS) absorbance have proven to be very successful in delivering consistent yield and purity. Online concentration and purity identification as presented here will help to shift the process design from timed to data-based fractionation or column switching and therefore give a greater certainty to match purity and yield targets, thus reducing the risk of batch failure. Also, the safety margins for data based fractionation can be smaller, leading to higher yield and productivity.

Furthermore, the knowledge of concentrations of all components online throughout the chromatographic run will help during process design. At the moment, the chromatographic run has to be fractionated into a lot of small volumes and analyzed offline to identify the actual concentration profiles. This is cost intensive as well as time consuming and, in addition, carries a significant risk of product degeneration of sensitive proteins because of long analysis times. The same problem and solution respectively apply for model parameter determination and model validation for a simulation-based design process [2,3].

Hence, a lot of research has been undertaken to achieve a deconvolution of chromatographic peaks. In general, the approaches can be split into inline and offline methods.

For offline or at-line peak deconvolution in particular two different approaches can be found. A classical at-line method is the division of the complete run into small fractions. These fractions are then investigated by a suitable analytical method afflicted with the method specific failure [4–8]. Although analysis time might be rather short, online sampling always results in a rather large response time. Especially the use of gas or liquid chromatographic analysis often has to deal with overlapping peaks itself due to selectivity variances [9].

Another offline or delayed online approach is a full mathematical analysis of the chromatogram. This analysis assumes that every peak will follow a mathematical function, e.g., Gaussian or modified Gaussian, and estimates the function parameters. This assumes a Gaussian or modified Gaussian shape might be approximately right for analytical chromatography, but is rather uncommon for preparative separations. The identification of peaks occurs by first, second or higher order derivatives of the chromatographic signal [10–12].

To identify a component and determine the parameters for its Gaussian function, the peak must be processed to a certain point. In most cases, at least the first inflection point has to be reached. More often, the peak maximum and second inflection point have to be detected already. Hence, this peak deconvolution method cannot be performed in real-time.

For preparative separations, an improvement can be achieved by the use of process modelling. Having a valid process model implemented during process design, the real behavior and elution of the components can be monitored [13–15].

Spectroscopy is among the most common methods of detection. Hence, major progress was achieved in terms of a multicomponent analysis using ultraviolet (UV), visible (VIS) or infrared spectral data. Mid-infrared spectroscopy (MIR) was used for host-cell protein quantification [16],

UV/VIS spectroscopy for determining the protein and nucleic acid content of viruses [17] as well as for a variety of proteins in a multicomponent mixture [18–20].

According to the Beer–Lambert law, the UV-extinction E_λ of a component at a given wavelength λ is the product of the concentration c, the path length d and a component specific coefficient called extinction coefficient ε_λ as shown in Equation (1) [21,22]:

$$lg\left(\frac{I_{0,\lambda}}{I_{t,\lambda}}\right) = E_{\lambda,i} = \varepsilon_{\lambda,i}\cdot c_i\cdot d. \tag{1}$$

Technically, this law applies to highly diluted mixtures only. Nevertheless, the deviations are often negligible.

The UV/VIS extinction over the wavelengths, viz. the UV/VIS spectrum, is unique for almost every component. Thus, the sum spectrum of a mixture can be disassembled into the single component spectra. It can be found that the absorbance of a mixture of n components sums up from the single component extinctions according to Equation (2) [23,24]:

$$E_\lambda = \sum_{i=1}^{n} \varepsilon_{\lambda,i}\cdot c_i\cdot d. \tag{2}$$

A diode array-based UV/VIS measurement provides as many extinction values as there are diodes in the detector, often 256 or 1024. Each diode represents one specific wavelength sector. Hence, Equation (2) can be formulated for each diode leading to a large set of linear expressions. With prior knowledge of the extinction coefficients of each component $\varepsilon_{\lambda,i}$, this set of linear equations can be solved for the concentrations c_i. This can be done with several mathematical methods like the least-squares or non-negative least-squares (NNLS) [25,26] algorithm. In theory, the experimental effort to measure the extinction coefficients $\varepsilon_{\lambda,i}$, is low. For each single component one injection with known concentration is sufficient. There is no need to calibrate a large set of mixtures with different compositions and concentrations. However, it might be necessary to measure the extinction coefficients $\varepsilon_{\lambda,i}$ for different concentrations of the single components. It can be shown that for higher concentrations, peaks appear in the UV/VIS spectrum that are not visible at lower concentrations. This is due to detector sensitivity only.

The first example in this paper shows the application of the NNLS-algorithm by measuring the concentrations of three proteins from an analytical ion exchange chromatography.

Another approach for UV/VIS-diode array detector (DAD) based concentration measurements was introduced by Brestrich et al. [18,27,28]. Partial least-squares regression is used to create a statistical model. The PLS regression compresses a set of even highly collinear predictor data X into a set of latent variables T. With these orthogonal latent variables observations can be fitted to depended variables Y. In this case, X is the UV/VIS spectra and Y represent the concentrations. For a better understanding of PLS, see [29–31].

In both the work of Brestrich et al. [27] and this work, the SIMPLS-algorithm [30] is used. This does not solve the set of linear equations spanned by Equation (2), but creates a statistic model. This model has to be trained by a set of experiments. Contrary to the non-negative least-squares approach, it is not sufficient to only calibrate for single components. The experimental design has to account for different compositions and different concentrations of each component present in the mixture that should be analyzed later. Thus, the amount of experiments increases dramatically with the number of components. Again, the detector sensitivity has a major impact, as does the detector type, age and utilization status.

The second example in this paper shows the application of the SIMPLS-algorithm for inline and real-time monomer and dimer concentration measurements of monoclonal antibody IgG.

Although the used algorithm is the same, this work differs from other work by a simpler setup. Instead of different programs for each task, only one self-written program is used to do the data acquisition, all calculations, data storage and communication with the programmable logic controller (PLC). Therefore, there is no software bottleneck allowing for very fast measurements. The PLC controls the pumps and valves of a continuous chromatography prototype that was not used in this work. This work is rather a major milestone to achieving a fully automated and self-optimizing system for the prototype, enabling life pooling, purity-based column switching and advanced quality control.

2. Materials and Methods

2.1. Model Proteins, Buffers and Columns

All experiments with proteins were carried out in 20 mM NaPi buffer at pH 6.0. For ion exchange chromatographic separations, this buffer was used as equilibration buffer A. For elution buffer B, 1 M NaCl was added. For analytical size exclusion chromatography (SEC), a buffer containing 100 mM sodium sulfate and 100 mM NaPi was used at pH 6.6. All salts were obtained from Merck KGaA, Darmstadt, Germany.

For the three component mixture experiments Chymotrypsinogen A, Lysozyme (AppliChem GmbH, Darmstadt, Germany) and Cytochrome C (Merck KGaA, Darmstadt, Germany) were used.

IgG was obtained from our own cell culture with an industrial Chinese Hamster Ovary (CHO) cell line and purified by protein A chromatography prior to the experiments.

Ion exchange separations were performed on prepacked strong cation exchange columns with Fractogel® EMD SO_3^- (M) (5–50, 1 mL, Atoll GmbH, Weingarten, Germany).

Analytical size exclusion columns Yarra® SEC-3000 (3 μm, 300 × 4.6 mm) were obtained from Phenomenex® Inc., Torrance, CA, USA.

Protein A chromatography was performed with PA ID Poros® Protein A Sensor Cartridges (Applied Biosystems, Waltham, MA, USA).

2.2. Devices and Instruments

The experimental setup consisted of a standard VWR-Hitachi LaChrom Elite® HPLC system with a quaternary gradient pump L-2130, Autosampler L-2200 and diode array detector L-2455 (VWR International, Radnor, PA, USA). The later was not used for the ICM but for comparative measurements. For the ICM measurements, a Smartline DAD 2600 with 10 mm, 10 μL flow cell from Knauer Wissenschaftliche Geräte GmbH, Berlin, Germany was used. Experimental validations were based on SEC analysis after online fractionation with a Foxy Jr.® from Teledyn Isco, Lincoln, NE, USA.

2.3. Inline Concentration Measurements

The inline concentration measurements are based on UV/VIS spectra measured with a diode array detector (Smartline DAD 2600 from Knauer Wissenschaftliche Geräte GmbH, Berlin, Germany) with 256 diodes and a wavelength range of 190 to 510 nm. The selectable bandwidth is 4 to 25 nm. The highest sampling rate is 10 Hz, which is 100 ms [32]. Data collection and analyses were performed by a conventional Windows desktop computer, which uses a standard EIA RS-232 serial port for the communication with the detector. Since the communication between different applications and programs tends to be a major bottleneck, a self-written program was used. An object-oriented, concurrent and class-based programming language [33] was used (Java). Java runs on its own Java Virtual Machine (JVM), which is available for a variety of platforms and computer architectures. Hence, programming in Java follows the "write once, run anywhere" idea. This makes a program written in Java easily applicable on different machines [33]. The ICM application handles the communication between the DAD and the computer, processes the data, displays the results in different charts and stores the data in "comma separated values" (*.csv) files. The user can choose from several algorithms to implement. Amongst those are the least squares, non-negative least squares [25,26] and SIMPLS (a partial least squares variant) [30], the simplex and powell algorithm and some more. It should be noted that these are not only different algorithm, but different approaches. The non-negative least squares algorithm is used to solve the equation system described earlier (Equation (2)). However, PLS provides a statistical model that is related to the spectral data. Which algorithm should be used depends on the complexity of the given sample. As a starting point, the single-component spectra of each component should be compared. In this work, an application for the non-negative least squares and one for the SIMPLS is shown.

2.4. ICM Examples

2.4.1. Protein Test Mixture on Ion Exchange Column under Analytical Conditions with NNLS

To show the power of ICM for analytical separations, a separation of three proteins on an ion exchange column was performed. Fractogel® EMD SO_3^- (M) was used in prepacked 1-mL columns (5–50, Atoll GmbH, Weingarten, Germany).

The binding buffer A was 20 mM NaPi buffer with a pH of 6.0. For elution, buffer B 1 M NaCl was added. The chromatographic run started with 100% buffer A and proceeded with a 10 CV gradient to 100% buffer B. A flow rate of 1 mL/min was used. This method is meant not to achieve baseline separation, but produce widely overlapping peaks.

The test mixture contained Chymotrypsinogen A, Cytochrome C and Lysozyme. 10 mg of each protein were dissolved separately in 1-mL binding buffer, leading to three samples with a concentration of 10 g/L each. To identify the differences in UV/VIS spectra, 20 µL of each sample was injected onto the column and measured with the DAD detector at a certain peak height corresponding to 0.01 g/L.

The single component spectra are shown in Figure 1. It can be seen that Chymotrypsinogene A and Lysozyme have similar spectra. Cytochrome C, however, is relatively unique. Nevertheless, the differences are big enough not to need PLS.

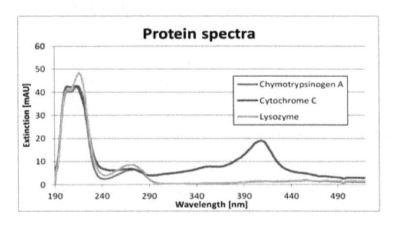

Figure 1. Single-component spectra of Chymotrypsinogene A, Cytochrome C and Lysozyme.

The inline concentration measurements were done by solving the set of linear equations (Equation (2)) for the concentrations with the non-negative least-squares algorithm. Hence, the extinction coefficients $\varepsilon_{\lambda,i}$ for the three proteins were needed.

The extinction coefficients $\varepsilon_{\lambda,i}$ were measured separately for each component. The proteins were dissolved in buffer A separately and injected onto the ion exchange column as described previously. The resulting chromatogram at 280 nm wavelength was converted from extinction to concentration course according to Equation (3):

$$c_i(t) = F \cdot E_{\lambda=280}(t).$$ (3)

The conversion factor F was obtained with Equation (4):

$$F = \frac{m_{i,inj}}{\dot{V} \cdot \int_0^t E_\lambda(t)dt}.$$ (4)

Now, the concentration is known for every time point of the chromatogram. Thus, the extinction coefficients $\varepsilon_{\lambda,i}$, are the only unknown variable left in Equation (2). In this work, Equation (2) was solved for the coefficients at a time point corresponding to 0.1 g/L protein concentration. This calibration has to be done for each protein.

One problem of this approach is the superposition of the protein spectrum with any other spectrum of co eluting components. This might result from UV/VIS active compounds in the chromatographic buffer or from leachables/extractables of the column itself. To overcome this problem, a blank run can be done before the actual measurements to perform a baseline correction.

For some components, one might find that different concentrations lead to different spectra. Physically speaking, this is not possible. However, for rising concentrations, peaks in the spectrum might appear that were not present at lower concentrations. These peaks were simply not visible at lower concentrations due to low detector sensitivity. In this case, it is best to analyze the peak at different concentrations, hence obtaining extinction coefficient values at different concentrations. This should be equal except for these cases where detector sensitivity comes into account. For those coefficients, a spline interpolation over the concentration is done.

The actual separation for testing the peak deconvolution was performed with the same column under the same conditions. The test mixture contained all three proteins.

Quantitative analysis is usually performed based on peak areas. The peak area is a function of the amount of protein injected. To produce the exact same peak areas in the three-component run compared to the single component runs, the same amount of each protein must be injected. Thus, the sample was produced by mixing 0.5 mL of each of the protein solutions used previously. Therefore, this sample has exactly one third of the concentration of each protein compared to the single component samples. Hence, 60 µL were injected to the column.

The peak areas of the single component runs are easily calculated. The corresponding areas from the mixture experiment were obtained by three different methods. First by integrating the concentration curve obtained with the inline concentration measurements. Second, by the perpendicular method. As a typical chromatographic approach, the extinction curve is integrated. The areas between two peaks were divided by a vertical line at the local minima. These areas have to be compared to a calibration curve. The third method is a typical offline peak deconvolution method. The real peak shape is approximated by assuming Gaussian or modified Gaussian behavior. These peaks can then again be integrated and compared to a calibration curve.

2.4.2. Immunoglobulin G (IgG) Monomer and Dime with SIMPLS

A mixture of IgG monomer and dimer was used to show the potential for pharmaceutical production. Both molecules have almost identical UV/VIS spectra. To distinguish between both is therefore relatively hard. Nevertheless, from a product quality point of view, it is very important to know the concentrations of IgG oligomers.

Since the differences in UV/VIS spectra are low, the SIMPLS algorithm was used. This must be calibrated with a training set of data containing different IgG monomer and dimer concentrations.

The monoclonal antibody IgG came from our own fed batch fermentation of an industrial cell culture line. The cell culture was clarified with centrifugation (3000 g) and filtration (0.2 µm syringe filter, VWR International, Radnor, PA, USA). Afterwards, purification was done with protein A chromatography (PA ID Sensor Cartridges, Applied Biosystems, Waltham, MA, USA). The protein A product peak was then loaded to a size exclusion column (Yarra® SEC-3000, 3 µm, 300 × 4.6 mm, Phenomenex Inc., Torrance, CA, USA). Here, only the upper 50% of the dimer and the monomer peak were fractionated. Hence, the overlapping region of monomer and dimer was not used. After protein A and size exclusion chromatography, no other protein besides IgG and no other contaminates are present. We did not find a fixed equilibrium between the monomer and dimer concentration. However, conversions from one form into the other occur, so that there was no pure dimer or monomer. The concentration in the SEC monomer fraction after some conversion time (overnight) was roughly

0.5 mg/mL monomer and 0.02 mg/mL dimer. The dimer fraction contained 0.2 mg/mL monomer and 0.1 mg/mL dimer.

Out of these two fractions, 11 mixtures were created to calibrate the statistic model. Therefore, different volumetric mix ratios were prepared, starting with 100 vol.% monomer and 0 vol.% dimer. The ratios decreased respectively increased with a 10 vol.% step size to 0 vol.% monomer and 100 vol.% dimer. From eleven mixtures, nine were used as a training set and the other three as validation sets, namely 80 vol.% monomer, 50 vol.% monomer and 20 vol.% monomer.

For each sample, analytical size exclusion chromatography was performed again to get the actual monomer and dimer concentrations.

The experiments itself were performed by injecting 0.1 mL into a small stirred tank of 2 mL total volume. The inlet stream consisted of chromatographic buffer A with a volumetric flow of 1 mL/min. The outlet stream, also 1 mL/min, was directly connected to the Smartline DAD 2600. After the DAD, the stream was fractionated with a Foxy Jr.® (Teledyn Isco, Lincoln, NE, USA) fraction collection module. 0.5 min fractions were taken and this 0.5 mL fractions were analyzed offline with the size exclusion chromatography already mentioned.

This setup represents a worst-case scenario, since no column or separation takes place. With moderately overlapping peaks, one might enhance your result by applying some mathematical assumptions; this cannot be done here. Furthermore, this experiment simulates conditions one would find in several other, non-chromatographic unit operations within the downstream of monoclonal antibodies, like filtration. This shows the applicability for inline quality control for example in the last filtration step.

3. Results and Discussion

The presented inline concentration measurement method shows wide, almost general applicability whenever UV/VIS active component mixtures are involved. In this work, the ability to enhance the accuracy of analytical measurements, and to make real time pooling decisions based on real time data could be shown. For the latter case, the calculation time is of major interest. Since only one program is used for data collection and processing, no time delay could be found throughout all experiments. The UV/VIS diode array detector was run with a sampling rate of 100 ms. The data transfer and all calculations were finished prior to the measurement of the next data point. Thus, one ICM concentration measurement lasts less than 100 ms.

It should be noted that every method or calibration comes with a systematic error itself. In this case, impurities present in the assumed to be pure calibration mixture could not be detected later on. This applies for example for low level impurities in the protein standard or in the IgG fractions after size exclusion chromatography.

3.1. Protein Test Mixture on Ion Exchange Column under Analytical Conditions with NNLS

One chromatogram and the corresponding inline concentration measurements are displayed in Figure 2. The reference extinction is 280 nm. It is important to understand that the protein concentrations (light blue, red, green) do not have to match the reference extinction plot (dark blue). The proportions would match only if all three proteins had the same extinction coefficient at 280 nm which is obviously not the case.

Prior to the injection of the three component mixture, the exact same amount of each component was injected separately as described earlier. The comparisons between the single component injections with the ICM peak of the same component in the three component run are shown in Figure 3. It can be seen that the Chymotrypsinogene-A peak in the mixture is pushed a little bit to an earlier elution. The mean residence time shifts from 6.07 min to 5.96 min. Although, the dilution front of this peak is sharper. This is in good agreement with the displacement theory of chromatography. The Cytochrome-C peak has mainly the same shape in both experiments, but tends to co-elute with both neighboring components slightly. The Lysozyme peak is in both cases more or less the same.

For both later proteins, there are only minor changes in the residence time. All values are displayed in Table 1.

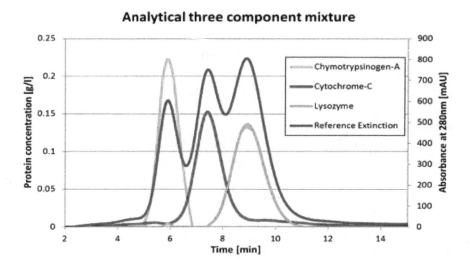

Figure 2. Inline concentration measurement of a three component protein mixture.

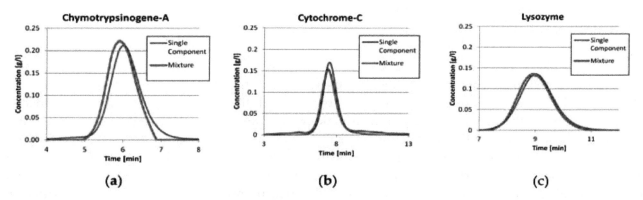

Figure 3. Comparison between the single component injection (blue line) and the deconvoluted peak (red line) of the same component in the mixture for the three proteins Chymotrypsinogene-A (**a**); Cytochrome-C (**b**) and Lysozyme (**c**).

Table 1. Deviation from single component to mixture measurement.

Protein	Mean Residence Time	
	Single Component (min)	Mixture (min)
Chymotrypsinogene-A	6.07	5.96
Cytochrome-C	7.62	7.63
Lysozyme	9.03	9.01

The chromatograms in Figure 3 allow for an easy comparison of the total amount of protein in both experiments. Since the ICM method measures concentrations not extinction, the deviations for this method are calculated comparing the total protein amount measured for single component injections to the three component system. This is calculated from feed concentration and injection volume. The mean deviation for the ICM method used for the chromatogram in Figure 2 is 0.02% with a standard deviation of 0.58% compared to $-16.99\% \pm 7.01\%$ for the perpendicular, $17.58\% \pm 15.82\%$ for the Gaussian and $21.27\% \pm 15.54\%$ for the modified Gaussian approach. The results for each component are listed in Table 2.

Table 2. Deviation from single component to mixture measurement.

Protein	ICM (%)	Perpendicular (%)	Gaussian (%)	Modified Gaussian (%)
Chymotrypsinogen-A	−0.63	−7.09	9.92	12.71
Cytochrom-C	0.50	−22.37	3.21	8.02
Lysozyme	0.19	−21.52	39.62	43.09
Mean Value	0.02	−16.99	17.58	21.27
Standard deviation	0.48	7.01	15.82	15.54

It should be noted that the ICM measurements might be sensitive to the gradient. Some gradients, more specific some modifier, are UV/VIS active itself. Even if the gradient does not become visible in the chromatogram at a specific wavelength, there might be an effect to the measurement. When the calibration is done with chromatographic runs of the single components as described, most of this problem is already solved since the gradient is already present in the calibration measurements. Otherwise, a blank run should be made before the measurements. The UV data measured during the actual run are than corrected by subtracting the blank run UV/VIS data.

Figure 4 shows the course of the different peak deconvolution methods. The peak in the middle is left out for clarity. It can be seen that the perpendicular area determination is always neglecting some area. On the other hand, both Gaussian functions (grey and light grey) overestimate the real behavior. It can be seen that the mathematical fits show the first and third peak to be overlapping, which is not the case in reality. The ICM method represents the real behavior best. Because it is not based on some model assumptions, the ICM method further has the potential to also identify tag along effects.

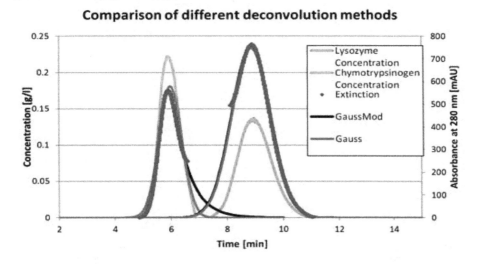

Figure 4. Comparison of the different peak deconvolution methods.

The mathematical methods can only be applied after the run or with huge delay, since the peak needs to be fully developed or at least needs to be developed past the maximum. The ICM measurements presented above were performed inline and with 100 ms between each data point. Since the self-written program is capable of communication with PLC, the data can be used to do live pooling or process optimization during a production run.

The results above were produced with extinction coefficients known beforehand. Similar results could be obtained without knowing the coefficients beforehand. An analysis of the complete run can calculate the extinction coefficients and deconvolute the overlapping peaks by assuming pure components at the beginning and end of the first or last peak respectively. The coefficients for the second component can be calculated by knowing the first and second component coefficients and the total spectra. This would deconvolute the peaks, but not give the exact concentration, since the link between concentration, extinction coefficients and the spectra is missing. In combination with known extinction coefficients for known components, this approach can be used to detect unknown components and give their concentration as a pseudo concentration linked to a known component.

3.2. Immunoglobulin G (IgG) Monomer and Dimer with SIMPLS

As mentioned before, eleven different ratios of IgG monomer and dimer were measured from which nine were used for the SIMPLS calibration and three for the validation. The corresponding UV/VIS spectra for the mixture with the highest and lowest monomer content are shown in Figure 5a. The spectra are standardized (z-score) to emphasize the differences. One statistic model was created to calculate both IgG monomer and dimer concentration at the same time as opposed to creating two models, one for each component. The Variable Importance on Projections (VIP) can be found in Figure 5b. Both Figure 5a,b show, that there are only minor differences in UV/VIS absorption for IgG monomer and dimer. The most important region is from 200 to 290 nm. This predication is supported by Figure 6a, which shows the loadings for each latent variable over wavelength. Again, the highest values are in the region from 200 to 290 nm. The region beyond 390 nm might be dominated by noise. Figure 6b shows the importance of each latent variable for the concentration results (Y-matrix). As expected, the first latent variables are the most important. But especially for the dimer concentration, variables 5 to 7 also show significant contribution.

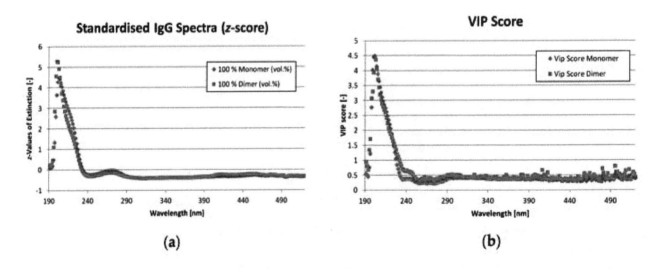

Figure 5. (a) Ultraviolet/Visible light (UV/VIS) spectra of the trainings data with the highest and lowest Immunoglobulin G (IgG) monomer content. The red dots represent the mixture with 100 vol.% monomer, the green dots with 100 vol.% dimer, respectively. However, this does not mean pure monomer or dimer since a conversion from one into the other takes place; (b) Variable Importance on Projections (VIP) scores for monomer (red) and dimer (green).

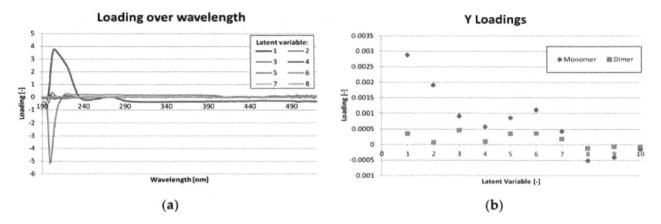

Figure 6. (a) Loading over wavelength diagram for the first eight latent variables. The higher the absolute value, the more important is this wavelength for the latent variable; (b) loadings of the Y results over latent variables. The higher the absolute value, the higher is the importance of this latent variable for the concentration calculation of monomer or dimer respectively.

As expected, the percentage of explained variance in the response increases with the number of latent variables used in the algorithm. For three latent variables, the percentage of explanation is 80%, for six variables it is over 93%. It maxes out at 98% with eight or more latent variables. Thus, eight latent variables where used for the validation measurements. The root mean square error of calibration (RSMEC) for eight latent variables is 0.14 mg/L for the IgG monomer and 0.025 mg/L for IgG dimer.

Figures 7a and 4b show the results for two of the validation measurements. These experiments represent the injection of the sample with 80 vol.% monomer/20 vol.% dimer (Figure 4a) and 20 vol.% monomer/80 vol.% dimer (Figure 4b), respectively. Again, these numbers represent the volumetric mixing ratio of the SEC fractions as described earlier. Due to conversion of either monomer to dimer or vice versa the mixing ratio does not match the concentration ratio.

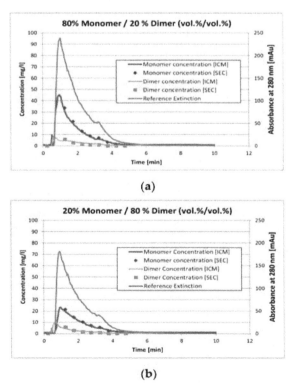

Figure 7. Concentration measurements over time of IgG monomer and dimer after injecting into a continuous stirred-tank reactor: (a) Volumetric mixing ratio of 80% monomer and 20% dimer; (b) Volumetric mixing ratio of 20% monomer and 80% dimer.

The solid lines represent the ICM measurements whereas the squares with the same color represent the corresponding SEC analysis. The later are done by fractionation the stirred tank outlet with an interval of 0.5 min. The ICM measurements however are continuous. To compare the results, the ICM values for the 0.5 min interval were not averaged. Instead, the ICM concentration value for the corresponding time at the middle of the fractionation interval was used.

The comparison for all validation experiments is shown in Figure 8:

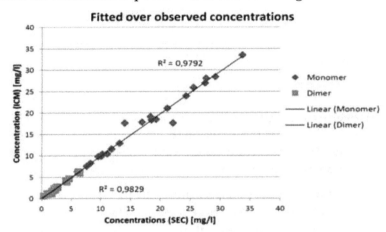

Figure 8. Concentrations based on fractionation and size exclusion chromatography (SEC) analyses compared to concentrations measured with inline concentration measurements (ICM).

The results in Figures 7 and 8 show that the ICM measurements are in good agreement with the SEC measurements. The overall coefficient of determination R^2 is 0.98 for both IgG monomer and dimer. The root mean square error of prediction (RMSEP) is 0.13 mg/L for the IgG monomer and 0.019 mg/L for IgG dimer.

The ICM measurements provide the concentrations and therefore composition of the outlet stream. This can be used to calculate the purity of the product stream in almost real time (100 ms). Purity calculation based on ICM measurements compared to the corresponding offline SEC gives a mean derivation of 0.15%. Within the 24 data points, the minimum deviation was 0.01% and the maximum deviation was 6%.

Since the SIMPLS-algorithm reduces the UV/VIS spectra to a statistic model, it is possible that it only finds a certain fixed distribution between the two components. This would presumably give the same multiplier between both concentrations. Figure 4a,b however show that this is not the case. The extinction values for the 20 vol.% monomer run are roughly 25% lower than for the 80 vol.% monomer run. The IgG monomer concentration however is more than 50% lower and the dimer concentration is 15% higher. Hence, it is reasonable to assume that the algorithm determines the concentrations correctly instead of just splitting the extinction with a fixed proportion.

Since the test mixture was prepared with IgG samples after Protein A and SEC, the purity of the IgG was relatively high. For in-process measurements, for example after protein A, more components and impurities have to be taken into account. Depending on the impurities, the distinction between the IgG monomer and dimer might become more challenging. However, it is hypothesized that at least the distinction between IgG in total and other impurities should be possible.

4. Conclusions

The proposed inline concentration measurement based on UV/VIS spectral data is a new and comparatively easy method for the real time quantification of UV/VIS active components. This indicates a huge potential for analytical as well as preparative and production-scale chromatography as well as for other unit operations. It is a key-enabling methodology for process development by aid of process modelling in order to determine model parameters efficiently—which is currently the major obstacle preventing a general use of simulation instead of empirics in industry for piloting and operation of almost any unit operation in regulated industry under Process Analytical Technology (PAT) and QbD design methods.

The inherent problem of overlapping peaks in analytical chromatography is reduced significantly by applying ICM. The accuracy of the quantitative determination of proteins could be shown to be improved to more than 99% compared to under 85% for conventional, state-of-the-art techniques.

The analysis time is less than 100 ms, so that the rate-limiting step is the data acquisition done by the detector itself. This enables a variety of process control options like live pooling and online optimization of the chromatographic process.

In the case of preparative separations, even for very similar components the purity can be measured at approximately 99.8% accuracy. This is an enormous advantage, since the real-time concentrations and purities are completely unknown for current process analytics. This leads to new possibilities for process control strategies. For example, batch chromatography could perform real-time pooling decisions based on the ICM data, leading to less batch failure and a higher product quality. Since product-related purity data are measured inline, there is a huge potential for cost and time savings by reducing offline analytics. The derived method overcomes obstacles in industrial application resulting from the dependency of extinction coefficients on detector type, age and signal strength by adopting reliable self-adjusting methods based on optimization algorithms, which provide mathematically proven quantitative reliability.

New process control options of multicolumn chromatography processes like Simulated Moving Bed (SMB) and their derivatives, e.g., integrated counter current chromatography (see [34]) based on the ICM-approach will be presented in the near future.

Acknowledgments: The authors thank the ITVP lab team especially Frank Steinhäuser and Volker Strohmeyer for their effort and support. Special thanks are also addressed to Fabian Mestmäcker, Dominik Stein and Thorsten Roth for excellent laboratory work.

Author Contributions: Steffen Zobel-Roos conceived and designed the experiments as well as wrote the paper. Mourad Mouellef wrote the program code and evaluated the experimental results. Christian Siemers substantively revised the work and contributed know-how in process automation. Jochen Strube is responsible for conception and supervision.

References

1. Degerman, M.; Westerberg, K.; Nilsson, B. Determining Critical Process Parameters and Process Robustness in Preparative Chromatography—A Model-Based Approach. *Chem. Eng. Technol.* **2009**, *32*, 903–911. [CrossRef]

2. Borrmann, C.; Helling, C.; Lohrmann, M.; Sommerfeld, S.; Strube, J. Phenomena and Modeling of Hydrophobic Interaction Chromatography. *Sep. Sci. Technol.* **2011**, *46*, 1289–1305. [CrossRef]

3. Helling, C.; Strube, J. Modeling and Experimental Model Parameter Determination with Quality by Design for Bioprocesses. In *Biopharmaceutical Production Technology*; Subramanian, G., Ed.; Wiley-VCH: Weinheim, Germany, 2012; pp. 409–443.

4. Fahrner, R.L.; Blank, G.S. Real-time control of antibody loading during protein an affinity chromatography using an on-line assay. *J. Chromatogr. A* **1999**, *849*, 191–196. [CrossRef]

5. Kaltenbrunner, O.; Lu, Y.; Sharma, A.; Lawson, K.; Tressel, T. Risk-benefit evaluation of on-line high-performance liquid chromatography analysis for pooling decisions in large-scale chromatography. *J. Chromatogr. A* **2012**, *1241*, 37–45. [CrossRef] [PubMed]

6. Proll, G.; Kumpf, M.; Mehlmann, M.; Tschmelak, J.; Griffith, H.; Abuknesha, R.; Gauglitz, G. Monitoring an antibody affinity chromatography with a label-free optical biosensor technique. *J. Immunol. Methods* **2004**, *292*, 35–42. [CrossRef] [PubMed]

7. Rathore, A.S.; Wood, R.; Sharma, A.; Dermawan, S. Case study and application of process analytical technology (PAT) towards bioprocessing: II. Use of ultra-performance liquid chromatography (UPLC) for making real-time pooling decisions for process chromatography. *Biotechnol. Bioeng.* **2008**, *101*, 1366–1374. [CrossRef] [PubMed]

8.   Rathore, A.S.; Parr, L.; Dermawan, S.; Lawson, K.; Lu, Y. Large scale demonstration of a process analytical technology application in bioprocessing: Use of on-line high performance liquid chromatography for making real time pooling decisions for process chromatography. *Biotechnol. Prog.* **2010**, *26*, 448–457. [CrossRef] [PubMed]

9.   Gey, M. *Instrumentelle Analytik und Bioanalytik. Biosubstanzen, Trennmethoden, Strukturanalytik, Applikationen*; Springer: Berlin/Heidelberg, Germany, 2008.

10. Kong, H.; Ye, F.; Lu, X.; Guo, L.; Tian, J.; Xu, G. Deconvolution of overlapped peaks based on the exponentially modified Gaussian model in comprehensive two-dimensional gas chromatography. *J. Chromatogr. A* **2005**, *1086*, 160–164. [CrossRef] [PubMed]

11. Vivó-Truyols, G.; Torres-Lapasió, J.R.; van Nederkassel, A.M.; Vander Heyden, Y.; Massart, D.L. Automatic program for peak detection and deconvolution of multi-overlapped chromatographic signals part I: Peak detection. *J. Chromatogr. A* **2005**, *1096*, 133–145. [CrossRef] [PubMed]

12. Vivó-Truyols, G.; Torres-Lapasió, J.R.; van Nederkassel, A.M.; Vander Heyden, Y.; Massart, D.L. Automatic program for peak detection and deconvolution of multi-overlapped chromatographic signals part II: Peak model and deconvolution algorithms. *J. Chromatogr. A* **2005**, *1096*, 146–155. [CrossRef] [PubMed]

13. Helling, C.; Dams, T.; Gerwat, B.; Belousov, A.; Strube, J. Physical characterization of column chromatography: Stringent control over equipment performance in biopharmaceutical production. *Trends Chromatogr.* **2013**, *8*, 55–71.

14. Osberghaus, A.; Drechsel, K.; Hansen, S.; Hepbildikler, S.K.; Nath, S.; Haindl, M.; von Lieres, E.; Hubbuch, J. Model-integrated process development demonstrated on the optimization of a robotic cation exchange step. *Chem. Eng. Sci.* **2012**, *76*, 129–139. [CrossRef]

15. Osberghaus, A.; Hepbildikler, S.; Nath, S.; Haindl, M.; von Lieres, E.; Hubbuch, J. Optimizing a chromatographic three component separation: A comparison of mechanistic and empiric modeling approaches. *J. Chromatogr. A* **2012**, *1237*, 86–95. [CrossRef] [PubMed]

16. Capito, F.; Skudas, R.; Kolmar, H.; Stanislawski, B. Host cell protein quantification by Fourier transform mid infrared spectroscopy (FT-MIR). *Biotechnol. Bioeng.* **2013**, *110*, 252–259. [CrossRef] [PubMed]

17. Porterfield, J.Z.; Zlotnick, A. A simple and general method for determining the protein and nucleic acid content of viruses by UV absorbance. *Virology* **2010**, *407*, 281–288. [CrossRef] [PubMed]

18. Dismer, F.; Hansen, S.; Oelmeier, S.A.; Hubbuch, J. Accurate retention time determination of co-eluting proteins in analytical chromatography by means of spectral data. *Biotechnol. Bioeng.* **2013**, *110*, 683–693. [CrossRef] [PubMed]

19. Hansen, S.K.; Skibsted, E.; Staby, A.; Hubbuch, J. A label-free methodology for selective protein quantification by means of absorption measurements. *Biotechnol. Bioeng.* **2011**, *108*, 2661–2669. [CrossRef] [PubMed]

20. Hansen, S.K.; Jamali, B.; Hubbuch, J. Selective high throughput protein quantification based on UV absorption spectra. *Biotechnol. Bioeng.* **2013**, *110*, 448–460. [CrossRef] [PubMed]

21. Otto, M. *Analytische Chemie*; WILEY-VCH: Weinheim, Germany, 2011.

22. Wedler, G. *Lehrbuch der Physikalischen Chemie*; VCH Verlagsgesellschaft: Weinheim, Germany, 1985.

23. Atkins, P.W.; de Paula, J. *Physikalische Chemie*; Wiley-VCH: Weinheim, Germany, 2012.

24. Sawyer, D.T.; Heinemann, W.R.; Beebe, J.M. *Chemistry Experiments for Instrumental Methods*; Wiley: New York, NY, USA, 1984.

25. Bro, R.; de Jong, S. A fast non-negativity-constrained least squares algorithm. *J. Chemom.* **1997**, *11*, 393–401. [CrossRef]

26. Lawson, C.L.; Hanson, R.J. *Solving Least Squares Problems*; Society for Industrial and Applied Mathematics: Philadelphia, PA, USA, 1995.

27. Brestrich, N.; Briskot, T.; Osberghaus, A.; Hubbuch, J. A tool for selective inline quantification of co-eluting proteins in chromatography using spectral analysis and partial least squares regression. *Biotechnol. Bioeng.* **2014**, *111*, 1365–1373. [CrossRef] [PubMed]

28. Brestrich, N.; Sanden, A.; Kraft, A.; McCann, K.; Bertolini, J.; Hubbuch, J. Advances in inline quantification of co-eluting proteins in chromatography: Process-data-based model calibration and application towards real-life separation issues. *Biotechnol. Bioeng.* **2015**, *112*, 1406–1416. [CrossRef] [PubMed]

29. Andersson, M. A comparison of nine PLS1 algorithms. *J. Chemom.* **2009**, *23*, 518–529. [CrossRef]

30. De Jong, S. SIMPLS: An alternative approach to partial least squares regression. *Chemom. Intell. Lab. Syst.* **1993**, *18*, 251–263. [CrossRef]

31. Wold, S.; Sjöström, M.; Eriksson, L. PLS-regression: A basic tool of chemometrics. *Chemom. Intell. Lab. Syst.* **2001**, *58*, 109–130. [CrossRef]

32. KNAUER. *Smartline UV Detector 2600 Manual/Handbuch*; KNAUER: Berlin, Germany, 2007.

33. Gosling, J. *The Java Language Specification, Java SE 7 Edition*, 4th ed.; Addison-Wesley: Upper Saddle River, NJ, USA, 2013.

34. Zobel, S.; Helling, C.; Ditz, R.; Strube, J. Design and Operation of Continuous Countercurrent Chromatography in Biotechnological Production. *Ind. Eng. Chem. Res.* **2014**, *53*, 9169–9185. [CrossRef]

6

Modular Chimeric Antigen Receptor Systems for Universal CAR T Cell Retargeting

Ashley R. Sutherland [1], Madeline N. Owens [1] and C. Ronald Geyer [2,*]

[1]   Department of Biochemistry, Microbiology and Immunology, University of Saskatchewan,
      Saskatoon, SK S7N 5E5, Canada; ashley.sutherland@usask.ca (A.R.S.); mno167@usask.ca (M.N.O.)
[2]   Department of Pathology and Laboratory Medicine, University of Saskatchewan, Saskatoon, SK S7N 5E5, Canada
*   Correspondence: ron.geyer@usask.ca

Abstract: The engineering of T cells through expression of chimeric antigen receptors (CARs) against tumor-associated antigens (TAAs) has shown significant potential for use as an anti-cancer therapeutic. The development of strategies for flexible and modular CAR T systems is accelerating, allowing for multiple antigen targeting, precise programming, and adaptable solutions in the field of cellular immunotherapy. Moving beyond the fixed antigen specificity of traditional CAR T systems, the modular CAR T technology splits the T cell signaling domains and the targeting elements through use of a switch molecule. The activity of CAR T cells depends on the presence of the switch, offering dose-titratable response and precise control over CAR T cells. In this review, we summarize developments in universal or modular CAR T strategies that expand on current CAR T systems and open the door for more customizable T cell activity.

Keywords: chimeric antigen receptor (CAR T); universal CAR T; modular CAR T; universal immune receptor; CAR adaptor; adoptive immunotherapy; antibody; split CAR

1. Introduction

Engineering T cells to express chimeric antigen receptors (CARs) has shown wide-ranging potential as a potent anti-cancer therapeutic. Characteristically, CARs consist of an extracellular antigen-binding single-chain antibody variable fragment (scFv) and hinge region linked to transmembrane and intracellular signaling regions. This engineered construct fuses the specificity of an antibody to T cell-effector functions, allowing for target cell lysis, release of cytokines, and T cell proliferation [1,2]. In clinical trials, CAR T cell therapy has shown remarkable success in treating hematological malignancies by targeting B cell antigen CD19. Numerous studies showed high remission rates, rapid tumor eradication, and durable responses in patients with refractory disease, raising expectations for expanding the types of cancers that can be treated with CAR therapy [3–5]. Although these results are encouraging, several challenges exist that inhibit the broad application of this treatment. Firstly, tumor heterogeneity is a complication that hinders CAR T development. Conventional CAR T cells have a fixed, single-antigen targeting ability, making the therapy vulnerable to antigen-loss relapse due to downregulation or antigen deletion [6,7]. CAR T therapy targeting a single antigen may initially demonstrate tumor regression; however, many cases have been reported in clinical trials of antigen-negative relapse after CD19 CAR T therapy due to tumor antigen escape [8,9]. Engineering of CAR T cells against a variety of tumor-associated antigens (TAAs) is a method to overcome tumor immunoediting, yet this approach comes with its own set of challenges. Further clinical success of CARs would necessitate the engineering of T cells tailored for each patient targeting various TAAs. However, significant technical requirements and financial costs involved in the generation and optimization of CARs directed at individual antigens limit this approach's usefulness. To circumvent the technical and economic challenges of individually manufacturing and testing each new CAR, creating a platform using 'universal' redirected T cells against virtually any cell surface antigen is of particular importance for the rapid screening in pre-clinical models and the broad application of CAR T therapy.

The ability to generate modular or universal CARs hinges on the separation of targeting and signaling elements. Modular CAR T cells are not targeted at the tumor antigen itself; instead, the CAR is directed at an adaptor or switch element (Figure 1). This adaptor serves as the targeting element, binding to the tumor antigen, and is required to bridge the immunological synapse. The firing of the CAR T should occur only in the presence of the switch, and swapping out the adaptor molecule allows for redirection of the T cell without the need for re-engineering and time-consuming remanufacturing. This modular treatment approach offers the possibility for flexibility in tumor targeting in the clinic; adapting with the patient's tumor by adjusting treatment based on the cancer's changing antigen expression could be envisioned. Fixed antigen targeting often hinders cancer treatment, with this modular CAR T approach driving an already innovative biological therapy into truly tailored cancer therapy.

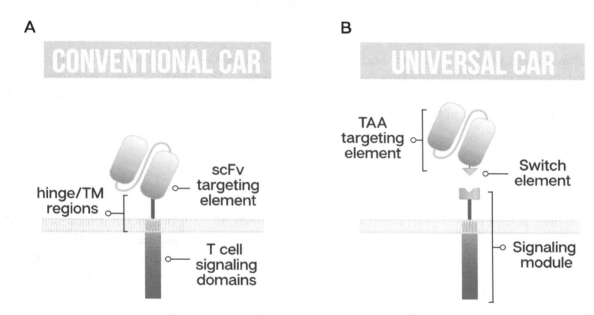

Figure 1. Schematic representation of a conventional CAR T cell and a universal or modular CAR T cell (**A**) Conventional CAR T cells have a single-chain antibody fragment (scFv) targeting element, expressed in tandem with signaling domains derived from the T cell receptor and costimulatory domains such as 4-1BB and CD28 connected through a transmembrane (TM) domain and a flexible spacer or hinge region; (**B**) a universal CAR T cell has a split design containing a tumor-associated antigen (TAA) targeting element, usually derived from a monoclonal antibody, a switch element and the signaling module, consisting of the T cell signaling domains and an extracellular region which interacts with the switch element.

In the toolkit of building modular CARs, the number of adaptors has been increasing, with components such as immunoglobulin (IgG)-based adaptors such as scFvs (single-chain variable fragment), Fabs (antigen-binding fragment), nanobodies, and full-length IgGs being the most established. Both antibody-based and targeting ligand adaptors have been redirected using tags attached either genetically or post-translationally and include peptide tags such as neo-epitopes, SpyTag, leucine zippers, biotin and fluorescein isothiocyanate (FITC). Repurposing clinically approved IgGs and adding redirecting tags could reduce the regulatory hurdles and allow for a suite of targeting elements that clinicians could employ for a wide variety of cancer indications.

Improving the safety profile of CAR T therapy is a rapidly developing area of research with the goal of expanding the therapy to treat a broader range of cancer patients. With the promise of CAR T therapy comes life-threatening side effects, including severe cytokine release syndrome

(CRS), neurological toxicities and organ failure, resulting from the unrestrained proliferation of CAR T cells [10,11]. Toxicities related to on-target off-tumor reactions can occur when low levels of the targeted cancer antigen found on normal tissue are targeted by the engineered T cells. When toxicities become severe enough, administration of high-dose corticosteroids is required, decreasing the T cell numbers [10–12]. Research in the area of 'next-generation' CAR T cells has incorporated methods such as suicide genes or switches as a means to eliminate T cells. These 'emergency stop' methods may avert a lethal outcome to the patient; however, the drawback is that the CAR T cells are eliminated, and with it any therapeutic response—a bad ending for a costly and time-consuming therapy. Universal or modular CAR T strategies that require administration of an adaptor may fit the criteria for better control of engineered T cells. The ability to titrate on adaptors could facilitate the 'turning off' of CAR T cells by halting administration of the adaptor, possibly enhancing their safety profile without the need to destroy the T cells. Additionally, this tunable response could better manage side effects as well as fine tuning of CAR T activity. These approaches for CAR T generation allow for conjugation of the tagged targeting element with the anti-tag CAR T. This enables targeting multiple TAAs and flexibility in administration of the targeting element, a step towards overcoming current clinical limitations of CAR T therapy.

In this review, we summarize emerging systems developed to overcome the limitations of CARs with fixed antigen specificity using universal CAR T strategies. This modular approach using adaptors to 'turn on' CARs enables targeting multiple TAAs with one receptor, imparting near-limitless antigen specificity and fine tuning of CAR activity.

2. Modular CAR T Platforms

2.1. Biotin-Binding Immune Receptors

Exploiting one of nature's strongest non-covalent bonds, the avidin–biotin interaction has been used to generate a universal tumor-targeting system, biotin-binding immunoreceptor (BBIR) (Figure 2A). BBIRs constructed by Urbanska et al. [13] consist of an extracellular modified dimeric avidin (dcAv) linked to an intracellular T cell signaling domain. This split design allows for easy target modification and targeting of multiple antigens. Monomeric avidin was unable to elicit an effector response, most likely due to the decreased affinity between biotin and monomeric avidin.

Tumor cells in vitro are either pre-targeted or co-administered with biotinylated antigen-targeting molecules (IgG antibodies, scFvs, or other tumor-specific ligands), and T cells expressing BBIRs bound specifically to exert effector cell functions. In vitro functioning of dcAv BBIR is comparable to traditional CAR T for cell lysis and cytokine secretion, illustrating this system's utility to target cells and perform effector functions. Significantly, BBIR cells generated a dose-dependent response with the addition of adaptors. When tested against a panel of cells with variable TAAs, BBIRs could target antigens both simultaneously or sequentially, showing the tunability of CAR response and their utility in antigen escape scenarios. Furthermore, the authors proposed a platform using BBIRs to screen candidate antibodies or other targeting elements in vitro for rapid pre-clinical screening. BBIRs performed similarly in vivo in a xenograft mouse model of human ovarian cancer. As CAR safety is essential for moving into the clinic, BBIRs were exposed to supraphysiological levels of biotin and showed no antigen-independent activation. Interestingly, T cells could not be 'pre-armed' with the biotinylated targeting element; the adaptor had to be either pre-targeted to coat the tumor surface or co-administered with BBIR T cells.

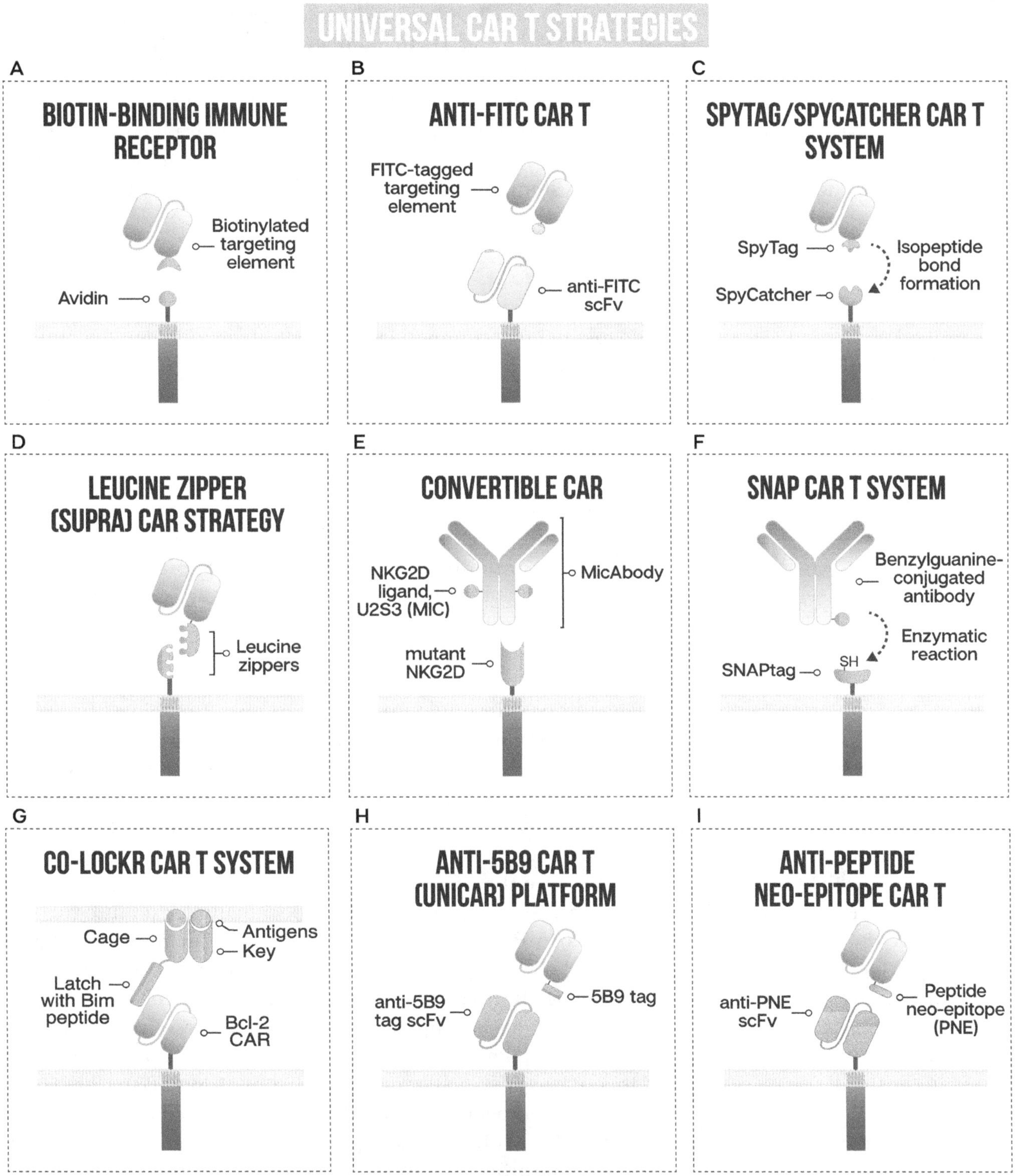

Figure 2. A schematic of strategies used in universal CAR T design: (**A**) biotin-binding immune receptor; (**B**) anti-FITC CAR T; (**C**) the SpyTag/SpyCatcher CAR T system; (**D**) leucine zipper or SUPRA CAR T; (**E**) convertibleCAR or modified NKG2D CAR T; (**F**) SNAP CAR T enzymatic CAR labeling system; (**G**) the co-localization-dependent protein switch (Co-LOCKR) CAR T system; (**H**) UniCAR or anti-5B9 peptide CAR platform; (**I**) anti-peptide neo-epitope (PNE) CAR T.

Lohmueller et al. [14] drew on this system and further affinity enhanced streptavidin, designing a biotin-binding domain where monomeric streptavidin could be used in the CAR system with higher affinity to biotin than the dimeric form. This affinity-enhanced form, mSA2, has a more compact structure than the dimeric form employed previously, possibly increasing the type of antigens able to be targeted by this system. The mSA2 CARs were able to distinguish antigen-positive cells precoated with biotinylated antibody in vitro and produce a specific effector response. Antigen-negative tumor cells did not elicit an effector response, neither did non-binding biotinylated antibody, showing that in order for CAR T cells to be turned on, the antibody must be bound to the target cells. The mSA2 CAR T cells showed potent effector functions; however, its potential immunogenicity could hamper its adoption in the clinic. With the BBIR system, excess biotin does not impart an inhibitory effect, and therefore could not be used as a potential 'off switch' for added safety.

2.2. Anti-FITC CAR Strategy

Fluorescein isothiocyanate (FITC), derived from fluorescein, is a fluorescent label commonly used to tag antibodies. Tamada et al. [15] first exploited this common labeling method and generated anti-FITC CAR T cells able to be directed by FITC-tagged antibodies (Figure 2B). The extracellular portion of the CAR is comprised of an anti-FITC scFv that recognizes FITC-labeled cetuximab (anti-EGFR), trastuzumab (anti-HER2), and rituximab (anti-CD20), antibodies that are already employed clinically. Redirected CAR T cells were found to be effective both in vitro and in vivo to specifically bind their respective tumor cells and exert anti-tumor effects. This system showed effectiveness at targeting multiple TAAs to better address heterogenous cancer populations. Additionally, the use of anti-FITC CAR T cells was shown to restore the usefulness of monoclonal antibodies to additional cancer types. They discuss that in patients with Kras mutations, cetuximab does not provide therapeutic benefits; however, when cetuximab is utilized with anti-FITC CAR T cells, anti-tumor effects are shown, as illustrated with the SW480 cell line that containing a Kras mutation. The anti-FITC CAR T system was applied using trastuzumab—Cao et al. conjugated FITC to trastuzumab in a site-specific manner compared to another strategy where a peptide neo-epitope (PNE) was fused to trastuzumab [16]. Both antibody tagging methods showed a dose-titratable immune response, capable of completely clearing HER2-positive tumors in vivo. The first clinical use of trastuzumab incorporated into a CAR T resulted in a serious adverse event, with the patient developing on-target, off-tumor toxicity related to the redirection of CAR T cells to lung epithelium, proving fatal [17]. Since this initial trial, many groups have investigated safer ways to target HER2, reviewed by Liu et al. [18], with the modular anti-FITC CAR T technology, a contender to address the safety issues with targeting this cancer-associated antigen.

Expanding the targeting elements to more than full-length antibodies, Zhang et al. employed switchable CAR-engineered T cells using anti-tumor peptides that specifically target integrin avβ3 through an 18-amino acid sequence fused to FITC [19]. This peptide adaptor molecule, termed FITC-HM-3, specifically targeted tumor cells and regulated CAR T cell activity. Demonstrating that low-molecular-weight switch molecules can be effective at redirecting engineered T cells, Lee et al. [20] employed a cocktail of small bifunctional molecules in conjunction with anti-fluorescein CAR T cells to target cancer cells in vitro and in vivo. The bifunctional molecules, called CAR T cell adapter molecules (CAMs), consist of fluorescein linked to a tumor-specific ligand through a hydrophilic spacer. The use of a mixture of CAMs enables the targeting of heterogenous solid tumors and broadens the applicability of CAR T cell therapy by using small molecules, which could improve tumor penetration, as opposed to larger full-length antibodies. Additionally, improved safety is offered by the short half-life (~90 min) of small molecules, allowing them to rapidly clear from receptor-negative tissue.

Optimizing the complex between the CAR T cell, switch, and tumor antigen is essential for optimal CAR T activation and cell killing. Using the modular CAR system, Ma et al. [21] utilized anti-FITC CARs to target both CD19 and CD22, whereby antibody fragments were site-specifically modified with FITC through genetically encoded non-canonical amino acids. This allowed for the incorporation of FITC to optimize of the geometry of the immunological synapse. Compared head to head, the optimized anti-FITC CAR T targeting CD19 performed similarly to conventional CD19-targeting CAR T, necessary for moving this technology forward into the clinic. Furthermore, excess FITC at 10 μM was shown to dampen CAR T activity in vitro, a feature that could be used to improve safety in the clinic. Others have shown that the addition of FITC-labeled non-specific antibodies could also be used to attenuate CAR T cells [15].

The targeting of folate receptors using anti-FITC CARs has been demonstrated by several groups [22–24]. Lu et al. [23], using FITC conjugated to folic acid as the switch molecule, modeled severe cytokine release syndrome and determined that CRS could be alleviated through the titration of the folate FITC adaptor or by intermittent dosing. Reversal of severe CRS could be achieved by intravenous sodium fluorescein to transiently interrupt CARs, without destroying the engineered T cells. With the ability to shut down the CAR T response through the addition of FITC [21], FITC labeled non-specific antibodies [15] or sodium fluorescein [23,24], this system with its added 'safety switches' could allow for engineered immune cell deactivation if toxicity develops, possibly being able to salvage the therapy by re-administering the switch molecules. While encouraging, the possible immunogenicity of FITC adaptors in the context of CAR T systems requires further study.

2.3. The SpyTag-SpyCatcher Universal CAR T System

The SpyTag/SpyCatcher protein ligation system employs a unique peptide: protein ligation reaction to link the tagged targeting element to the immune receptor. In 2012, Zackeri et al. reported a fibronectin-binding protein from *Streptococcus pyogenes* that, upon splitting it into two parts, followed by rational engineering, an N-terminal protein fragment (SpyCatcher) and a C-terminal 13-amino acid peptide (SpyTag) were produced [25]. The two parts will spontaneously reconstitute to form an isopeptide bond without the need for co-factors, enzymes, or specific conditions. Minutolo et al. exploited this system to generate a SpyCatcher immune receptor [26] (Figure 2C). This immune receptor contains the SpyCatcher protein as the extracellular domain, linked to intracellular signaling regions. TAA-specific targeting ligands, such as IgG antibodies, are site-specifically labeled with SpyTag. This post-translational covalent assembly allows for the redirection of T cells to multiple TAAs to exert targeted effector cell functions. The SpyCatcher immune receptor activity depends on the presence of both target antigen and SpyTag-labeled targeting element, allowing for titratable control of the engineered T cells. Arming the SpyCatcher CAR T cells with SpyTagged antibodies showed receptor levels decreasing over time, with complete loss observed after 96 h. SpyCatcher CAR T cells were shown to become functional upon the addition of SpyTag targeting element and lyse antigen-expressing target cells in vitro. Using an immunodeficient mouse xenograft model, the authors showed that HER2-positive xenografts could be targeted with SpyCatcher CAR T cells pre-armed with SpyTagged Herceptin. Additional targeting ligand was administered every three days, and administration throughout treatment was shown to be necessary for tumor clearance. The SpyTag/SpyCatcher system was tested using targeting elements against HER2, EGFR, EpCAM and CD20 and Liu et al. expanded the range of targetable antigens by demonstrating SpyCatcher immune receptors could be constructed to target the hepatocellular carcinoma antigen, human glypican-3 (hGPC3) using a SpyTagged anti-hGPC3 scFv [27].

Potential immunogenicity is an issue that may hamper SpyCatcher immune receptor adoption in the clinic. Owing to its bacterial origin, the Tag/Catcher system may be vulnerable to recognition by the patient's immune system. Work has been performed in developing SpyCatcher/SpyTag variants with truncations aimed at reducing potential immunogenicity [28] and tested using immunocompetent mice, but further study is needed to determine the likelihood of adverse reactions in humans.

2.4. Leucine Zippers to Retarget CAR T

Cho and colleagues developed a split, universal, and programmable (SUPRA) CAR system that allows for a modular platform to tune the specificity and activation of CAR T cells [29] (Figure 2D). The system consists of two parts: (1) a universal receptor (zipCAR) expressed on T cell surfaces (2) and a tumor-targeting scFv adaptor (zipFv). The zipCAR component consists of intracellular signaling domains linked through a transmembrane domain to an extracellular leucine zipper. The zipFv is a fusion protein consisting of an scFv and a leucine zipper that can interact with the leucine zipper of the zipCAR.

The split CAR design has several variables that can be manipulated to modify the specificity and adjust the SUPRA CAR T cells' activity. The leucine zipper pairs' affinity correlated with cellular activation as determined by cytokine secretion and target cell killing efficiency. Cells with higher zipCAR expression showed greater cytokine secretion upon activation. The authors showed that SUPRA CAR T cell activity could be inhibited using competitive zipFvs with leucine zipper domains that bind the original zipFv but not the zipCAR, thus preventing the activation of zipCARs. The activation level of SUPRA CAR T cells could be further modified by changing the competitive zipFv's leucine zipper's affinity for the original zipFv. SUPRA CAR T cells can also be used to increase tumor specificity through combinatorial antigen sensing, wherein more than one zipFv is introduced. Different signaling domains could be controlled by orthogonal SUPRA CARs, where zipCARs consisting of different intracellular signaling domains and leucine zipper components to specifically activate certain pathways upon antigen binding. The in vitro and in vivo effectiveness of the zipCAR platform was demonstrated; however, further studies, including clinical trials, are needed to confirm its efficacy and safety.

2.5. ConvertibleCAR Strategy Using Modified NKG2D Extracellular Domain

This modular CAR T cell variant, termed *convertible*CAR T cells, uses an inert form of the NKG2D extracellular domain as the ectodomain of the CAR [30] (Figure 2E). NKG2D, an activating receptor expressed on NK cells and some myeloid and T cells, was mutated in its ectodomain such that it cannot engage naturally occurring ligands. This mutant is deemed inert and referred to as inert NKG2D (iNKG2D). Orthogonal ligands were selected that specifically engaged iNKG2D but not WT NKG2D. Antibodies were fused to the orthogonal ligand, U2S3, to generate bispecific MicAbodies, which can specifically direct and activate iNKG2D-CAR-expressing T cells upon binding the respective antigen on a target cell surface. This modular system allows *convertible*CAR T cells to be redirected to different antigen-positive target cells. Additionally, the U2S3 ligand can be fused to payloads, such as cytokines to be delivered to iNKG2D-CAR-expressing cells, promoting their expansion. Expanding the repertoire of modular CAR T systems to more than cancer, Herzig et al. demonstrated that a *convertible*CAR T approach can be utilized to effectively and specifically kill HIV-infected CD4 cells [31]. Despite the advances in antiretroviral therapy, the primary obstacle to curing HIV-positive individuals is latently infected cells that persist. In an effort to target this reservoir of HIV-infected cells, the authors employed *convertible*CAR T cells armed with anti-HIV antibodies fused to an orthogonal MIC ligand. This allowed for the specific killing of HIV-infected primary CD4 T cells in vitro, only when the *convertible*CAR T cells and MicAbodies were bound. The use of a modified human activating receptor, NKGD2, may reduce the chance of an immunogenic reaction in the clinic, but *convertible*CAR system's safety has yet to be established.

2.6. SNAP CAR Strategy: Enzymatic Self-Labeling CARs

As one of the newest methods to be utilized for the generation of modular CAR Ts, an enzymatic strategy to link adaptor to CAR signaling regions is employed, where the CAR's extracellular domain contains the self-labeling SNAPtag enzyme [32] (Figure 2F). Antibodies are conjugated with benzylguanine (BG), with which the SNAP enzyme can react and form a covalent bond. SNAPtag is a modified human O-6-methylguanine-DNA methyltransferase, engineered to react with BG. Potent effector cell activity was shown when SNAP-CAR T cells were co-cultured with antigen-positive target cells, both with BG-conjugated full-length IgG antibodies and Fab fragment. An advantage to this anti-tag CAR system is the formation of a covalent bond between the SNAP enzyme and the BG moiety on the antibody.

Along with the SpyTag/SpyCatcher system, SNAP CARs are distinct from the other anti-tag systems, which rely on a transient interaction between antibody-tag conjugate and the CAR-modified cells. Additionally, the SNAP protein is of human origin and thus is unlikely to be immunogenic. A similar system was designed using the synthetic Notch receptor (synNotch) instead of the T cell receptor, wherein upon antigen binding, the Notch core protein is cleaved by endogenous proteases and releases a transcription factor from the cell membrane where it then travels to the nucleus to carry out its transcriptional regulation function. The generated self-labeling synNotch receptor, containing the SNAPtag protein covalently fused to the adaptor antibody, similar to the SNAP CAR system, functions as modular platforms for switchable CAR T activity.

2.7. The Co-Localization-Dependent Protein Switch (Co-LOCKR) CAR T System

Utilizing a novel logic-gated system, Lajoie et al. designed a protein switch system termed co-localization-dependent protein switch (Co-LOCKR), whereby the switch is engaged through a conformational change only when conditions are met, allowing for the implementation of AND, OR and NOT logic gates for precision target cell killing [33] (Figure 2G). The switch consists of a 'cage' protein, which sequesters a functional 'latch' peptide in an inactive conformation. The binding of a separate 'key' protein will induce a conformational change such that an effector protein or CAR T cell can interact. The authors employed a Bim-Bcl-2 interacting pair where the CAR contains a Bcl-2 binder which interacts with the Bim contained on the latch peptide. Using designed ankyrin repeat protein (DARPin) domains to target the cage element to HER2 and two key domains to EGFR and EpCAM, only cells that co-express both antigens (either HER2 + EGFR or HER2 + EpCAM) will activate Co-LOCKR. The cage domain containing the latch with Bim peptide will only be exposed once the key element interacts, initiating Bcl-2 CAR binding and subsequent T cell activation. Using target cells that express combinations of HER2, EGFR and EpCAM in a mixed population, a HER2-EpCAM Co-LOCKR showed that it would preferentially kill cells expressing both HER2 and EpCAM, and not those expressing HER2 and EGFR, or only HER2 or only EpCAM. The same experiments were performed with HER2-EGFR Co-LOCKR showing target cell killing by Bcl-2 CAR was restricted to only cells containing both HER2 and EGFR. These experiments demonstrated that CAR T cells were engaged specifically when in the presence of target cells co-expressing the correct pair of antigens and the degree of CAR expansion correlated with the density of antigen. The authors showed that between 2.5 nM and 20 nM of Co-LOCKR could be used without causing off-target CAR T cell killing, and the sensitivity of the switch could be further tuned through altering the cage-latch and cage-key affinities.

This method has the ability to reduce off-target effects and precisely direct CAR T activity towards specific target antigens. Additionally, decoy proteins fused to a targeting domain against an antigen to be avoided could be created, allowing for a CAR T 'off switch', where NOT logic is employed as the decoy sequesters the key, preventing cage activation and CAR T firing. In vivo experimentation is needed to evaluate the system's efficacy, and further studies on the potential immunogenicity of the designed proteins are required to broaden the application of this modular CAR T system.

2.8. Anti-5B9 Tag CAR: The UniCAR Platform

Using a unique peptide derived from an autoantigen to redirect CAR T cells, a novel modular CAR system, termed UniCAR, was developed [34] (Figure 2H). The system consists of two components: (1) a CAR with an anti-La protein scFv and (2) specific targeting modules (TMs) that redirect UniCAR T cells to targeted tumor cells. The anti-La protein recognizes a short non-immunogenic peptide motif of ten aa (5B9 tag) derived from the human nuclear autoantigen La/SS-B. TMs consist of a binding domain, such as a tumor-specific scFv, fused to the 5B9 tag that is recognized by the scFv portion of the UniCAR. UniCAR T cells are inactive when TMs are absent, providing an 'on' and 'off switch' to effector cell activity. The variety of antigens targeted by this system illustrates the flexibility of this approach; CD33, CD98, CD123, FLT3, EGFR, STn, GD2, PSMA, and PSCA [34–43] have all been targeted with the UniCAR platform. An advantage of the UniCAR system is the inherent safety switch by halting the infusion of TMs, and the flexibility that can enable targeting of tumor escape variants by using bispecific targeting agents.

Cartellieri et al. used the UniCAR system to target acute myeloid leukemia (AML), a heterogenous leukemic disease [34]. A previous analysis showed that nearly all AML blasts are positive for

CD33, CD123, or both, and scFv-based TMs were designed to target these antigens. Additionally, a dual-specific TM was engineered to target CD33 and CD123 and was shown in a cytotoxicity assay to lyse AML cell lines more effectively than equal molar ratios of each monospecific TM. Using this bispecific strategy may help reduce the risk of tumor escape variants. In the absence of TMs, the UniCAR T cells remained inert in vivo and did not show signs of toxicity.

As a more 'off-the-shelf' therapeutic approach, Mitwasi et al. demonstrated that UniCAR platform could be adapted to the NK-92 cell line [44]. The TM targeted the disialoganglioside GD2. Two types of TMs were explored: an scFv form as previously described, and a novel homodimeric format wherein the E5B9 epitope is connected to the GD2-specific antibody domain via an IgG4 Fc region. This novel TM format was used due to its longer half-life compared to the scFv version; the longer half-life was desired to be closer to that of the NK-92 lifespan due to their limited in vivo persistence. Therefore, they do not require a fast safety switch and the longer half-life of the adaptor reduces the need for continuous infusion. Both versions of the TM led to efficient and specific cell lysis of GD2+ neuroblastoma cells in vitro and in vivo. The use of the NK-92 cell line provides advantages such as lower side effect risk due to their restricted lifespan. Although the 5B9 peptide is derived from an autoantigen, studies completed examining the immune response against the La autoantigen demonstrated anti-La antibodies were not developed and an immune response was not mounted against the 5B9 peptide, as reviewed by Bachmann [45], which would indicate that UniCAR TMs are likely not immunogenic.

Albert et al. examined whether other antibody derivatives could be employed in the UniCAR platform [37]. They incorporated a nanobody targeting EGFR as the targeting module, which effectively retargeted UniCAR T cells to EGFR+ tumor cells and mediated specific cell lysis in vitro and in vivo. The anti-EGFR nanobody was subsequently radiolabeled with ^{64}Cu and ^{68}Ga, and biodistribution, clearance and stability of the targeting module-UniCAR complex were measured. The experiments established that TMs could be released from the UniCAR and dissociated both in vitro and in vivo in a dose-dependent manner, demonstrating its ability to act as a self-limiting switch. The rapid elimination of the nanobody-based TM could improve its safety profile. This work, along with Loureiro et al. [38] and Ardnt et al. [42], demonstrated the potential for UniCARs to be used for targeted immunotherapy and simultaneously as a PET imaging tool to track CAR T therapy. The PET tracer PSMA-11, which binds prostate-specific membrane antigen, was converted into a UniCAR-TM having a dual function as a CAR retargeting element as well as a non-invasive PET imaging reagent, making this a member of a new class of theranostics.

2.9. Anti-PNE CARs: Redirecting T Cells Using Peptide Neo-Epitope Tagging

Similar to the UniCAR platform, anti-PNE CARs take advantage of a peptide tag to redirect CAR T cells. Rodgers et al. first engineered an antibody-based bifunctional switch to be compatible with anti-peptide neo-epitope (PNE) CAR T cells, called switchable CAR-T cells (sCAR T) [46] (Figure 2I). The switch molecule is a 14 amino acid peptide neo-epitope derived from a yeast transcription factor that was shown to have a low probability of inducing an antibody response. The sCAR T cells form an immunological synapse through a PNE engrafted Fab to specifically direct T cell activity to the targeted cells using an anti-PNE scFv CAR. The authors created sCAR T cells directed against CD19 and CD20 and used the system to target B cell malignancies. The switch molecules were systematically optimized, focusing on spatial interactions, to achieve the most efficacious effector/target cell interaction. The authors show that sCAR-T cell activity is titratable, dose-dependent, and strictly dependent on the presence of the switch molecule; all of these characteristics contribute to improved safety compared to that of conventional CAR T cell therapy. Additionally, the codelivery of anti-CD19 and -CD20 switch molecules may prevent antigen escape to more effectively eliminate heterogenous B cell cancers. Viaud and colleagues further studied CD19-directed switchable CARs by examining the factors determining the induction of memory and expansion of sCAR T cells [47]. The formation of a memory population is important to consider, as a naïve, persistent central memory phenotype has been correlated with prolonged remissions in acute lymphoblastic leukemia patients. Conventional CAR T cell therapy cannot achieve the "rest" period required to stimulate a memory phenotype as they are constitutively "on" and interact with antigen. sCAR T cells targeted against CD19+ B cell lymphomas in a competent murine host showed that the timing and dosage of the anti-CD19 switch molecule could promote the expansion and contraction as well as the phenotype of the sCAR T cell population. It was established that a "rest" period used in conjunction with cyclical dosing of switch molecules could induce the production of a memory population, showing potential for enhancing the efficiency and persistence of CAR engineered T cells.

In addition to hematological cancers, anti-PNE CARs have been developed to target solid tumors expressing HER2 [16,48]. Pancreatic ductal adenocarcinoma (PDAC) was targeted with switchable CAR T cells using an anti-HER2 Fab-based switch molecule engrafted with a PNE tag. Using patient-derived xenografts obtained from patients with advanced stage, difficult-to-treat pancreatic tumors, durable remission was achieved by a single injection of switchable CAR T cells and five doses of the switch molecules. Switch molecules were further administered for 10–14 injections, resulting in long-term remission for all animals involved. Switchable CAR T cells persisted even after switch injections were halted, demonstrating switchable CAR T cells have the potential to be effective in safely treating aggressive and disseminated disease. The ability to modulate the dosage of the switchable CAR T may allow for safer targeting of HER2 and other antigens in the clinic.

3. Conclusions and Future Perspectives

CAR T cell therapy has already proven itself in the clinic as a powerful anti-cancer therapeutic. Needed to further its expansion into a wider array of cancers types is both identification of new targets combined with innovative CAR T design. For CAR T therapy to realize its potential in solid tumors, addressing tumor heterogenicity is paramount to its adoption in the clinic, along with a means to better modulate CAR activity to enhance its safety profile. An adaptable system such as modular CAR Ts conceivably could address these issues by tailoring CARs to a patient's specific cancer and adapting treatment using a toolkit of adaptor targeting elements. Simultaneous or sequential targeting of multiple TAAs through universal CARs could mitigate antigen escape, all without the time-consuming and expensive re-engineering of T cells.

Essential for the success of any CAR T approach is the ability to mitigate side effects. Modular CAR activity can be dialed in for enhanced control of engineered T cells and interruption of switch molecules administration, or in some cases using titratable 'off switches', able to dampen side effects associated with T cell proliferation. The use of adaptors to redirect CAR T cells expands on the repertoire of possible targeting elements such as using full-length IgGs; elements that are not possible through traditional CAR genetic engineering approaches. Although the adaptor format is near-limitless, the expense of generating CAR switch molecules and the requirement of continuous or multiple infusions of adaptors could curb its clinical implementation. CAR switch molecules rely on the addition of exogenous components; infusion of elements with non-endogenous origin could prove immunogenic, and the effect on patients remains untested.

The versatile nature of modular CARs and the ability for intelligent antigen targeting makes it an attractive candidate for CAR T therapy to be accessible to a wider range of cancer indications. Combining modular CAR T technology with new approaches in allogeneic CAR T treatment or natural killer (NK) cell engineering could create an extremely versatile product and a truly "off-the-shelf" therapy. Modular CAR T technology advances precision controllable engineered T cells and offers a more sophisticated approach to an already potent anti-cancer immunotherapy.

Author Contributions: A.R.S., writing—original draft preparation; M.N.O., writing; C.R.G., supervision. All authors have read and agreed to the published version of the manuscript.

Abbreviations

CAR	Chimeric antigen receptor
TAA	Tumor-associated antigen
IgG	Immunoglobulin
Fab	Antigen-binding fragment
scFv	Single-chain variable fragment
FITC	Fluorescein isothiocyanate
CRS	Cytokine release syndrome
BBIR	Biotin-binding immune receptor
dcAv	Dimeric avidin
PNE	Peptide neo-epitope
CAM	CAR T cell adapter molecule
hGPC3	Human glypican-3
SUPRA	Split, universal, and programmable
iNKG2D	Inert NKG2D
BG	Benzylguanine
synNotch	Synthetic Notch receptor
TM	Targeting modules
AML	Acute myeloid leukemia
sCAR T	Switchable CAR T
PDAC	Pancreatic ductal adenocarcinoma
NK	Natural killer

References

1. Sadelain, M.; Brentjens, R.; Rivière, I. The Basic Principles of Chimeric Antigen Receptor Design. *Cancer Discov.* **2013**, *3*, 388–398. [CrossRef]

2. Shirasu, N.; Kuroki, M. Functional Design of Chimeric T-Cell Antigen Receptors for Adoptive Immunotherapy of Cancer: Architecture and Outcomes. *Anticancer Res.* **2012**, *32*, 2377–2383.

3. Brentjens, R.J.; Davila, M.L.; Riviere, I.; Park, J.; Wang, X.; Cowell, L.G.; Bartido, S.; Stefanski, J.; Taylor, C.; Olszewska, M.; et al. CD19-Targeted T Cells Rapidly Induce Molecular Remissions in Adults with Chemotherapy-Refractory Acute Lymphoblastic Leukemia. *Sci. Transl. Med.* **2013**, *5*, 177ra38. [CrossRef]

4. Lee, D.W.; Kochenderfer, J.N.; Stetler-Stevenson, M.; Cui, Y.K.; Delbrook, C.; Feldman, S.A.; Fry, T.J.; Orentas, R.; Sabatino, M.; Shah, N.N.; et al. T cells expressing CD19 chimeric antigen receptors for acute lymphoblastic leukaemia in children and young adults: A phase 1 dose-escalation trial. *Lancet* **2015**, *385*, 517–528. [CrossRef]

5. Kochenderfer, J.N.; Dudley, M.E.; Feldman, S.A.; Wilson, W.H.; Spaner, D.E.; Maric, I.; Stetler-Stevenson, M.; Phan, G.Q.; Hughes, M.S.; Sherry, R.M.; et al. B-cell depletion and remissions of malignancy along with cytokine-associated toxicity in a clinical trial of anti-CD19 chimeric-antigen-receptor–transduced T cells. *Blood* **2012**, *119*, 2709–2720. [CrossRef]

6. Xu, X.; Sun, Q.; Liang, X.; Chen, Z.; Zhang, X.; Zhou, X.; Li, M.; Tu, H.; Liu, Y.; Tu, S.; et al. Mechanisms of Relapse After CD19 CAR T-Cell Therapy for Acute Lymphoblastic Leukemia and Its Prevention and Treatment Strategies. *Front. Immunol.* **2019**, *10*, 2664. [CrossRef]

7. Kailayangiri, S.; Altvater, B.; Wiebel, M.; Jamitzky, S.; Rossig, C. Overcoming Heterogeneity of Antigen Expression for Effective CAR T Cell Targeting of Cancers. *Cancers* **2020**, *12*, 1075. [CrossRef]

8. Maude, S.L.; Laetsch, T.W.; Buechner, J.; Rives, S.; Boyer, M.; Bittencourt, H.; Bader, P.; Verneris, M.R.; Stefanski, H.E.; Myers, G.D.; et al. Tisagenlecleucel in Children and Young Adults with B-Cell Lymphoblastic Leukemia. *N. Engl. J. Med.* **2018**, *378*, 439–448. [CrossRef]

9. Park, J.H.; Rivière, I.; Gonen, M.; Wang, X.; Sénéchal, B.; Curran, K.J.; Sauter, C.; Wang, Y.; Santomasso, B.; Mead, E.; et al. Long-Term Follow-up of CD19 CAR Therapy in Acute Lymphoblastic Leukemia. *N. Engl. J. Med.* **2018**, *378*, 449–459. [CrossRef]

10. Chen, H.; Wang, F.; Zhang, P.; Zhang, Y.; Chen, Y.; Fan, X.; Cao, X.; Liu, J.; Yang, Y.; Wang, B.; et al. Management of cytokine release syndrome related to CAR-T cell therapy. *Front. Med.* **2019**, *13*, 610–617. [CrossRef]

11. Brudno, J.N.; Kochenderfer, J.N. Recent advances in CAR T-cell toxicity: Mechanisms, manifestations and management. *Blood Rev.* **2019**, *34*, 45–55. [CrossRef] [PubMed]

12. Thakar, M.S.; Kearl, T.J.; Malarkannan, S. Controlling Cytokine Release Syndrome to Harness the Full Potential of CAR-Based Cellular Therapy. *Front. Oncol.* **2020**, *9*, 1529. [CrossRef] [PubMed]

13. Urbanska, K.; Lanitis, E.; Poussin, M.; Lynn, R.C.; Gavin, B.P.; Kelderman, S.; Yu, J.; Scholler, N.; Powell, D.J. A Universal Strategy for Adoptive Immunotherapy of Cancer through Use of a Novel T-cell Antigen Receptor. *Cancer Res.* **2012**, *72*, 1844–1852. [CrossRef] [PubMed]

14. Lohmueller, J.J.; Ham, J.D.; Kvorjak, M.; Finn, O.J. mSA2 affinity-enhanced biotin-binding CAR T cells for universal tumor targeting. *OncoImmunology* **2018**, *7*, e1368604. [CrossRef] [PubMed]

15. Tamada, K.; Geng, D.; Sakoda, Y.; Bansal, N.; Srivastava, R.; Li, Z.; Davila, E. Redirecting Gene-Modified T Cells toward Various Cancer Types Using Tagged Antibodies. *Clin. Cancer Res.* **2012**, *18*, 6436–6445. [CrossRef]

16. Cao, Y.; Rodgers, D.T.; Du, J.; Ahmad, I.; Hampton, E.N.; Ma, J.S.Y.; Mazagova, M.; Choi, S.; Yun, H.Y.; Xiao, H.; et al. Design of Switchable Chimeric Antigen Receptor T Cells Targeting Breast Cancer. *Angew. Chem. Int. Ed.* **2016**, *55*, 7520–7524. [CrossRef]

17. Morgan, R.A.; Yang, J.C.; Kitano, M.; Dudley, M.E.; Laurencot, C.M.; Rosenberg, S.A. Case Report of a Serious Adverse Event Following the Administration of T Cells Transduced With a Chimeric Antigen Receptor Recognizing ERBB2. *Mol. Ther.* **2010**, *18*, 843–851. [CrossRef]

18. Liu, X.; Zhang, N.; Shi, H. Driving better and safer HER2-specific CARs for cancer therapy. *Oncotarget* **2017**, *8*, 62730–62741. [CrossRef]

19. Zhang, E.; Gu, J.; Xue, J.; Lin, C.; Liu, C.; Li, M.; Hao, J.; Setrerrahmane, S.; Chi, X.; Qi, W.; et al. Accurate control of dual-receptor-engineered T cell activity through a bifunctional anti-angiogenic peptide. *J. Hematol. Oncol.* **2018**, *11*, 44. [CrossRef]

20. Lee, Y.G.; Marks, I.; Srinivasarao, M.; Kanduluru, A.K.; Mahalingam, S.M.; Liu, X.; Chu, H.; Low, P.S. Use of a Single CAR T Cell and Several Bispecific Adapters Facilitates Eradication of Multiple Antigenically Different Solid Tumors. *Cancer Res.* **2019**, *79*, 387–396. [CrossRef]

21. Ma, J.S.Y.; Kim, J.Y.; Kazane, S.A.; Choi, S.-H.; Yun, H.Y.; Kim, M.S.; Rodgers, D.T.; Pugh, H.M.; Singer, O.; Sun, S.B.; et al. Versatile strategy for controlling the specificity and activity of engineered T cells. *Proc. Natl. Acad. Sci. USA* **2016**, *113*, E450–E458. [CrossRef] [PubMed]

22. Chu, W.; Zhou, Y.; Tang, Q.; Wang, M.; Ji, Y.; Yan, J.; Yin, D.; Zhang, S.; Lu, H.; Shen, J. Bi-specific ligand-controlled chimeric antigen receptor T-cell therapy for non-small cell lung cancer. *Biosci. Trends* **2018**, *12*, 298–308. [CrossRef] [PubMed]

23. Lu, Y.J.; Chu, H.; Wheeler, L.W.; Nelson, M.; Westrick, E.; Matthaei, J.F.; Cardle, I.I.; Johnson, A.; Gustafson, J.; Parker, N.; et al. Preclinical Evaluation of Bispecific Adaptor Molecule Controlled Folate Receptor CAR-T Cell Therapy With Special Focus on Pediatric Malignancies. *Front. Oncol.* **2019**, *9*, 151. [CrossRef] [PubMed]

24. Kim, M.S.; Ma, J.S.Y.; Yun, H.; Cao, Y.; Kim, J.Y.; Chi, V.; Wang, D.; Woods, A.; Sherwood, L.; Caballero, D.; et al. Redirection of Genetically Engineered CAR-T Cells Using Bifunctional Small Molecules. *J. Am. Chem. Soc.* **2015**, *137*, 2832–2835. [CrossRef]

25. Zakeri, B.; Fierer, J.O.; Celik, E.; Chittock, E.C.; Schwarz-Linek, U.; Moy, V.T.; Howarth, M. Peptide tag forming a rapid covalent bond to a protein, through engineering a bacterial adhesin. *Proc. Natl. Acad. Sci. USA* **2012**, *109*, E690–E697. [CrossRef]

26. Minutolo, N.G.; Sharma, P.; Poussin, M.; Shaw, L.C.; Brown, D.P.; Hollander, E.E.; Smole, A.; Rodriguez-Garcia, A.; Hui, J.Z.; Zappala, F.; et al. Quantitative Control of Gene-Engineered T-Cell Activity through the Covalent Attachment of Targeting Ligands to a Universal Immune Receptor. *J. Am. Chem. Soc.* **2020**, *142*, 6554–6568. [CrossRef]

27. Liu, X.; Wen, J.; Yi, H.; Hou, X.; Yin, Y.; Ye, G.; Wu, X.; Jiang, X. Split chimeric antigen receptor-modified T cells targeting glypican-3 suppress hepatocellular carcinoma growth with reduced cytokine release. *Ther. Adv. Med. Oncol.* **2020**, *12*, 1–16. [CrossRef]

28. Liu, Z.; Zhou, H.; Wang, W.; Tan, W.; Fu, Y.-X.; Zhu, M. A novel method for synthetic vaccine construction based on protein assembly. *Sci. Rep.* **2014**, *4*, 7266. [CrossRef]

29. Cho, J.H.; Collins, J.J.; Wong, W.W. Universal Chimeric Antigen Receptors for Multiplexed and Logical Control of T cell Responses. *Cell* **2018**, *173*, 1426–1438. [CrossRef]

30. Landgraf, K.E.; Williams, S.R.; Steiger, D.; Gebhart, D.; Lok, S.; Martin, D.W.; Roybal, K.T.; Kim, K.C. convertibleCARs: A chimeric antigen receptor system for flexible control of activity and antigen targeting. *Commun. Biol.* **2020**, *3*, 296. [CrossRef]

31. Herzig, E.; Kim, K.C.; Packard, T.A.; Vardi, N.; Schwarzer, R.; Gramatica, A.; Deeks, S.G.; Williams, S.R.; Landgraf, K.; Killeen, N.; et al. Attacking Latent HIV with convertibleCAR-T Cells, a Highly Adaptable Killing Platform. *Cell* **2019**, *179*, 880–894. [CrossRef] [PubMed]

32. Lohmueller, J.; Butchy, A.A.; Tivon, Y.; Kvorjak, M.; Miskov-Zivanov, N.; Deiters, A.; Finn, O.J. Post-Translational Covalent Assembly of CAR and Synnotch Receptors for Programmable Antigen Targeting; Synthetic Biology. 2020. Available online: https://www.biorxiv.org/content/10.1101/2020.01.17 (accessed on 28 March 2020).

33. Lajoie, M.J.; Boyken, S.E.; Salter, A.I.; Bruffey, J.; Rajan, A.; Langan, R.A.; Olshefsky, A.; Muhunthan, V.; Bick, M.J.; Gewe, M.; et al. Designed protein logic to target cells with precise combinations of surface antigens. *Science* **2020**, *369*, eaba6527. [CrossRef] [PubMed]

34. Cartellieri, M.; Feldmann, A.; Koristka, S.; Arndt, C.; Loff, S.; Ehninger, A.; von Bonin, M.; Bejestani, E.P.; Ehninger, G.; Bachmann, M.P. Switching CAR T cells on and off: A novel modular platform for retargeting of T cells to AML blasts. *Blood Cancer J.* **2016**, *6*, e458. [CrossRef] [PubMed]

35. Fasslrinner, F.; Arndt, C.; Feldmann, A.; Koristka, S.; Loureiro, L.R.; Schmitz, M.; Jung, G.; Bornhaeuser, M.; Bachmann, M. Targeting the FMS-like Tyrosin Kinase 3 with the Unicar System: Preclinical Comparison of Murine and Humanized Single-Chain Variable Fragment-Based Targeting Modules. *Blood* **2019**, *134*, 5614. [CrossRef]

36. Albert, S.; Arndt, C.; Feldmann, A.; Bergmann, R.; Bachmann, D.; Koristka, S.; Ludwig, F.; Ziller-Walter, P.; Kegler, A.; Gärtner, S.; et al. A novel nanobody-based target module for retargeting of T lymphocytes to EGFR-expressing cancer cells via the modular UniCAR platform. *Oncoimmunology* **2017**, *6*, e1287246. [CrossRef]

37. Albert, S.; Arndt, C.; Koristka, S.; Berndt, N.; Bergmann, R.; Feldmann, A.; Schmitz, M.; Pietzsch, J.; Steinbach, J.; Bachmann, M. From mono- to bivalent: Improving theranostic properties of target modules for redirection of UniCAR T cells against EGFR-expressing tumor cells in vitro and in vivo. *Oncotarget* **2018**, *9*, 25597–25616. [CrossRef]

38. Loureiro, L.R.; Feldmann, A.; Bergmann, R.; Koristka, S.; Berndt, N.; Máthé, D.; Hegedüs, N.; Szigeti, K.; Videira, P.A.; Bachmann, M.; et al. Extended half-life target module for sustainable UniCAR T-cell treatment of STn-expressing cancers. *J. Exp. Clin. Cancer Res.* **2020**, *39*, 77. [CrossRef]

39. Loureiro, L.R.; Feldmann, A.; Bergmann, R.; Koristka, S.; Berndt, N.; Arndt, C.; Pietzsch, J.; Novo, C.; Videira, P.; Bachmann, M. Development of a novel target module redirecting UniCAR T cells to Sialyl Tn-expressing tumor cells. *Blood Cancer J.* **2018**, *8*, 81. [CrossRef]

40. Mitwasi, N.; Feldmann, A.; Bergmann, R.; Berndt, N.; Arndt, C.; Koristka, S.; Kegler, A.; Jureczek, J.; Hoffmann, A.; Ehninger, A.; et al. Development of novel target modules for retargeting of UniCAR T cells to GD2 positive tumor cells. *Oncotarget* **2017**, *8*, 108584–108603. [CrossRef]

41. Feldmann, A.; Arndt, C.; Bergmann, R.; Loff, S.; Cartellieri, M.; Bachmann, D.; Aliperta, R.; Hetzenecker, M.; Ludwig, F.; Albert, S.; et al. Retargeting of T lymphocytes to PSCA- or PSMA positive prostate cancer cells using the novel modular chimeric antigen receptor platform technology "UniCAR". *Oncotarget* **2017**, *8*, 31368–31385. [CrossRef]

42. Arndt, C.; Feldmann, A.; Koristka, S.; Schäfer, M.; Bergmann, R.; Mitwasi, N.; Berndt, N.; Bachmann, D.; Kegler, A.; Schmitz, M.; et al. A theranostic PSMA ligand for PET imaging and retargeting of T cells expressing the universal chimeric antigen receptor UniCAR. *Oncoimmunology* **2019**, *8*, 1659095. [CrossRef] [PubMed]

43. Bachmann, D.; Aliperta, R.; Bergmann, R.; Feldmann, A.; Koristka, S.; Arndt, C.; Loff, S.; Welzel, P.; Albert, S.; Kegler, A.; et al. Retargeting of UniCAR T cells with an in vivo synthesized target module directed against CD19 positive tumor cells. *Oncotarget* **2018**, *9*, 7487–7500. [CrossRef] [PubMed]

44. Mitwasi, N.; Feldmann, A.; Arndt, C.; Koristka, S.; Berndt, N.; Jureczek, J.; Loureiro, L.R.; Bergmann, R.; Máthé, D.; Hegedüs, N.; et al. "UniCAR"-modified off-the-shelf NK-92 cells for targeting of GD2-expressing tumour cells. *Sci. Rep.* **2020**, *10*, 2141. [CrossRef] [PubMed]

45. Bachmann, M. The UniCAR system: A modular CAR T cell approach to improve the safety of CAR T cells. *Immunol. Lett.* **2019**, *211*, 13–22. [CrossRef]

46. Rodgers, D.T.; Mazagova, M.; Hampton, E.N.; Cao, Y.; Ramadoss, N.S.; Hardy, I.R.; Schulman, A.; Du, J.; Wang, F.; Singer, O.; et al. Switch-mediated activation and retargeting of CAR-T cells for B-cell malignancies. *Proc. Natl. Acad. Sci. USA* **2016**, *113*, E459–E468. [CrossRef]

47. Viaud, S.; Ma, J.S.Y.; Hardy, I.R.; Hampton, E.N.; Benish, B.; Sherwood, L.; Nunez, V.; Ackerman, C.J.; Khialeeva, E.; Weglarz, M.; et al. Switchable control over in vivo CAR T expansion, B cell depletion, and induction of memory. *Proc. Natl. Acad. Sci. USA* **2018**, *115*, E10898–E10906. [CrossRef]

48. Raj, D.; Yang, M.-H.; Rodgers, D.; Hampton, E.N.; Begum, J.; Mustafa, A.; Lorizio, D.; Garces, I.; Propper, D.; Kench, J.G.; et al. Switchable CAR-T cells mediate remission in metastatic pancreatic ductal adenocarcinoma. *Gut* **2019**, *68*, 1052–1064. [CrossRef]

7

Epitope Sequences in Dengue Virus NS1 Protein Identified by Monoclonal Antibodies

Leticia Barboza Rocha [1,†], Rubens Prince dos Santos Alves [2,†], Bruna Alves Caetano [1],
Lennon Ramos Pereira [2], Thais Mitsunari [1], Jaime Henrique Amorim [2,‡],
Juliana Moutinho Polatto [1], Viviane Fongaro Botosso [3], Neuza Maria Frazatti Gallina [4],
Ricardo Palacios [5], Alexander Roberto Precioso [5], Celso Francisco Hernandes Granato [6],
Danielle Bruna Leal Oliveira [7], Vanessa Barbosa da Silveira [7], Daniela Luz [1],
Luís Carlos de Souza Ferreira [2] and Roxane Maria Fontes Piazza [1,*]

[1] Laboratório de Bacteriologia, Instituto Butantan, São Paulo, 05503-900 SP, Brazil;
leticia.rocha@butantan.gov.br (L.B.R.); bruna.caetano@butantan.gov.br (B.A.C.);
thais.mitsunari@butantan.gov.br (T.M.); juliana.yassuda@butantan.gov.br (J.M.P.);
daniedaluz@yahoo.com.br (D.L.)
[2] Laboratório de Desenvolvimento de Vacinas, Instituto de Ciências Biomédicas, Universidade de São Paulo,
São Paulo, 05508-000 SP, Brazil; rubens.bmc@gmail.com (R.P.d.S.A.); lennon_rp@usp.br (L.R.P.);
jh.biomedico@gmail.com (J.H.A.); lcsf@usp.br (L.C.d.S.F.)
[3] Laboratório de Virologia, Instituto Butantan, São Paulo, 05503-900 SP, Brazil;
viviane.botosso@butantan.gov.br
[4] Divisão de Desenvolvimento Tecnológico e Produção; Instituto Butantan, São Paulo, 05503-900 SP, Brazil;
neuza.gallina@butantan.gov.br
[5] Divisão de Ensaios Clínicos e Farmacovigilância, Instituto Butantan, São Paulo, 05503-900 SP, Brazil;
ricardo.palacios@butantan.gov.br (R.P.); alexander.precioso@butantan.gov.br (A.R.P.)
[6] Departamento de Medicina, Disciplina de Doenças Infecciosas e Parasitárias,
Universidade Federal de São Paulo, São Paulo, 04023-062 SP, Brazil; celso.granato@grupofleury.com.br
[7] Laboratório de Virologia Molecular e Clínica, Departamento de Microbiologia, Instituto de Ciências
Biomédicas, Universidade de São Paulo, São Paulo, 05508-000 SP, Brazil; danibruna@gmail.com (D.B.L.O.);
vanessa.silveirabio@gmail.com (V.B.d.S.)
* Correspondence: roxane@butantan.gov.br
† These authors contributed equally to the present work.
‡ Present address: Laboratório de Microbiologia, Centro das Ciências Biológicas e da Saúde, Universidade
Federal do Oeste da Bahia, Barreiras, 47805-100. Bahia, Brazil.

Abstract: Dengue nonstructural protein 1 (NS1) is a multi-functional glycoprotein with essential functions both in viral replication and modulation of host innate immune responses. NS1 has been established as a good surrogate marker for infection. In the present study, we generated four anti-NS1 monoclonal antibodies against recombinant NS1 protein from dengue virus serotype 2 (DENV2), which were used to map three NS1 epitopes. The sequence [193]AVHADMGYWIESALNDT[209] was recognized by monoclonal antibodies 2H5 and 4H1BC, which also cross-reacted with Zika virus (ZIKV) protein. On the other hand, the sequence [25]VHTWTEQYKFQPES[38] was recognized by mAb 4F6 that did not cross react with ZIKV. Lastly, a previously unidentified DENV2 NS1-specific epitope, represented by the sequence [127]ELHNQTFLIDGPETAEC[143], is described in the present study after reaction with mAb 4H2, which also did not cross react with ZIKV. The selection and characterization of the epitope, specificity of anti-NS1 mAbs, may contribute to the development of diagnostic tools able to differentiate DENV and ZIKV infections.

Keywords: dengue virus; NS1; Zika virus; mAbs; antibody recognition; amino acid sequences

1. Introduction

Dengue fever is an important mosquito-borne and the most prevalent and costly arbovirus affecting humans, caused by one of the four serotypes of dengue virus (DENV 1–4) [1]. In the last decade, a large number of dengue epidemics have occurred, which resulted in enormous economic and human loss in parts of Asia and South America [2,3]. Considering Brazil only, more than three million cases of confirmed dengue infections occurred between 2015 and 2017, with 70 cases per 100,000 inhabitants [4].

The DENV genome is composed of a single positive-sense RNA that encodes a single viral polyprotein that is further processed by viral and host proteases into three structural proteins (C, prM/M, and E) and seven nonstructural proteins (NS1, NS2A, NS2B, NS3, NS4A, NS4B, and NS5). NS1 is the first nonstructural protein to be translated and is essential to virus replication [5]. It is a conserved N-linked glycoprotein with a variable molecular mass of 46–55 kDa, which depends on its glycosylation status [6]. The NS1 protein can be found as a dimer associated with vesicular compartments within the cell, where it plays an important role as an essential cofactor in the virus replication process [7]. Alternatively, NS1 can be secreted into the extracellular space as a hexameric lipoprotein particle [8] that interacts with several plasma proteins [9,10].

The recent introduction of the Zika virus (ZIKV) to the American continent represented a regional and worldwide public health challenge [11]. The close evolutionary relationship between DENV and ZIKV is reflected by the high sequence conservation of both structural and non-structural proteins [12]. In this aspect, the identification of monoclonal antibodies (mAbs) able to react specifically with DENV or cross-react with ZIKV proteins is a relevant feature for the validation of the diagnostic tools based on the NS1 protein.

In pioneering work by Falconar et al. [8], the immunogenic regions of DENV2 NS1 employing mAbs were extensively studied. Recently, certain studies have been using new methods to predict the binding epitopes of proteins to specific antibodies [13,14]. This approach was also applied to identify binding epitopes of DENV NS1 protein serotypes [15–17]. Also, the crystal structure of the DENV2 NS1 protein (PDB code: 4O6B) has been solved in both dimeric and hexameric configurations [6], which provides a useful guide for the selection of potential epitopes for therapy and vaccine strategies.

In the present study, recombinant DENV2 NS1 was used to immunize mice and generate murine mAbs. Four mAbs were isolated, purified, characterized and tested for reactivity with native NS1 produced by all DENV serotypes in Vero-infected cells and also for cross-reactivity with ZIKV NS1.

2. Results

2.1. Isolation and Characterization of NS1-Specific DENV mAbs

Fusion of popliteal lymph node cells, from mice immunized with DENV2 rNS1, with a non-Ig-secreting or synthesizing line derived from a cell line created by fusing a BALB/c mouse spleen cell and the mouse myeloma P3X63Ag8 (SP2/O-Ag14) mouse myeloma cells, generated 25 secretory hybridomas. Among them, four hybridomas were selected by enzyme-linked immunosorbent assay (ELISA) and sub cloned by limiting dilution and named as 4F6, 4H2, 4H1BC, and 2H5. The clones were expanded, supernatants collected and mAbs purified for further characterization. Accordingly, mAbs 4F6 and 4H2 were characterized as IgG2a (immunoglobulin G), and 2H5 and 4H1BC as IgG1. The affinity constants were similar (10^{-8} M) as well as their reactivity with and limits of detection of NS1 (Table 1).

Table 1. Characteristics of the monoclonal antibodies (mAbs) against dengue virus (DENV) nonstructural protein 1 (NS1).

Name	4F6	4H2	2H5	4H1BC
IgG Subtype [a]	IgG2a	IgG2a	IgG1	IgG1
DENV2 NS1 reactivity [b]	Yes	Yes	Yes	Yes
Dissociation Constant (KD) [c]	1.1×10^{-8} M	6.2×10^{-8} M	7.3×10^{-8} M	8.4×10^{-8} M
Detection limit [d]	16 ng/mL	32 ng/mL	32 ng/mL	32 ng/mL
Epitope sequence [e]	[25]VHTWTEQYKFQPES[38]	[127]ELHNQTFLIDGPETAEC[143]	[193]AVHADMGYWIESALNDT[209]	[193]AVHADMGYWIESALNDT[209]
DENV (1–4) reactivity [f]	No	Yes	No	No
ZIKV reactivity [g]	No	No	Yes	Yes

[a] The Ig isotype and IgG subtypes were performed by enzyme-linked immunosorbent assay (ELISA) using anti-IgA, anti-IgM, anti-IgG1, anti-IgG2a, anti-IgG2b and anti-IgG3 coated onto microplates; [b] The Dengue virus serotype 2 (DENV2) NS1 reactivity was evaluated by indirect ELISA and immunoblotting using rNS1; [c] Dissociation constant was performed by ELISA [18]; [d] Detection limit was evaluated by ELISA using different concentrations of rNS1; [e] The conservancy of DENV2 NS1 epitopes recognized by specific mAbs in a peptide array was analyzed among the four serotypes of DENV, using three samples of NS1 amino acid sequences as representative of each DENV serotype; [f,g] DENV (1–4) and Zika virus (ZIKV) reactivity was evaluated by immunofluorescence in Vero cells infected with the specific virus strains.

The recognition pattern of the four NS1 mAbs was evaluated by ELISA using either intact or heat-denaturated rNS1. All NS1 mAbs recognized the intact rNS1 protein, and although mAb 4F6 reacted similarly with the intact and the heated-treated rNS1 (Figure 1A), the other three mAbs (4H2, 2H5 and 4H1BC) reacted more efficiently with the intact protein (Figure 1B–D, respectively), which indicated that the recognized epitopes were, at least, partially represented by conformational structures. All four MAbs also recognized rNS1 in an immunoblot assay (Figure S1).

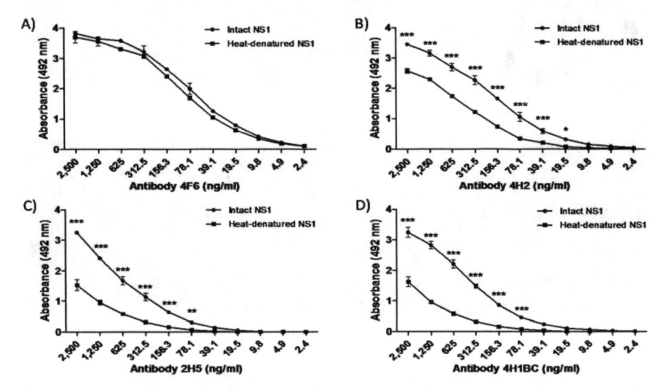

Figure 1. Characterization of nonstructural protein 1-specific (NS1) monoclonal antibodies (mAbs) reactivity by enzyme-linked immunosorbent assay (ELISA). Reactivity of mAbs to heated-treated or intact rNS1, as solid phase-bound antigens. The mAbs 4F6 (**A**), 4H2 (**B**), 2H5 (**C**) and 4H1BC (**D**) were serially diluted (log2) from an initial concentration of 2.5 μg/mL. Each well was adsorbed with 400 ng of rNS1. Heat denaturation was performed at 100 °C for 10 min. Statistical analyses were performed by two-way variance analysis followed by Bonferroni's post-test. (*** $p < 0.01$; ** $p < 0.1$; * $p < 0.5$).

2.2. Detection of Native DENV2 NS1 and Epitope Mapping

After selection, mAbs were tested by immunofluorescence assays using fixed DENV2-infected Vero cells. All four mAbs recognized the native viral NS1 expressed in infected cells, as shown in Figure 2. To localize the specific mAbs binding sites/epitopes, peptide mapping array experiments were performed (Figure S2). The results showed that mAb 4F6 reacted with the peptide corresponding to the sequence [25]VHTWTEQYKFQPES[38] of NS1 (Table 1), which is located in an external loop of the protein 3D structure (Figure 3). The 4H2 mAb recognized the peptide corresponding to the sequence [127]ELHNQTFLIDGPETAEC[143] of NS1 (Table 1), which is located in beta-sheets in an external region of the protein 3D structure (Figure 4). The other two mAbs (2H5 and 4H1BC) showed the same binding specificity and recognized the peptide [193]AVHADMGYWIESALNDT[209] (Table 1). This sequence was also located in a beta-sheet structure, located in an internal region of the protein (Figure 5). The analysis of epitope conservancy in several strains of DENV serotypes as well as Zika strains is detailed in Table S1.

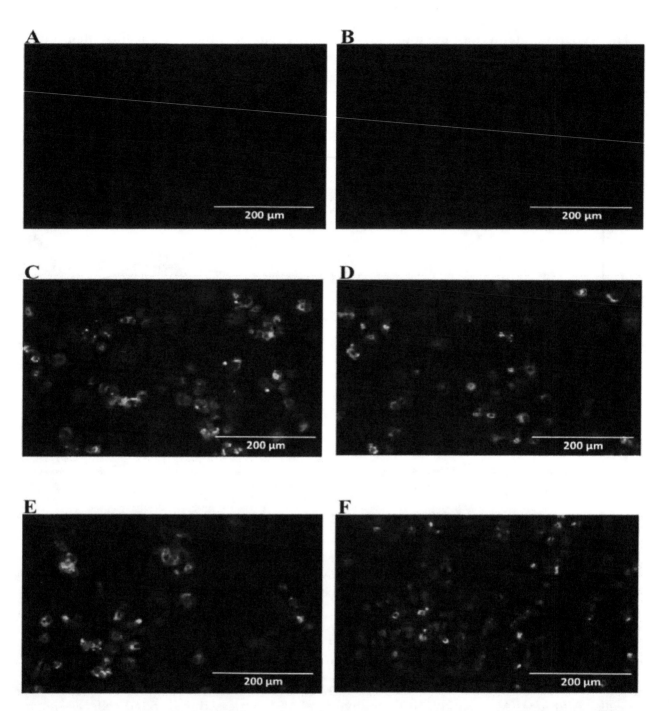

Figure 2. Reactivity of NS1-specific mAbs to dengue-serotype 2-infected Vero cells. Cells were infected with a multiplicity of infection (MOI) of 0.5, fixed, permeabilized and treated with each of the tested mAbs 48 h post infection. Then, cells were labeled with Alexa fluor® conjugated goat-anti mouse IgG. The negative controls: Mock-infected cells treated with a pool of mAbs anti-NS1 (**A**) and DENV2-infected cells labeled only with secondary antibody (**B**); Tested mAbs: (**C**) 4F6; (**D**) 4H2; (**E**) 2H5 and (**F**) 4H1BC. Magnification of 200×.

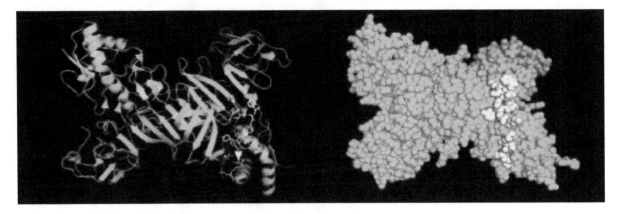

Figure 3. Three-dimensional structural model of a NS1 dimer and regions corresponding to epitopes recognized by 4F6 mAb. The NS1 3D model was generated by the program Python Molecular (PyMOL) in green. The sequence ^{25}VHTWTEQYKFQPES^{38} is highlighted in yellow.

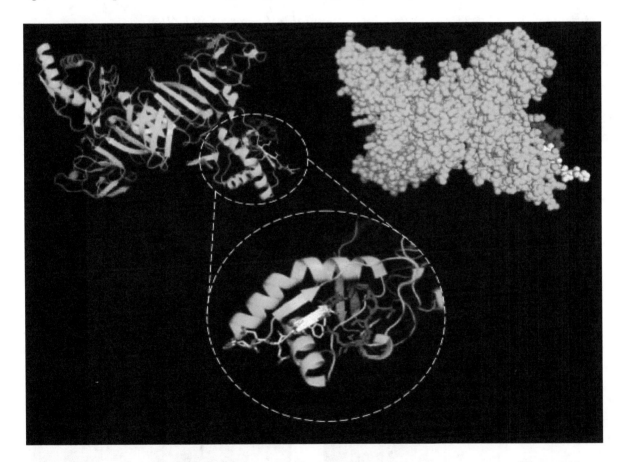

Figure 4. Three-dimensional structural model of a NS1 dimer and regions corresponding to epitopes recognized by 4H2 mAb. The NS1 3D model was generated by the program PyMOL in green. The sequence ^{127}ELHNQTFLIDGPETAEC^{143} is highlighted in red and white. In the detail the red structure represents the novel nine-amino acid sequence described herein.

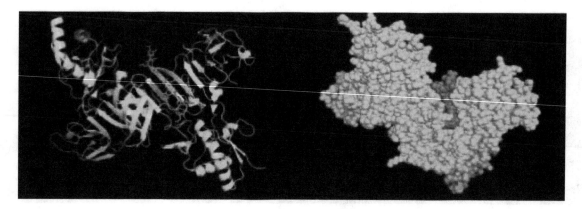

Figure 5. Three-dimensional structural model of a NS1 dimer and regions corresponding to epitopes recognized by 2H5 and 4H1BC mAbs. The NS1 3D model was generated by the program PyMOL in green. The sequence [193]AVHADMGYWIESALNDT[209] is highlighted in blue.

2.3. Analyses of mAbs' Cross-Reactivity with Different DENV Serotype and ZIKV

Since NS1 shares a high homology with amino acid sequences found among different flavivirus, the selected mAbs were tested for recognition of native ZIKV NS1 by immunofluorescence assay, using fixed ZIKV-infected Vero cells. In Figure 6, two mAbs are observed to cross-react with native ZIKV-NS1 in this test (2H5 and 4H1BC) (Figure 6C,D, Table 1). The other two mAbs (4F6 and 4H2) were specific for DENV NS1 (Figure 6A,B, Table 1). We also tested in vitro the reactivity of 4F6 and 4H2 mAbs with DENV serotypes, other than DENV2, and only the 4H2 mAb reacted with all four DENV serotypes (Figure 7, Table 1).

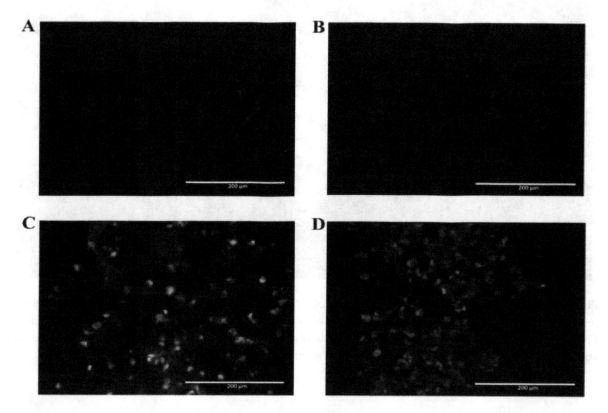

Figure 6. Reactivity of NS1-specific mAbs to zika virus-infected Vero cells. Cells were infected with a MOI of 0.05. 72 h post infection, cells were fixed, permeabilized and treated with each of the tested mAbs. Then, cells were labeled with FITC-conjugated goat-anti mouse IgG. Tested mAbs: (**A**) 4F6; (**B**) 4H2; (**C**) 2H5 and (**D**) 4H1BC. Magnification of 200×.

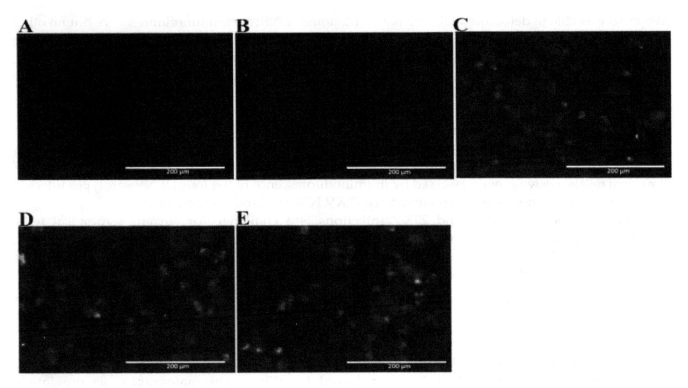

Figure 7. Reactivity of 4H2 mAb to Vero cells infected with DENV of different serotypes. Vero cells were infected with a MOI of 0.5, fixed, permeabilized and treated with mAb 4H2 48 h post infection. Then, cells were labeled with Alexa fluor® conjugated goat-anti mouse IgG. The negative controls: (**A**) Mock infected cells treated with a pool of mAbs anti-NS1 and (**B**) DENV-infected cells labeled only with secondary antibody; Tested DENV serotypes: (**C**) DENV1; (**D**) DENV3 and (**E**) DENV4. Magnification of 200×.

3. Discussion

The DENV NS1 has been used as a target antigen against dengue infection either for vaccines, antiviral drug design or diagnostic methods. Indeed, this protein is secreted by infected cells during the acute phase and circulates in the blood at high concentrations [19]. Nevertheless, the NS1 shares parts of its amino acid sequence among flavivirus. In the present study, we generated four mAbs against DENV2 recombinant NS1 and analyzed their reactivity with the dimeric-NS1 form. The mAbs were also reactive with the native NS1 produced in infected cells but showed different features. The epitope sequences recognized by different mAbs have been recently described and been considered the strategic point for understanding these interactions [15–17].

The mAbs 2H5 and 4H1BC showed a similar recognition pattern and share the same epitope binding, ^{193}AVHADMGYWIESALNDT^{209}. This epitope has been reported as one of the immunodominant B cell epitopes in DENV2 NS1 [20]. This sequence was described in silico and is buried in a beta-sheet structure [15,17]. The recognition of the heat-denatured rNS1 was lower for these mAbs when compared with the non-denatured rNS1, suggesting that these mAbs recognize mainly a conformational epitope. Indeed, by immunofluorescence, both 2H5 and 4H1BC mAbs reacted with dengue virus serotype 2 infected Vero cells. However, they cross-reacted with native ZIKV NS1 in Vero infected cells. The in silico analyses of the similarity of this peptide sequence between different flaviviruses showed that this epitope is highly conserved in these virus but not Yellow fever, Japanese encephalitis and West Nile viruses (Table S2).

The mAb 4F6 recognizes the DENV2 complex-conserved LD2 epitope ^{25}VHTWTEQYKFQPES^{38}, located on the surface of NS1 fusion loop [8,15,17]. A previous study showed a mAb that binds in this motif is able to recognize the purified NS1 hexamer from all four DENV serotypes [21]. However,

4F6 mAb was able to detect only DENV2 native monomeric NS1 by immunofluorescence but no other serotypes. The divergent results may be accounted to methodological issues, since immunofluorescence is less sensitive and aims to detect infected cells expressing mainly monomeric intracellular NS1, while the purified hexamers were used in an ELISA-based detection system. Hence, this epitope may be exposed depending on the NS1 oligomeric level and the DENV serotype.

The fourth mAb obtained, 4H2, recognized the amino acid sequence [127]ELHNQTFLIDGPET AEC[143]. A preceding work described a shorter sequence, [125]STESHNQTFL[134] exposed in the same loop of DENV2 NS1 [15]. Interestingly, the sequence herein described has nine additional amino acids not previously reported as a B cell epitope and shifting the exposed region to a beta-sheet structure. It recognizes the native protein assessed by immunofluorescence of the four DENV serotypes infected Vero cells, but it did not cross-react with native ZIKV NS1 in Vero-infected cells.

Differentiation of DENV and ZIKV infections is a challenge for current serological tests, particularly in areas where both viruses circulate and co-infection can occur. Thus, mAbs, like 4H2, may be particularly useful for the development of an immunofluorescence based-assay that minimizes the risks associated with false positive results among ZIKV-infected subjects.

4. Materials and Methods

4.1. Viral Strains and Viral Antigen

The obtention of purified DENV2 NS1 dimers was achieved after denaturation/refolding steps of the protein expressed in *E. coli* followed by affinity chromatography, as previously reported [22]. This recombinant protein was utilized as an antigen for monoclonal antibody development and characterization. Four dengue serotypes and one Zika virus strain were used for further characterization of the mAbs obtained: a dengue virus serotype 2 JHA1 strain [23,24], a rDEN1Δ30 vaccine strain obtained by Δ30 deletion in 3′UTR of DENV1 Western Pacific strain [25], a rDEN3Δ30/31-7164 vaccine strain obtained by Δ30 and Δ31 deletions in 3′ untranslated region (UTR) of DENV3 Slemann/78 strain [26], a rDEN4Δ30 vaccine strain obtained by Δ30 deletion in 3′ UTR of DENV4 Dominica/81 strain [27], and a Brazilian Zika virus strain (ZIKVBR) (Evandro Chagas Institute, Belem, PA, Brazil).

4.2. Dengue NS1 Monoclonal Antibody (mAb) Production

Four to six week-old female BALB/c mice were immunized via footpad route with 10 µg rNS1 adsorbed to 1 µg recombinant heat-labile toxin (rLT) [22] as adjuvant. The immunization protocols consisted of three booster injections of the rNS1 and rLT in 0.01 M phosphate buffered saline (PBS), pH 7.4 at 15 days intervals. The mouse with the highest antibody titer was boosted with 10 µg of rNS1 three days prior to cell fusion. The popliteal lymph node cells were fused to SP2/O-Ag14 mouse myeloma cells (2:1) using polyethylene glycol 1500 (Sigma Aldrich, St Louis, MO, USA) [28], with modifications [29]. The supernatant fluids were screened for specific antibodies by indirect ELISA in which 100 µL of hybridoma supernatant was added to a 96-well MaxiSorp microplates (Nunc®, Rochester, NY, USA) previously coated with 1 µg/mL of purified rNS1 to screen cultures for antibody production. Antibody-secreting cells were expanded and cloned at limiting dilution [29]. This study was carried out in accordance with the recommendations of Ethical Principles in Animal Research, adopted by the Brazilian College of Animal Experimentation. The protocol was approved by the Ethical Committee for Animal Research of Butantan Institute (995/12).

4.3. Dengue NS1 mAbs Characterization

Hybridoma supernatants were incubated with each of the anti-isotype (anti-IgG1, anti-IgG2a, anti-IgG2b, anti-IgG3, anti-IgA and anti-IgM antibodies) previously coated at MaxiSorp microplates followed by incubation with horseradish peroxidase-conjugated rabbit anti-mouse-IgG+A+M+ (1:1000) (Zymed, San Francisco, CA, USA) [27]. The supernatants from selected clones were filtered (0.45 µm) and purified by protein G affinity chromatography (GE-Healthcare, Freiburg, Germany). MAb purity was observed in a 12% polyacrylamide gel electrophoresis containing sodium dodecyl sulphate (SDS-PAGE) staining with Coomassie blue R-250.

The detection limit was established using rNS1 concentrations from 1 to 512 ng coated on microplates, followed incubation with 10 μg/mL of NS1 mAb and with goat anti-mouse peroxidase-conjugated antibody (Invitrogen, Carlsbad, CA, USA) diluted 1:5000. The three-step ELISA was employed to determine the dissociation constants (KD) of antigen-antibody interactions under equilibrium conditions [28].

ELISA assay was also applied in order to observe the reactivity of mAb NS1 against intact and denatured rNS1. For this, MaxiSorp microplates (Thermo Fischer Scientific, Waltham, MA, USA) were coated with 4 μg/mL of Dengue virus serotype 2 (DENV2) rNS1 heat-treated (100 °C for 10 min) or non-heated. The NS1 mAbs were serially diluted (log2) in an initial concentration of 2.5 μg/mL followed by incubation with goat anti-IgG mouse conjugated with horseradish peroxidase (1:10,000).

The reactivity of NS1 mAb against intact and denatured rNS1 was also analyzed by immunoblotting. Thus, 1 μg or 0.5 μg of rNS1 denatured (heat-treated for 10 min at 100 °C) or intact (non-heated) were separated by electrophoresis in denaturing condition polyacrylamide gel containing sodium dodecyl sulphate (SDS-PAGE) 15%. Nitrocellulose membranes (GE-Healthcare, Freiburg, Germany) containing the transferred proteins were tested with NS1 mAbs at a final concentration of 200 ng/mL. Thus, the membranes were incubated with goat anti-IgG mouse conjugated with peroxidase (1:10,000). The reactive protein bands were identified by exposing membranes to a solution of luminol-hydrogen peroxide according to the manufacturer's instructions (Sigma Aldrich, St Louis, MO, USA). Images were captured by Image Lab™ software (Bio-Rad, Hercules, CA, USA).

4.4. Epitope Characterization and Structure Analysis

Peptide mapping was performed using CelluSpot Peptide Array (Intavis, Heidelberg, Germany) following the manufacturer's recommendations. The slides were produced with dots containing 11 amino acids with overlapping of eight amino acids. Briefly, the slides were blocked, followed by incubation with 30 μg/mL mAb. Next, the slides were incubated with anti-mouse horseradish peroxidase conjugate (1:5000). After washing, diaminobenzidine and hydrogen peroxide were added and the reaction was stopped by the addition of distilled water.

We employed PyMol program (DeLano Scientific LLC, San Carlos, CA, USA, 2009) to predict the structure and the epitope of NS1. For the NS1 structure, we used the available PDB file from Protein Data Bank (code: 4O6B) [6]. For the structure of monoclonal antibodies, we first performed the prediction with Phyre [30].

4.5. NS1 Sequences Database Building

One database consisting of amino acid sequences of the NS1 protein in FASTA format was built. Sequences were retrieved from the National Center for Biotechnology Information (NCBI) protein database. Sequences from serotype 1 of DENV have the following accession numbers: ABG75766, ABG75761 and AFN54943. Sequences from serotype 2 of DENV have the following accession numbers: AIE17400, ABK51383 and AFZ40226. Sequences from serotype 3 of DENV have the following accession numbers: ADM63678, AAT79552 and ALI16137. Sequences from serotype 4 of DENV have the following accession numbers: AGI95993, ALB78116 and AFD53008. Sequences from ZIKV isolates have the following accession numbers: AMR39836, AMD61710, ASK51714, ARB07991, AMD16557 and ARB07967.

4.6. Conservancy Analysis

The IEDB conservancy analysis was used to determine the conservancy of epitopes for monoclonal antibodies 4F6, 4H2, 2H5 and 4H1BC. A sequence identity threshold of ≥20% was applied.

4.7. NS1 mAbs Reactivity to Dengue Virus Serotypes and Zika Virus

Vero cells grown on six-well plates were infected with the viral strains at a MOI of 0.5 for 48 h for DENV and at a MOI of 0.05 for 72 h for ZIKV. The cells were fixed with 1% formaldehyde for 10 min at 4 °C and then permeabilized with 0.5% saponin in PBS for DENV and with cold acetone at −20 °C for ZIKV. The cells were then blocked with PBS containing 10% bovine fetal serum for 30 min. Both cells were treated with mAbs diluted in permeabilization buffer at a concentration of 10 μg/mL for 1 h at room temperature for DENV and 37 °C for 30 min for ZIKV. After three washing steps with PBS, the cells were further treated with Alexa fluor488® (Thermo Fisher, Waltham, MA, USA) conjugated goat anti-mouse IgG at room temperature for 1 h. After another washing period (five times) with PBS, cells were examined using an EVOS digital inverted microscope. Mock infected and cell infected marked with just secondary antibody was the negative control. Also, Vero cells infected with ZIKVBR were tested in order to determine the cross reactivity of the mAbs.

5. Conclusions

In the present study we generated four monoclonal antibodies against the nonstructural protein 1 (NS1) of dengue virus serotype 2. One of them (4H2 mAb) recognizes by immunofluorescence the four-dengue virus serotype and did not cross react to zika virus. Thus, the selection and characterization of the epitope, specificity of anti-NS1 mAbs, may contribute to the development of diagnostic tools able to differentiate DENV and ZIKV infections.

Acknowledgments: We would like to thank Pedro Vasconcelos, from Evandro Chagas Institute, Belém, PA, Brazil for providing a lyophilized ZIKVBR seed. This work was supported by grants from São Paulo Research Foundation (FAPESP): 2009/53894-3; 2011/51761-6; 2014/17595-0 to L.C.S.F. 2013/06589-6; 2013/50955-7 to R.M.F.P and from Conselho Nacional de Desenvolvimento Científico e Tecnológico (CNPq) awarded to R.M.F.P. LBR was a recipient of post-doctoral FAPESP fellowship (2012/09096-8).

Author Contributions: L.B.R., R.P.d.S.A., L.R.P., V.F.B., D.B.L.O., L.C.d.S.F. and R.M.F.P. conceived and designed the experiments; L.B.R., R.P.d.S.A., B.A.C., L.R.P., T.M. and J.M.P. performed the experiments; L.B.R., R.P.d.S.A., B.A.C., L.R.P., T.M., D.B.L.O., D.L., L.C.d.S.F. and R.M.F.P. analyzed the data; J.H.A., N.M.F.G., R.P., A.R.P., C.F.H.G., L.C.d.S.F. and R.M.F.P. contributed reagents/materials/analysis tools; L.B.R., R.P.d.S.A., B.A.C., D.L., L.C.d.S.F. and R.M.F.P. wrote the paper.

References

1.   Guzman, M.G.; Halstead, S.B.; Artsob, H.; Buchy, P.; Farrar, J.; Gubler, D.J.; Hunsperger, E.; Kroeger, A.; Margolis, H.S.; Martínez, E.; et al. Dengue: A continuing global threat. *Nat. Rev. Microbiol.* **2010**, *8*, S7–S16. [CrossRef] [PubMed]

2.   Bhatt, S.; Gething, P.W.; Brady, O.J.; Messina, J.P.; Farlow, A.W.; Moyes, C.L.; Drake, J.M.; Brownstein, J.S.; Hoen, A.G. The global distribution and burden of dengue. *Nature* **2013**′ *496*, 504–507. [CrossRef] [PubMed]

3.   Daep, C.A.; Muñoz-Jordán, J.L.; Eugenin, E.A. Flaviviruses, an expanding threat in public health: Focus on dengue, West Nile, and Japanese encephalitis virus. *J. Neurovirol.* **2014**, *6*, 539–560. [CrossRef] [PubMed]

4.   Secretaria de Vigilância em Saúde, Ministério da Saúde. *Bol. Epidemiol.* **2017** *48*, 1–9.

5.   Chambers, T.J.; Hahn, C.S.; Galler, R.; Rice, C.M. Flavivirus genome organization, expression, and replication. *Annu. Rev. Microbiol.* **1990**, *44*, 649–688. [CrossRef] [PubMed]

6.   Akey, D.L.; Brown, W.C.; Dutta, S.; Konwerski, J.; Jose, J.; Jurkiw, T.K.; DelProposto, J.; Ogata, C.W.; Skiniotis, G.; Kuhn, R.J.; et al. Flavivirus NS1 structures reveal surfaces for associations with membranes and the immune system. *Science* **2014**, *343*, 881–885. [CrossRef] [PubMed]

7. Mackenzie, J.M.; Jones, M.K.; Young, P.R. Immunolocalization of the dengue virus nonstructural glycoprotein NS1 suggests a role in viral RNA replication. *Virology* **1996**, *1*, 232–240. [CrossRef] [PubMed]

8. Falconar, A.K.; Young, P.R.; Miles, M.A. Precise location of sequential dengue virus subcomplex and complex B cell epitopes on the nonstructural-1 glycoprotein. *Arch. Virol.* **1994**, *137*, 315–326. [CrossRef] [PubMed]

9. Silva, E.M.; Conde, J.N.; Allonso, D.; Nogueira, M.L.; Mohana-Borges, R. Mapping the interactions of dengue virus NS1 protein with human liver proteins using a yeast two-hybrid system: Identification of C1q as an interacting partner. *PLoS ONE* **2013**, *8*, e57514. [CrossRef] [PubMed]

10. Muller, D.A.; Young, P.R. The flavivirus NS1 protein: Molecular and structural biology, immunology, role in pathogenesis and application as a diagnostic biomarker. *Antivir. Res.* **2013**, *98*, 192–208. [CrossRef] [PubMed]

11. Gyawali, N.; Bradbury, R.S.; Taylor-Robinson, A.W. The global spread of Zika virus: Is public and media concern justified in regions currently unaffected? *Infect. Dis. Poverty* **2016**, *19*, 5. [CrossRef] [PubMed]

12. Kochakarn, T.; Kotanan, N.; Kümpornsin, K.; Loesbanluechai, D.; Thammasatta, M.; Auewarakul, P.; Wilairat, P.; Chookajorn, T. Comparative genome analysis between Southeast Asian and South American Zika viruses. *Asian Pac. J. Trop. Med.* **2016**, *9*, 1048–1054. [CrossRef] [PubMed]

13. Zhang, X.; Sheng, J.; Plevka, P.; Kuhn, R.J.; Diamond, M.S.; Rossmann, M.G. Dengue structure differs at the temperatures of its human and mosquito hosts. *Proc. Natl. Acad. Sci. USA* **2013**, *110*, 6795–6799. [CrossRef] [PubMed]

14. Jiao, Y.; Legge, F.S.; Zeng, X.; Treutlein, H.R.; Zeng, J. Antibody recognition of Shiga toxins (Stxs): Computational identification of the epitopes of Stx2 subunit A to the antibodies 11E10 and S2C4. *PLoS ONE* **2014**, *2*, e88191. [CrossRef] [PubMed]

15. Jones, M.L.; Legge, F.S.; Lebani, K.; Mahler, S.M.; Young, P.R.; Watterson, D.; Treutlein, H.R.; Zeng, J. Computational Identification of Antibody Epitopes on the Dengue Virus NS1 Protein. *Molecules* **2017**, *22*, 607. [CrossRef] [PubMed]

16. Lebani, K.; Jones, M.L.; Watterson, D.; Ranzoni, A.; Traves, R.J.; Young, P.R.; Mahler, S.M. Isolation of serotype-specific antibodies against dengue virus non-structural protein 1 using phage display and application in a multiplexed serotyping assay. *PLoS ONE* **2017**, *12*, e0180669. [CrossRef] [PubMed]

17. Chaudhury, S.; Gromowski, G.D.; Ripoll, D.R.; Khavrutskii, I.V.; Desai, V.; Wallqvist, A. Dengue virus antibody database: Systematically linking serotype-specificity with epitope mapping in dengue virus. *PLoS Negl. Trop. Dis.* **2017**, *11*, e0005395. [CrossRef] [PubMed]

18. Friguet, B.; Chaffotte, A.F.; Djavadi-Ohaniance, L.; Goldberg, M.E. 1985. Measurements of the true affinity constant in solution of antigen-antibody complexes by enzyme-linked immunosorbent assay. *J. Immunol. Methods* **1985**, *77*, 305–319. [CrossRef]

19. Vaughn, D.W.; Green, S.; Kalayanarooj, S.; Innis, B.L.; Nimmannitya, S.; Suntayakorn, S.; Rothman, A.L.; Ennis, F.A.; Nisalak, A. Dengue in the early febrile phase: Viremia and antibody responses. *J. Infect. Dis.* **1997**, *76*, 322–330. [CrossRef]

20. Jiang, L.; Zhou, J.M.; Yin, Y.; Fang, D.Y.; Tang, Y.X.; Jiang, L.F. Selection and identification of B-cell epitope on NS1 protein of dengue virus type 2. *Virus Res.* **2010**, *150*, 49–55. [CrossRef] [PubMed]

21. Gelanew, T.; Poole-Smith, B.K.; Hunsperger, E. Development and characterization of mouse monoclonal antibodies against monomeric dengue virus non-structural glycoprotein 1 (NS1). *J. Virol. Methods* **2015**, *222*, 214–223. [CrossRef] [PubMed]

22. Amorim, J.H.; Porchia, B.F.M.M.; Balan, A.; Cavalcante, R.C.M.; da Costa, S.M.; de Barcelos Alves, A.M.; de Souza Ferreira, L.C. Refolded dengue virus type 2 NS1 protein expressed in Escherichia coli preserves structural and immunological properties of the native protein. *J. Virol. Methods* **2010**, *167*, 186–192. [CrossRef] [PubMed]

23. Salvador, F.S.; Amorim, J.H.; Alves, R.P.S.; Pereira, S.A.; Ferreira, L.C.S.; Romano, C.M. Complete Genome Sequence of an Atypical Dengue Virus Serotype 2 Lineage Isolated in Brazil. *Genome Announc.* **2015**, *3*, e00779-15. [CrossRef] [PubMed]

24. Amorim, J.H.; Pereira Bizerra, R.S.; dos Santos Alves, R.P.; Sbrogio-Almeida, M.E.; Levi, J.E.; Capurro, M.L.; de Souza Ferreira, L.C. A genetic and pathologic study of a DENV2 clinical isolate capable of inducing encephalitis and hematological disturbances in immunocompetent mice. *PLoS ONE* **2012**, *7*, e44984. [CrossRef] [PubMed]

25. Whitehead, S.S.; Falgout, B.; Hanley, K.A.; Blaney, J.E., Jr.; Markoff, L.; Murphy, B.R. A live, attenuated Dengue virus type 1 vaccine candidate with a 30-nucleotide deletion in the 3′ untranslated region is highly attenuated and immunogenic in monkeys. *J. Virol.* **2003**, *77*, 1653–1657. [CrossRef] [PubMed]

26. Blaney, J.E., Jr.; Sathe, N.S.; Goddard, L.; Hanson, C.T.; Romero, T.A.; Hanley, K.A.; Murphy, B.R.; Whitehead, S.S. Dengue virus type 3 vaccine candidates generated by introduction of deletions in the 3′ untranslated region (3′-UTR) or by exchange of the DENV-3 3′-UTR with that of DENV-4. *Vaccine* **2008**, *26*, 817–828. [CrossRef] [PubMed]

27. Blaney, J.E., Jr.; Johnson, D.H.; Manipon, G.G.; Firestone, C.Y.; Hanson, C.T.; Murphy, B.R.; Whitehead, S.S. Genetic basis of attenuation of Dengue virus type 4 small plaque mutants with restricted replication in suckling mice and in SCID mice transplanted with human liver cells. *Virology* **2002**, *300*, 125–139. [CrossRef] [PubMed]

28. Khöler, G.; Milstein, C. Continuous cultures of fused cells secreting antibody of predefined specificity. *Biotechnology* **1975**, *24*, 524–526.

29. Rocha, L.B.; Luz, D.E.; Moraes, C.T.P.; Caravelli, A.; Fernandes, I.; Guth, B.E.C.; Horton, D.S.P.Q.; Piazza, R.M.F. Interaction between Shiga toxin and monoclonal antibodies: Binding characteristics and in vitro neutralizing abilities. *Toxins (Basel)* **2012**, *4*, 729–747. [CrossRef] [PubMed]

30. Kelley, L.A.; Mezulis, S.; Yates, C.M.; Wass, M.N.; Sternberg, M.J.E. The Phyre2 web portal for protein modeling, prediction and analysis. *Nat. Protoc.* **2015**, *10*, 845–858. [CrossRef] [PubMed]

8

Characterization of Co-Formulated High-Concentration Broadly Neutralizing Anti-HIV-1 Monoclonal Antibodies for Subcutaneous Administration

Vaneet K. Sharma [1,†](ID), Bijay Misra [2,†], Kevin T. McManus [3], Sreenivas Avula [1], Kaliappanadar Nellaiappan [2](ID), Marina Caskey [4], Jill Horowitz [4], Michel C. Nussenzweig [4,5], Michael S. Seaman [3], Indu Javeri [2] and Antu K. Dey [1,*](ID)

[1] IAVI, 125 Broad Street, New York, NY 10004, USA; VSharma@iavi.org (V.K.S.); SAvula@iavi.org (S.A.)
[2] CuriRx, Inc., 205 Lowell Street, Wilmington, MA 01887, USA; bjmisra@gmail.com (B.M.); nellaiappan@curirx.com (K.N.); Ijaveri@curirx.com (I.J.)
[3] Center for Virology and Vaccine Research, Beth Israel Deaconess Medical Center, Boston, MA 02215, USA; kmcmanu4@bidmc.harvard.edu (K.T.M.); mseaman@bidmc.harvard.edu (M.S.S.)
[4] Laboratory of Molecular Immunology, The Rockefeller University, New York, NY 10065, USA; mcaskey@mail.rockefeller.edu (M.C.); jhorowitz@mail.rockefeller.edu (J.H.); nussen@mail.rockefeller.edu (M.C.N.)
[5] Howard Hughes Medical Institute, The Rockefeller University, New York, NY 10065, USA
*   Correspondence: adey@iavi.org
†   Both authors contributed equally to the work.

Abstract: The discovery of numerous potent and broad neutralizing antibodies (bNAbs) against Human Immunodeficiency Virus type 1 (HIV-1) envelope glycoprotein has invigorated the potential of using them as an effective preventative and therapeutic agent. The majority of the anti-HIV-1 antibodies, currently under clinical investigation, are formulated singly for intra-venous (IV) infusion. However, due to the high degree of genetic variability in the case of HIV-1, a single broad neutralizing antibody will likely not be sufficient to protect against the broad range of viral isolates. To that end, delivery of two or more co-formulated bnAbs against HIV-1 in a single subcutaneous (SC) injection is highly desired. We, therefore, co-formulated two anti-HIV bnAbs, 3BNC117-LS and 10-1074-LS, to a total concentration of 150 mg/mL for SC administration and analyzed them using a panel of analytical techniques. Chromatographic based methods, such as RP-HPLC, CEX-HPLC, SEC-HPLC, were developed to ensure separation and detection of each antibody in the co-formulated sample. In addition, we used a panel of diverse pseudoviruses to detect the functionality of individual antibodies in the co-formulation. We also used these methods to test the stability of the co-formulated antibodies and believe that such an approach can support future efforts towards the formulation and characterization of multiple high-concentration antibodies for SC delivery.

Keywords: HIV/AIDS; co-formulation; high concentration; analytical characterization; antibody (s)

1. Introduction

The number of approved monoclonal antibodies (mAbs) for therapy against various cardiovascular, cancer, respiratory, hematology, and autoimmune diseases is continuously on the rise [1]. In addition to therapy against non-infectious diseases, monoclonal antibodies are also increasingly seen as potent prophylactic and therapeutic agents against several infectious pathogens [2–5], particularly those against which effective vaccines do not exist or are under arduous development. To date, over a hundred antibodies have been approved by various regulatory authorities; the majority of these antibody products are typically administered by intravenous (IV) infusion. IV administration, although a well-established route, is challenging to patients as well as to healthcare professionals. Subcutaneous (SC) administration, on the other hand, is increasingly becoming a clear patient preference due to time savings and potential for self-administration, including possibilities for healthcare professionals of administrating during home visits to patients [6,7].

The use of monoclonal antibodies as prophylactic and therapeutic options is particularly attractive against Human Immunodeficiency Virus type 1 (HIV-1) [8,9], a viral pathogen for which the development timeline for a prophylactic vaccine is uncertain [10–12]. Therefore, protection using passive administration of broadly neutralizing antibodies (bNAbs) against HIV-1 is being evaluated through multiple human clinical studies to test the validity of the approach. Broadly neutralizing (monoclonal) antibodies (bNAbs) such as VRC01 [13,14], 10-1074 [15]/10-1074-LS [16], 3BNC117 [17]/3BNC117-LS [18], VRC07-523-LS [19], PGT121 [20,21], and PGDM1400 [21] or their combinations are currently under investigation in multiple clinical trials. Recent studies by Bar-On et al. [22] and Mendoza et al. [23] showed that the combination of two bNAbs, 3BNC117 (directed to CD4-binding site epitope on HIV-1 surface envelope glycoprotein) [17,24] and 10-1074 (directed to V3-glycan epitope on HIV-1 surface envelope glycoprotein) [15,24], delivered by the intravenous (IV) route was well-tolerated and effective in maintaining virus suppression for extended periods in individuals harboring HIV-1 strains sensitive to the antibodies. These clinical studies, with safety, pharmacokinetics and viral load re-bound or decay as endpoints, have primarily used antibodies formulated for IV infusion. Moving forward, to overcome the high cost and burden of intra-venous administration, the high-concentration formulation of both antibodies (here referred to as co-formulation) for sub-cutaneous (SC) administration is planned. However, co-formulating two (or more) antibodies at high concentration is not only challenging due to the requirement to maintain their optimal quality attributes, low viscosity and stability in the chosen formulation condition but also in developing analytical methods that allow separation of individual antibodies to characterize their quality attributes and measure their individual and total stability [25]. Recently, Cao et al. reported the characterization of antibody charge variants and the development of "release" assays for co-formulated antibodies [26]. In another study, Patel et al. investigated the formulation of two anti-HIV bNAbs and through a series of analytical tools, including the mass spectrometry-based multi attribute method (MAM), the authors highlight the analytical challenges in the characterization of co-formulated antibodies [27].

Here, we describe the formulation of two high-concentration bnAbs, 3BNC117-LS and 10-1074-LS, to a final concentration of 150 mg/mL and characterize them through a panel of analytical methods to evaluate the suitability of the methods for future cGMP testing of the co-formulated drug product. Additionally, we show that the chromatography-based separation methods (RP-HPLC, SE-HPLC and IEX-HPLC) and virus-based neutralization assay are optimal to study each antibody in the co-formulated milieu and can potentially be used for "release" and "stability" testing of these materials.

2. Materials and Methods

2.1. Materials

2.1.1. Monoclonal Antibodies

3BNC117 is a monoclonal antibody of the IgG1κ isotype that specifically binds to the CD4 binding site (CD4bs) within HIV-1 envelope gp120. The bnAbs 10-1074 is of the IgG1λ isotype that specifically targets the V3 glycan supersite within HIV-1 envelope gp120. Both fully human parental monoclonal antibodies, 10-1074 and 3BNC117, were LS-modified, two amino acid substitutions, Methionine (M) to Leucine (L) at Fc position 428 (M428L) and Asparagine (N) to Serine (S) at Fc position 434 (N434S), to enhance the antibody binding affinity to the neonatal Fc receptor (FcRn) and prolong their half-life in mammals without impacting the antibody binding domain or its interaction with antigens [28,29]. The LS-modified monoclonal antibodies (MAbs) are referred to here as 3BNC117-LS and 10-1074-LS. The 3BNC117-LS and 10-1074-LS mAbs were produced at Celldex Therapeutics (Fall River, MA, USA).

Both antibodies were expressed via stable Chinese hamster ovary (CHO) cell line clones in a serum-free medium in a batch bioreactor using standard mammalian cell culture techniques. The harvested clarified supernatant was then used to purify the mAbs using a series of chromatographic steps that included MabSelect Sure, Sartobind Q, and SP Sepharose cation exchange column chromatography's. The SP Sepharose eluate was nano-filtered using Virosart HG filtration and concentrated to 150 mg/mL concentration by UFDF (Ultra-filtration Dia-filtration).

The 3BNC-117-LS monoclonal antibody concentrated to 150 mg/mL was formulated in a buffer containing 10 mM Methionine, 250 mM Trehalose, 0.05% Polysorbate 20, pH 5.2. The 10-1074-LS monoclonal antibody concentrated to 150 mg/mL was formulated in a buffer containing 5 mM Histidine, 250 mM Trehalose, 10 mM Methionine, 5 mM Sodium Acetate, 0.05% Polysorbate 20, pH 5.5.

For this study, 3BNC117-LS and 10-1074-LS, were co-formulated (1:1) by mixing at ambient conditions, and the buffer was exchanged such that the final formulation buffer was 5 mM Histidine, 250 mM Trehalose, 10 mM Methionine, 5 mM Sodium Acetate, 0.05% Polysorbate 20, pH 5.5.

2.1.2. Reagents

The hybridoma-based monoclonal anti-idiotype antibodies, used in the ELISA, were produced at Duke Human Vaccine Institute (Durham, NC, USA). The hybridomas were created by immunizing BALB/C mice with either 10-1074 Fab fragment or 3BNC117 Fab fragment. The generated anti-idiotype antibodies were chromatographically purified and concentrated to ~7 mg/mL in 1 × PBS pH 7.2, 0.22 μm filtered and stored at 4 °C until further use. The USP grade Histidine, Methionine, Polysorbate 20 were purchased from JT Baker Chemicals (Phillipsburg, NJ, USA) and Trehalose was purchased from Pfanstiehl, Inc. (Waukegan, IL, USA). All solutions were stored at 4 °C until used.

2.2. Methods

2.2.1. Reverse Phase High-Performance Liquid Chromatography (RP-HPLC)

RP-HPLC separation was performed on Agilent 1260 Infinity Quaternary LC coupled to a diode array detector (DAD). Best peak resolution was demonstrated using Agilent AdvanceBio RP-mAb Diphenyl, 2.1 × 100 mm column, 0.5 mL/min flow rate, with a column temperature of 60 °C and a step wise gradient (3 min washing at 35% B followed by 35% B to 39% B over 16 min). The eluted peaks were detected at 280 nm.

2.2.2. Ion Exchange (IEX)—HPLC

IEX-HPLC was performed on the Agilent 1260 Infinity Quaternary LC system equipped with a diode array detector (DAD) and coupled to ProPac WCX-10, 250 × 4 mm column (Thermo Scientific, Sunnyvale, CA, USA) maintained at 30 °C. Mobile phase A consisted of 20 mM Acetate, pH 5.2, while mobile phase B was 20 mM Acetate, 300 mM sodium chloride, pH 5.2. The pHs of both mobile phases was adjusted using 0.1 M NaOH solution. The flow rate was 0.7 mL/min and salt gradient separation, 50% to 100% B in 35 min, was performed. Peak detection was carried out at 280 nm and the peaks were integrated and percentage peak areas of each peak (as well as charge variants i.e., acidic/basic species) calculated corresponding to each mAbs.

2.2.3. Size-Exclusion High-Performance Liquid Chromatography (SE-HPLC)

SE-HPLC was performed on the Agilent 1260 Infinity Quaternary LC system equipped with a diode array detector (DAD) and coupled to TSKgel G3000SWXL, 5 μm, 7.8 mm × 30 cm column maintained at 30 °C. The mobile phase used was 10 mM histidine, 50 mM Arginine, 100 mM sodium sulfate, pH 6.0. The flow rate used was 1 mL/min. The eluted main and High-Molecular Weight (HMW) peaks were detected at 280 nm.

2.2.4. Enzyme-Linked Immunosorbent Assay (ELISA)

A sandwich ELISA was performed using 96-well Maxisorp plates coated over-night at 2–8 °C with 1 μg/mL of an anti-idiotypic antibody that specifically recognizes 3BNC117-LS (anti-ID monoclonal antibody) or 1 μg/mL of an anti-idiotypic antibody that specifically recognizes 10-1074-LS (anti-ID monoclonal antibody). After washing, plates were blocked with 200 μL Protein free blocking solution at 25 °C for 2 h at 200 RPM. Co-formulated antibody samples, quality controls and reference standards were added and incubated at room temperature. Subsequently, the plate was washed and 100 μL of 1:10,000 diluted peroxidase-conjugated AffiniPure F (ab') 2 Fragment Goat anti-Human IgG Fcγ Fragment specific (Jackson Immuno Research, West Grove, PA, USA) was added. The plate was incubated at room temperature for 60 ± 10 min at 200 RPM. The plate was washed, and the wells were incubated with 100 μL of SureBlue TMB substrate (Fisher Scientific, Somerset, NJ, USA) to develop the chromogenic signal (10 min at room temperature at 200 RPM). The reaction was stopped with the addition of 100 μL of 1% hydrochloric acid. The absorbance was measured at 450 nm using the Molecular Devices plate reader fitted with Softmax Pro software (Molecular Devices LLC, Sunnyvale, CA, USA). Titration curves for the reference standard and each test sample were created using 4-parameter logistic curve fitting to calculate EC50 values using GraphPad Prism software (version 7).

2.2.5. Virus Neutralization Assays

The virus neutralization assay was evaluated using a luciferase-based assay in TZM-bl cells, as previously described [30,31]. Briefly, antibody samples were tested using a starting concentration of 25 μg/mL with 5-fold serial dilutions against the panel of HIV-1 Env pseudoviruses. The selected panel of HIV-1 Env pseudoviruses were either 3BNC117 sensitive/10-1074 resistant ($n = 10$) or 3BNC117 resistant/10-1074 sensitive ($n = 10$). The IC50 and IC80 titers were calculated as the mAb concentration that yielded a 50% or 80% reduction in relative luminescence units (RLU), respectively, compared to the virus control wells after the subtraction of cell control RLUs. All assays were performed in a laboratory compliant with Good Clinical Laboratory Practice (GCLP) procedures.

2.2.6. FlowCAM® Imaging

FlowCAM® is an imaging particle analysis system that we used for imaging and analyzing particles, in the subvisible range, using flow microscopy. The FlowCAM® instrument (Fluid Imaging Technologies, Scarborough, ME, USA) was focused with 10 μm polystyrene beads at 3000/mL National Institute of Standards and Technology (NIST) standard. The samples were diluted by 4-fold by taking 200 μL of the sample in the corresponding buffer to a total volume of 0.8 mL, samples were analyzed at 0.08 mL/min through a 100 μm × 2 mm flow cell, and images of the particles were taken with a 10× optics system. Flash duration was set to 35.50 ms, and Camera Gain was set to 0. Visual-Spreadsheet software version 3.4.8 (DKSH Japan K.K., Tokyo, Japan) was used for data analysis.

2.2.7. Osmolality

Osmolality, a measurement of the total number of solutes in a liquid solution expressed in osmoles of solute particles per kilogram of solvent (mOsm/Kg), was measured in the antibody formulations using the industry-preferred freezing point depression method. The osmolality measurements were made using a Model 3340 single-sample freezing-point micro-osmometer (Advanced Instruments, Norwood, MA, USA), equipped with a 20 μL Ease Eject™ Sampler (Parts No. 3M0825 and 3M0828). The unit of measurement used was milliosmoles of the solute per 1 kg of pure solvent, expressed as mOsm/kg. The instrument was calibrated with 50 mOsm/kg (3MA005) and 850 mOsm/kg (3MA085) calibration standards and verified with a 290 mOsm/kg Clinitrol® Reference Solution (3MA029) prior to each analysis.

2.2.8. Dynamic Light Scattering (DLS)

Dynamic Light Scattering (DLS), which uses time-dependent fluctuations in the intensity of the scattered light to determine the effective size of a particle in nm range, was used to measure the particle size distribution in the antibody formulations. Dynamic light scattering was carried out at 25 °C, with a Malvern Zetasizer Nano Series instrument using a 633 nm/100 mW laser and a 90° detection angle. Particle size distribution (hydrodynamic diameter) by % intensity and % volume was determined along with the polydispersity index (PDI).

3. Results

Parental anti-HIV antibodies, 10-1074 and 3BNC117, were individually formulated at 20 mg/mL for IV administration [15,17]. Based on initial pK data from phase 1 clinical studies, the parental antibodies were LS modified (as described in the Materials section) to extend serum half-life. Thereafter, as a first step towards formulation to aid subcutaneous administration, the antibodies were concentrated 7.5-fold in a new formulation buffer with optimal viscosity to enable drug injection volumes of 2 mL. This resulted in 3BNC117-LS and 10-1074-LS as individually formulated bnAbs, at 150 mg/mL in respective buffers (described in the Materials and Methods section), for subsequent co-formulation studies.

These high-concentration individually formulated antibodies were extensively characterized using a wide range of analytical methods i.e., ELISA, SE-HPLC, RP-HPLC, IEX-HPLC, capillary isoelectric focusing (cIEF), CE-SDS (reduced and non-reduced), Sialic Acid analysis, intrinsic Tryptophan fluorescence spectroscopy, Isoquant analysis, dynamic light scattering (DLS), far and near UV circular dichroism (CD), differential scanning calorimetry (DSC), second derivative UV spectroscopy, N-terminal amino acid sequencing, HILIC based glycan profiling, liquid chromatography coupled with mass spectrometry (LC/MS), and peptide mapping by liquid chromatography coupled with tandem mass spectrometry (LC-MS/MS) (data not shown). In addition, both high-concentration bNAbs, in their respective formulation conditions, were found to be stable at 2–8 °C for ≥24 months (data not shown).

To address the need to co-formulate both the antibodies as a single drug product at a combined final concentration of 150 mg/mL for subcutaneous administration in clinical studies, a 1:1 mixture of both bNAbs (each at 75 mg/mL) was formulated in 5 mM Histidine, 250 mM Trehalose, 10 mM Methionine, 5 mM Sodium Acetate, 0.05% Polysorbate 20, pH 5.5 buffer and characterized using a series of methods to test for (positive) identity, purity, product qualities, and functionality.

3.1. Chromatographic Separation of Co-Formulated Monoclonal Antibodies

During analytical development, the aim was to select appropriate and optimal chromatographic techniques that could separate the two antibodies in their current co-formulation. Reverse phase high-performance liquid chromatography (RP-HPLC), ion exchange liquid chromatography (IEX), and size exclusion chromatography (SEC) were evaluated and found to achieve this separation goal. The separation efficiencies of each of these methods were challenged by the fact that both antibodies, 3BNC-117-LS and 10-1074-LS, are of the IgG1 subclass with similar molecular size and three-dimensional structure, and therefore significant method development and optimization of the chromatographic methods were necessary to achieve the desired separation goals.

3.2. Reverse Phase High-Performance Liquid Chromatography (RP-HPLC)

Reverse phase liquid chromatography (RP-HPLC), due to the denaturing effect of the low pH and high organic solvent mobile phase, was expected to separate and quantify the two bNAbs, in the co-formulated milieu, based on their differences in the relative hydrophobicity. Initial assessment was performed on the Agilent 1260 Infinity quaternary LC coupled to a DAD detector using two columns: AdvanceBio RP-mAb Diphenyl, 2.1 × 100 mm, 3.5 μm (Agilent) and Accucore 150-C4 2.6 μm, 100 × 2.1 mm (Thermo). These columns represent two different stationary phase chemistries, diphenyl offers alternative selectivity and Accucore C-4 wide pore (150 Å) offers lower hydrophobic retention. A generic method development strategy was followed using 0.1% TFA in acetonitrile as mobile phase B, 0.5 mL/minute flow rate. Since, the individually formulated antibodies did elute at 30–40% acetonitrile at elevated temperature (60 °C column temperature) (data not shown), the initial gradient conditions for developing the method was set at 34% to 41% mobile phase B for 7 min. As part of the method optimization, different chromatographic conditions were tested to increase peak resolution: increasing temperature (45, 60, 70, and 80 °C), different mobile phases or organic modifiers in acetonitrile (methanol as mobile phase B or methanol/ IPA (5% v/v) as organic modifier in acetonitrile mobile phase), and different gradient conditions (34% B to 38% B for 16 min and 35% B to 39% B for 16 min). Finally, a method with 34% to 41% mobile phase B, and a column temperature of 60 °C, was selected that resulted in two separate peaks, corresponding to each monoclonal antibody (Figure 1A). This RP-HPLC method was then tested for linearity, precision, accuracy, and specificity parameters. Linearity was evaluated for the total peak area of 10-1074-LS and 3BNC117-LS in a co-formulated sample by calculation of a regression line using the least squares method. (Figure 1B). Linearity for the 3BNC117-LS specific area (Figure 1C) and 10-1074-LS specific area (Figure 1D) were also calculated; the R^2 obtained was 1 for both analyses. Precision, for intra and inter day variability, was assessed by testing the repeatability of the target concentration of 2.5 μg (for each antibody) six times. The intra-assay precision for the total peak area ranged from 0.1% to 0.3% and the inter-assay precision was 0.3% for 3 experiments on separate days (days 1, 2, and 3) (Supplementary Table S1A). The intra- and inter-precisions for the individual peak areas, 10-1074-LS peak area and 3BNC117-LS peak area, were also similar. The intra- and inter-precisions for the 10-1074-LS peak area were ≤0.4% and ≤0.3%, respectively (Supplementary Table S1B). The intra- and inter-precisions for the 3BNC117-LS peak area were ≤0.2% and ≤0.2%, respectively (Supplementary Table S1C). Accuracy was tested by percentage recoveries of the mean of three determinations of six different concentrations (1 to 8 μg column load). Based on the percent recoveries, we concluded that the RP-HPLC method accuracy was within a variation of ≤2% relative standard deviation (RSD) (Supplementary Table S1D). These results indicate that this RP-HPLC method is suitable and, after appropriate method validation, can be used for future testing of the 3BNC117-LS + 10-1074-LS co-formulated drug product.

3.3. Ion Exchange High-Performance Liquid Chromatography (IEX-HPLC)

To allow the characterization of charge heterogeneity and high-resolution separation of each antibody (in the co-formulated sample), it was expected that the ion exchange (IEX) chromatography can separate the two bNAbs based on their charge differences. IEX chromatography is a non-denaturing technique and among the different IEX modes, since cation-exchange chromatography (CEX) is the preferred approach for characterizing antibody charge variants [32,33], it was chosen. The CEX method was developed on the Agilent 1260 Infinity quaternary LC system equipped with a solvent delivery pump, an autosampler, and a diode array detector (DAD). A ProPac WCX-10, 250 × 4 mm column (Thermo Scientific, Sunnyvale, CA, USA) was used for the method development. A "classical" salt gradient separation (50% to 100% B in 35 min) was performed using mobile phase A, composed of 20 mM Acetate buffer, pH 5.2, and mobile phase B, composed of 20 mM Acetate buffer containing 300 mM sodium chloride, pH 5.2. The flow rate was set to 0.7 mL/min and column temperature was maintained at 30 °C. Peak detection was carried out at 280 nm and after integration of peaks, the percentage peak areas of each peak (as well as charge variants i.e., main, acidic, basic peak) corresponding to each monoclonal antibody were calculated (Figure 2A). This weak cation exchange (CEX) chromatography method was used to perform qualitative and quantitative analysis of the charge variants for each of the separated antibodies. The optimized CEX-HPLC method was further tested for linearity, precision, accuracy, and specificity parameters. Linearity was evaluated for main peaks, pre-main peaks, post main peaks, and total peak areas of 10-1074-LS and 3BNC117-LS in a co-formulated sample by calculation of a regression line using the least squares method (Figure 2B–D). Precision, for intra- and inter-assay variability, of the total peak area was assessed by testing the repeatability of the target concentration of 100 μg (total) six times. The charge variants for both

10-1074-LS and 3BNC117-LS were within 2.2% for the total peak area with intra-assay precision within 1.1–2.2% and inter-assay precision within <2.2% (Supplementary Table S2A). The variability of the 10-1074-LS specific peak was similar, with intra-assay precision ≤ 2.1% and inter-assay precision ≤ 1.8% (Supplementary Table S2B). The variability of the 3BNC117-LS specific peak was slightly higher, although similar, with intra-assay precision ≤ 2.6% and inter-assay precision ≤ 2.7% (Supplementary Table S2C). The accuracy was tested by percentage recoveries of the mean of three determinations of six different concentrations (50 to 300 μg column load); the method accuracy was observed to be ≤2% relative standard deviation (RSD) (Supplementary Table S2D). Based on these results, this CEX-HPLC method is suitable and after appropriate method validation can be used for future testing of the 3BNC117-LS + 10-1074-LS co-formulated drug product.

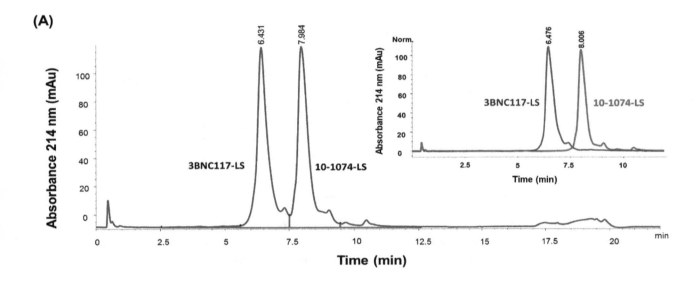

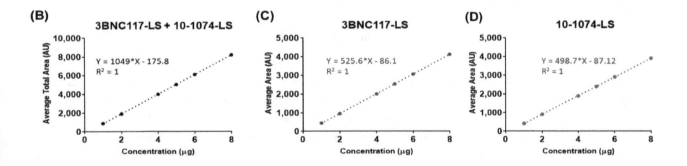

Figure 1. Reverse phase chromatogram with UV absorbance at 214 nm showing separation of two antibodies in the 1:1 co-formulated sample (total 150 mg/mL). (**A**) Peaks separated by reversed phase HPLC corresponding to the two antibodies are labeled. Inset shows the overlapped reverse phase chromatograms from the two-separate RP-HPLC run corresponding to the two antibodies, each at 150 mg/mL. The chromatography conditions were the same for the co-formulated and the individual antibody samples. Linearity analysis of concentration (in μg; x-axis) dependent increase in area under the curve (in Absorbance Units, AU; y-axis) for (**B**) total area (3BNC117-LS + 10-1074-LS), (**C**) 3BNC117-LS specific area, and (**D**) 10-1074-LS specific area.

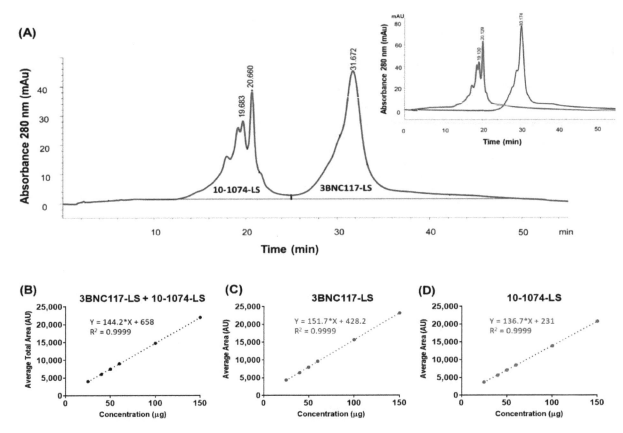

Figure 2. (**A**) Cation exchange chromatogram with UV absorbance at 280 nm showing separation of two antibodies in the 1:1 co-formulated sample (total 150 mg/mL). Peaks for each of the antibody are labeled. Inset shows the overlapped cation exchange chromatograms from the two separate chromatography runs corresponding to the two antibodies, each at 150 mg/mL. The chromatography conditions were the same for the co-formulated and the individual antibody samples. Linearity analysis of concentration (in μg; x-axis) dependent increase in area under the curve (in Absorbance Units, AU; y-axis) for (**B**) total area (3BNC117-LS + 10-1074-LS), (**C**) 3BNC117-LS specific area, and (**D**) 10-1074-LS specific area.

3.4. Size-Exclusion High-Performance Liquid Chromatography (SE-HPLC)

To separate the two antibodies (in the co-formulated sample) based on their molecular size and achieve separation through differential exclusion, we used Size Exclusion HPLC (SE-HPLC). SE-HPLC is widely used for determining the antibody purity, through the determination of percent monomer (and assessments of % HMW, High Molecular Weight, and % LMW, Low Molecular Weight, species), and therefore we were conscious of the possible limitation of the method to fully resolve the two similarly sized monoclonal antibodies in the co-formulated sample. When we evaluated two mobile phases (100 mM sodium acetate (pH 6.0) and 100 mM sodium sulfate (pH 6.0)) for the resolution of the antibodies in the co-formulated sample, we found that both phases resulted in one broad peak with no resolution of the two antibodies (data not shown). However, when we changed the mobile phase to 10 mM histidine, 50 mM arginine, 100 mM sodium sulfate, pH 6.0, a slight separation between the two peaks was observed (Figure 3A). When the salt (sodium sulfate) concentration was gradually increased from 100 to 550 mM sodium sulfate, to probe the effect of increasing salt on the separation of the two peaks (10-1074-LS and 3BNC117-LS peaks), we observed separation with greater resolution, despite the broadening of the late eluting 10-1074-LS peak. From the outset, since the intent of the SE-HPLC was not to resolve the two mAbs but to detect the levels of HMW (and LMW) species in the co-formulated sample and quantify aggregate levels (at the time of product release and during long-term storage) to ensure a means for measurement of percent monomeric antibody in the co-formulated milieu, this SE-HPLC method was accepted to be appropriate for use and tested further for linearity, precision, accuracy, and specificity parameters. Linearity was verified in a range of co-formulated samples with a R^2 of >0.99 (Figure 3B–D). The intra- and inter-precision at the target column load of 100 μg (total) for the main peak (monomer) area was within ≤0.2% (Supplementary Table S3A). The intra- and inter-precision at the target column load of 100 μg (total) for the % HMW peak area was within ≤0.7% and ≤4.3% (Supplementary Table S3B). However, the intra- and inter-precision at the target column load of 100 μg (total) for the % LMW peak area was higher, within ≤18.4% and ≤14% (Supplementary Table S3C); this higher % RSD was due to lower signal levels (lower levels of LMW), closer or below limit of quantification (LOQ). Accuracy was tested by percentage recoveries of the mean of three determinations of six different concentrations precisely prepared (50 to 300 μg column load); the method accuracy was observed to be within 2% RSD (Supplementary Table S3D). These results indicate that the SE-HPLC method is suitable and after appropriate method validation can be used for future testing of the 3BNC117-LS + 10-1074-LS co-formulated drug product.

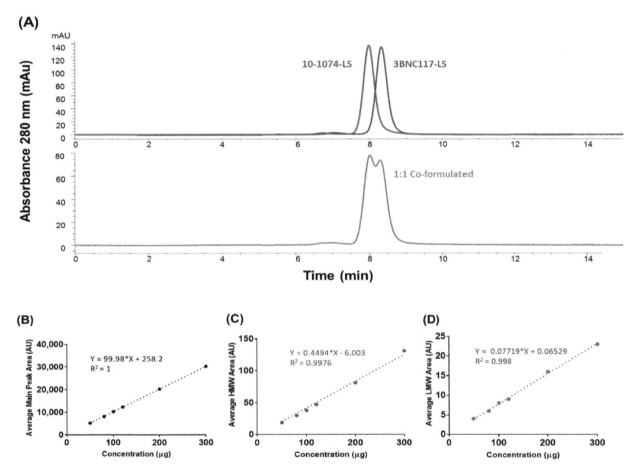

Figure 3. (**A**) Size exclusion chromatography profiles of 150 mg/mL for 10-1074-LS and 3BNC117-LS antibodies, individually formulated (top) and after co-formulation (1:1, 75 mg/mL each) (bottom) on the TSKgel column. Linearity analysis of concentration (in μg; x-axis) dependent increase in area under the curve (in Absorbance Units, AU; y-axis) for (**B**) average main peak (monomer) area (3BNC117-LS + 10-1074-LS monomer), (**C**) average High-Molecular Weight (HMW) peak area, and (**D**) average Low Molecular Weight peak area.

3.5. Positive Identification of Individual Antibody in the Co-Formulation Sample Using Anti-ID (Idiotype) Based ELISA

Since wildtype gp120-based ELISA would not be successful in differentiating the binding and the identity of the two antibodies, when present in a co-formulated sample, we generated a 10-1074 idiotype-specific antibody and a 3BNC117 idiotype-specific antibody to serve as reagents in a new ELISA that would utilize each antibody's identity based on their unique idiotype (ID). This format would provide a means for measuring the identity of an individual antibody in the co-formulated sample. After a series of optimization experiments, the anti-ID ELISA was successful to identify and differentiate both antibodies as well as detect their identity in the co-formulated sample (Figure 4). The anti-ID ELISA was tested for precision and accuracy (data not shown) and the overall variability, particularly inter-assay, was well within the 30–40% RSD, seen in bioassays (data not shown). These results indicate that the anti-ID based ELISA can be used for future testing of identity of the 3BNC117-LS + 10-1074-LS co-formulated drug product, after appropriate method validation.

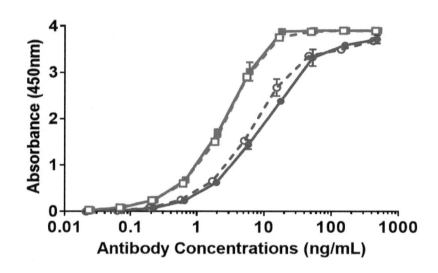

-o- **3BNC117-LS (Individual; Ref. Std.)** -●- **3BNC117-LS (Co-formulated)**

-□- **10-1074-LS (Individual; Ref. Std.)** -■- **10-1074-LS (Co-formulated)**

Figure 4. Test of identity of individual antibodies (3BNC117-LS and 10-1074-LS) in co-formulated sample (of 150 mg/mL total concentration) using anti-idiotypic (anti-ID) antibodies. Individual antibodies, 3BNC117-LS and 10-1074-LS at 150 mg/mL, were used as a reference standard. Open circle, dotted line—3BNC117-LS (150 mg/mL, reference standard), filled circle, filled line—3BNC117-LS (at 75 mg/mL in co-formulated sample), open square, dotted line—10-1074-LS (150 mg/mL, reference standard), filled square, filled line—10-1074-LS (at 75 mg/mL in co-formulated sample).

3.6. Potency Testing of Individual Antibody in the Co-Formulation Sample Using a Virus Neutralization Assay

A traditional HIV-1 pseudovirus neutralization assay was used to evaluate the functional activity or potency of the individual antibodies in the co-formulated sample. To do so, two panels of pseudoviruses (total $n = 20$) were selected: one panel ($n = 10$) for 3BNC117 and another ($n = 10$) for 10-1074. To test for 3BNC117 potency/functional activity, the panel involved ten 3BNC117 sensitive/10-1074 resistant viruses; to test for 10-1074 potency/functional activity, the panel involved ten 3BNC117 resistant/10-1074 sensitive viruses. Viruses were selected for having low/medium to high sensitivity to a single antibody based on historical data (data not shown). MuLV (Murine Leukemia Virus), a non-relevant virus, was used as a negative control and was not neutralized by either of the two control antibodies (data not shown). In comparison to the individual antibody (3BNC117 or 10-1074), used as control, the two co-formulated antibodies were potent and demonstrated their specific neutralization activity in their respective panels (Table 1A–D). Out of the 10 viruses sensitive to 3BNC117, 0013095-2.11 is not highly sensitive to 3BNC117; therefore, not only is the IC80 >25 μg/mL, the IC80 of the co-formulated 3BNC117-LS and 10-1074-LS is also higher when compared to IC80s for other viruses for the co-formulated product. (Table 1A). Despite this one virus, which could be replaced by another virus in future, based on these results, the pseudovirus neutralization assay using the defined panel of viruses can be used for future testing of the 3BNC117-LS + 10-1074-LS co-formulated drug product.

Table 1. Neutralization activity of co-formulated 3BNC117-LS and 10-1074-LS (total 150 mg/mL) using 2 panels of pseudoviruses in TZM-bl cells. One panel (**A,B**) is used to test potency/functional activity of 3BNC117 (3BNC117 sensitive/10-1074 resistant viruses ($n = 10$)) and the other panel (**C,D**) is used to test potency/functional activity of 10-1074 (10-1074 sensitive viruses/3BNC117 resistant ($n = 10$)). The pseudovirus strains are indicated at the top of the table and IC50 and IC80 values (in μg/mL) for each of the samples, against those viruses, are reported. Individual antibodies, 3BNC117 and 10-1074, are used as controls for each panel. LS—Leucine-Serine substitution.

(A)										
Samples	**ZM249M.PL1**		**Q461.e2**		**0013095-2.11**		**62357.14.D3.4589**		**ZM53M.PB12**	
	IC50	IC80	IC50	IC80	IC50	IC80	IC50	IC80	IC50	IC80
3BNC117.LS + 10-1074.LS DP	0.042	0.15	0.042	0.153	1.161	15.162	0.043	0.15	0.153	0.568
3BNC117.LS (control)	0.037	0.13	0.039	0.143	1.396	>25	0.036	0.17	0.214	0.796
10-1074.LS (control)	>25	>25	>25	>25	>25	>25	>25	>25	>25	>25

(B)										
Samples	**C2101.c01**		**C4118.c09**		**THRO4156.18**		**415.v1.c1**		**CNE5**	
	IC50	IC80	IC50	IC80	IC50	IC80	IC50	IC80	IC50	IC80
3BNC117.LS + 10-1074.LS DP	0.029	0.135	0.034	0.162	1.498	8.209	0.05	0.115	0.193	0.898
3BNC117.LS (control)	0.044	0.15	0.051	0.183	1.939	9.815	0.048	0.142	0.193	0.911
10-1074.LS (control)	>25	>25	>25	>25	>25	>25	>25	>25	>25	>25

(C)										
Samples	**1394C9_G1 (Rev-)**		**ZM247v1 (Rev-)**		**Du422.1**		**6631.v3.c10**		**377.v4.c9**	
	IC50	IC80	IC50	IC80	IC50	IC80	IC50	IC80	IC50	IC80
3BNC117.LS + 10-1074.LS DP	0.02	0.077	0.02	0.099	0.032	0.114	0.157	0.796	0.418	1.397
3BNC117.LS (control)	>25	>25	>25	>25	>25	>25	>25	>25	>25	>25
10-1074.LS (control)	0.033	0.119	0.036	0.162	0.045	0.161	0.189	0.968	0.433	1.515

(D)										
Samples	**20915593**		**T278-50**		**21197826-V1**		**Du151.2**		**19715820_A10_H2**	
	IC50	IC80	IC50	IC80	IC50	IC80	IC50	IC80	IC50	IC80
3BNC117-LS + 10-1074-LS DP	1.525	5.872	1.047	11.952	0.678	2.269	0.004	0.013	0.056	0.204
3BNC117-LS (Control)	>25	>25	>25	>25	>25	>25	>25	>25	>25	>25
10-1074-LS (control)	2.02	5.817	2.174	15.13	0.613	2.188	0.005	0.015	0.074	0.253

3.7. Stability Assessment of Co-Formulated Antibodies

To assess the stability of the co-formulated antibodies at high-concentration in the chosen formulation, we performed a 28 day short stability study that included both a real-time stability study in storage conditions (i.e., at 5 ± 3 °C) and a study of samples in accelerated (25 ± 2 °C/RH 60% ± 5%) and stressed (40 ± 2 °C/RH 75% ± 5%) conditions. RH here refers to Relative Humidity.

For the real-time stability study, we used 2.0 mL co-formulated samples in 3.0 mL Schott glass vials and incubated the samples at 5 ± 3 °C. For evaluation at accelerated and stressed conditions, we used similar sample volumes in 3.0 mL Schott vials and incubated them at 25 ± 2 °C/RH 60% ± 5% (accelerated conditions) and 40 ± 2 °C/RH 75% ± 5% (stressed conditions). Samples were analyzed at T = 0, before study start, and thereafter samples were collected on a weekly basis and analyzed for visual appearance, pH, total protein concentration by UV spectroscopy (280 nm), purity (by determining % monomer and HMW aggregates) by SE-HPLC, charge variants (i.e., relative levels of acidic and basic species) by CEX-HPLC, content of individual antibody by RP-HPLC, protein degradation by SDS-PAGE, sub-visible particles by *FlowCAM*® instrument, viscosity by Viscosizer TD, and (hydrodynamic) particle size by DLS. At real-time storage conditions, the antibodies were stable in the co-formulated milieu for up to 4 weeks across all test parameters (Table 2). In addition, the antibodies were also stable in the accelerated conditions, 25 ± 2 °C/RH 60% ± 5%, for up to 4 weeks across all test parameters (Supplementary Table S4). Furthermore, the co-formulated antibodies were stable up to 4 weeks at stressed conditions, 40 ± 2 °C/RH 75% ± 5%, (Supplementary Table S5).

Table 2. Summary of 28 day stability testing results of co-formulated antibodies, 3BNC117-LS and 10-1074-LS (total 150 mg/mL), evaluated at 0, 1, 2, 3, and 4 weeks, after incubation at storage conditions of 5 ± 3 °C. HMW = High Molecular Weight; d.nm = Diameter in nm; PDI = Polydispersity Index; P/mL = Particles/mL.

Test Attributes		Weeks				
		0	1	2	3	4
	pH	5.65	5.6	5.62	5.60	5.59
	A280 (mg/mL)	142	137	142	139	149
	Viscosity (cP)	10.70	11.08	12.09	11.16	12.89
	Osmolality (mOsm/Kg)	345	336	333	336	337
SE-HPLC	HMW (%)	2.98	3.11	3.14	3.58	3.52
	Main Peak (%)	96.90	96.81	96.84	96.41	96.46
CEX-HPLC 3BNC117-LS	Main Peak (%)	48.78	49.08	49.15	49.27	49.71
	Pre-Main Peaks (%)	47.68	46.40	46.04	44.74	44.97
	Post-Main Peaks (%)	3.54	4.52	4.81	5.99	5.32
CEX-HPLC 10-1074-LS	Main Peak (%)	32.68	35.04	35.22	35.99	37.72
	Pre-Main Peaks (%)	61.64	59.70	59.55	59.07	57.45
	Post-Main Peaks (%)	5.68	5.26	5.23	4.94	4.83
RP-HPLC	3BNC117-LS (mg/mL)	68.05	65.88	70.00	68.70	71.48
	10-1074-LS (mg/mL)	76.70	75.75	80.54	78.83	82.09
DLS	Z-Average (d.nm)	10.25	10.44	10.26	10.23	10.30
	PDI	0.18	0.21	0.19	0.18	0.19
FlowCAM	2–10 μm (P/mL)	191	101	253	126	475
	10–25 μm (P/mL)	31	23	46	36	107
	25–50 μm (P/mL)	15	16	8	9	8

In addition to the above analysis, a limited set of samples (T = 2 weeks and T = 4 weeks) from all 3 (real-time, accelerated, and stressed) conditions were tested for potency (functional activity) of the antibodies using pseudovirus neutralization assay. When compared to unincubated co-formulated samples (control) (Table 1A–D), all samples were found to neutralize the pseudoviruses with little to no change in IC50 and 1C80 values and hence found to be stable for up to 4 weeks (Supplementary Table S6A–D). These results indicate not only the utility of the various assays in monitoring antibody stability in the co-formulated sample but also highlight the stability and suitability of the formulation in co-formulating the two antibodies.

This initial stability assessment and identification of appropriate analytical assays support the clinical development of these co-formulated drug products for future clinical studies.

4. Discussion

After the initial evaluation of passive administration of first generation anti-HIV antibodies (4E10+2F5+2G12) [34], the identification of a large number of next-generation anti-HIV bNAbs with greater breadth and potency in the past decade has opened the possibility for antibody-based treatment and/or prevention of HIV-1 infection. Several bNAbs have recently progressed to clinical trials in humans: VRC01 [13,14]/VRC01LS, 10-1074 [15]/10-1074-LS [16], 3BNC117 [17]/3BNC117-LS [18], VRC07-523-LS [19], PGT121 [20,21], and PGDM1400 [21] or their combinations. These early (phase I) clinical studies, with safety, pharmacokinetics, and viral load re-bound or decay as endpoints, have primarily used antibodies formulated for IV infusion. However, to overcome the vast diversity of HIV-1 variants, it is becoming increasingly clear that combinations of (two or more) bNAbs targeting distinct epitopes on the viral envelope (Env) will likely be required [35]. To support the development of bNAb combinations as products for clinical studies, co-formulating two or more antibodies, targeting different Env epitopes, as a single drug product and using a subcutaneous (SC) route for administration, are under consideration in multiple clinical studies. To that end, not only the high-concentration formulation of two or more antibodies in a limited volume will be necessary, but methods to test their individual quality attributes (e.g., purity, charge variants, potency) of the individual antibody in the co-formulated milieu will be required [35].

In this study, two anti-HIV-1 antibodies, 3BNC117-LS and 10-1074-LS, were co-formulated in a 1:1 ratio to achieve a final concentration of 150 mg/mL in 5 mM Histidine, 250 mM Trehalose, 10 mM Methionine, 5 mM Sodium Acetate, 0.05% Polysorbate 20, pH 5.5 buffer. To support the high-concentration formulation and development of the two antibodies for subcutaneous administration, formulation optimizations and analytical test method development and optimizations were performed. Analytical characterization and separation of individual antibodies in the co-formulated sample was challenging due to the high degree of similarity in the physico-chemical properties of the two (3BNC117-LS, and 10-1074-LS) antibodies. Systematic analytical development was carried out, using several methodologies, to obtain separation of the two antibodies. Specifically, chromatographic methods were developed to resolve and assess the quality attributes of the individual antibody in the co-formulated drug product. RP-HPLC and CEX-HPLC methods resulted in baseline separation of the two antibodies (3BNC117-LS and 10-1074-LS) in the co-formulated sample, and the peak profiles compared well to the individually (high-concentration) formulated antibodies. The SE-HPLC method was used to assess the combined high molecular weight species of the two antibodies; the data showed partially separated peaks, corresponding to the two co-formulated antibodies, with no additional % HMW species at this stage. Further evaluation of all HPLC methods for specificity, purity, accuracy, precision, and repeatability confirms that the methods are suitable for future testing of the such co-formulated antibody-based drug product.

In addition to the HPLC methods, an anti-ID ELISA was developed to test identity of the individual antibodies in the co-formulated drug product. In addition, the utilization of a separate and well-defined pseudovirus panel in a virus neutralization assay provided a functional assay platform to not only evaluate the potency/functionality of the individual antibodies but also an approach to test two (or more) antibodies via this functional assay.

In summary, through demonstration of the high-concentration co-formulation of two anti-HIV-1 antibodies and the development of separation-based testing methods, we present several analytical tools to test physico-chemical and functional attributes of co-formulated antibodies, which can contribute to the clinical development of these high-concentration antibodies. Finally, the little to no inter-molecular protein–protein interaction between the antibodies, even at ≥150 mg/mL, and their stability profile ensure the possibility of the development of such high-concentration antibodies as products for HIV prevention and/or treatment.

Supplementary Materials
Table S1: Precision and accuracy of the reverse phase chromatography method during analysis of co-formulated antibodies. Intra- and Inter- assay precision of (A) total peak area (10-1074-LS and 3BNC117-LS peaks), (B) 10-1074-LS-specific peak area and (C) 3BNC117-LS-specific peak area from six replicate runs of co-formulated samples analyzed by reverse phase chromatography. (D) Accuracy determination from percent recovery of a range of co-formulated samples analyzed on three different days (day 1, 2 and 3); Table S2: Precision and accuracy of the cation-exchange chromatography method during analysis of co-formulated antibodies. Intra- and Inter- assay precision of (A) total peak area (10-1074-LS and 3BNC117-LS peaks), (B) 10-1074-LS-specific peak area and (C) 3BNC117-LS-specific peak area from six replicate runs of co-formulated samples analyzed by cation-exchange chromatography. (D) Accuracy determination from percent recovery of a range of co-formulated samples analyzed on three different days (day 1, 2 and 3) for 6 different concentrations (50, 80, 100, 120, 200 and 300 g); Table S3: Precision and accuracy of the size-exclusion chromatography method during analysis of co-formulated antibodies. Intra- and Inter- assay precision of (A) main peak area (10-1074-LS and 3BNC117-LS monomer), (B) High Molecular Weight (HMW) peak area and (C) Low Molecular Weight (LMW) peak area from six replicate runs of co-formulated samples analyzed by size-exclusion chromatography. (D) Accuracy determination from percent recovery of a range of co-formulated samples analyzed on three different days (day 1, 2 and 3) for 6 different concentrations (50, 80, 100, 120, 200 and 300 g); Table S4: Summary of 28-day stability testing results of co-formulated antibodies, 3BNC117-LS and 10-1074-LS (each at 75 mg/mL), evaluated at 0, 1, 2, 3, and 4 weeks, after incubation at accelerated conditions of 25 ± 2 °C/RH 60% ± 5%. HMW = High Molecular Weight; PDI = Polydispersity Index; P/mL = Particles/mL; Table S5: Summary of 28-day stability testing results of co-formulated antibodies, 3BNC117-LS and 10-1074-LS, evaluated at 0, 1, 2, 3, and 4 weeks, after incubation

at stressed conditions of 40 ± 2 °C/75 ± 5% RH. HMW = High Molecular Weight; PDI = Polydispersity Index; P/mL = Particles/mL; Table S6: Testing of functional activity of 3BNC117-LS and 10-1074-LS in the co-formulated samples from the 28-days stability study using pseudovirus neutralization assay. 2 weeks samples (T = 2 weeks) and 4 weeks samples (T = 4 weeks) were selected from all 3 conditions and analyzed against 2 panels of pseudoviruses in TZM-bl cells. One panel (A and B) is used to test functional activity of 3BNC117 [3BNC117 sensitive/10-1074 resistant viruses (n = 10)] and the other panel (C and D) is used to test functional activity of 10-1074 [3BNC117 resistant/10-1074 sensitive viruses (n = 10)]. Both IC50 and IC80 values (in g/mL) are reported.

Author Contributions: A.K.D. and I.J. designed the experiments and strategy. B.M., K.T.M., and K.N. performed the experiments. V.K.S., S.A., K.N., M.C., J.H., M.C.N., M.S.S., I.J., and A.K.D. reviewed the data. V.K.S., B.M., and A.K.D. wrote the manuscript. All authors have read and agreed to the published version of the manuscript.

Acknowledgments: We would like to thank Kirill Yakovlevsky, Charles McneTablemar, and Amina Soukrati (at CuriRx, Inc., 205 Lowell Street, Wilmington, MA 01887, USA) for excellent technical assistance. We are grateful to Pervin Anklesaria and Susan Barnett (BMGF) for their input and support in this project.

References

1. Singh, S.; Kumar, N.K.; Dwiwedi, P.; Charan, J.; Kaur, R.; Sidhu, P.; Chugh, V.K. Monoclonal Antibodies: A Review. *Curr. Clin. Pharmacol.* **2018**, *13*, 85–99. [CrossRef] [PubMed]
2. Marston, H.D.; Paules, C.I.; Fauci, A.S. Monoclonal Antibodies for Emerging Infectious Diseases—Borrowing from History. *N. Engl. J. Med.* **2018**, *378*, 1469–1472. [CrossRef] [PubMed]
3. Walker, L.M.; Burton, D.R. Passive immunotherapy of viral infections: 'super-antibodies' enter the fray. *Nat. Rev. Immunol.* **2018**, *18*, 297–308. [CrossRef] [PubMed]
4. Keeffe, J.R.; Van Rompay, K.K.A.; Olsen, P.C.; Wang, Q.; Gazumyan, A.; Azzopardi, S.A.; Schaefer-Babajew, D.; Lee, Y.E.; Stuart, J.B.; Singapuri, A.; et al. A Combination of Two Human Monoclonal Antibodies Prevents Zika Virus Escape Mutations in Non-human Primates. *Cell Rep.* **2018**, *25*, 1385–1394. [CrossRef] [PubMed]
5. Geevarghese, B.; Simoes, E.A. Antibodies for prevention and treatment of respiratory syncytial virus infections in children. *Antivir. Ther.* **2012**, *17*, 201–211. [CrossRef] [PubMed]
6. Bittner, B.; Richter, W.; Schmidt, J. Subcutaneous Administration of Biotherapeutics: An Overview of Current Challenges and Opportunities. *BioDrugs* **2018**, *32*, 425–440. [CrossRef]
7. Stoner, K.L.; Harder, H.; Fallowfield, L.J.; Jenkins, V.A. Intravenous versus subcutaneous drug administration. Which do patients prefer? A systematic review. *Patient* **2015**, *8*, 145–153. [CrossRef]
8. Stephenson, K.E.; Barouch, D.H. Broadly Neutralizing Antibodies for HIV Eradication. *Curr. HIV/AIDS Rep.* **2016**, *13*, 31–37. [CrossRef]
9. Pegu, A.; Hessell, A.J.; Mascola, J.R.; Haigwood, N.L. Use of broadly neutralizing antibodies for HIV-1 prevention. *Immunol. Rev.* **2017**, *275*, 296–312. [CrossRef]
10. Kwong, P.D.; Mascola, J.R. HIV-1 Vaccines Based on Antibody Identification, B Cell Ontogeny, and Epitope Structure. *Immunity* **2018**, *48*, 855–871. [CrossRef]
11. McMichael, A.J.; Haynes, B.F. Lessons learned from HIV-1 vaccine trials: New priorities and directions. *Nat. Immunol.* **2012**, *13*, 423–427. [CrossRef] [PubMed]
12. Haynes, B.F.; McElrath, M.J. Progress in HIV-1 vaccine development. *Curr. Opin. HIV AIDS* **2013**, *8*, 326–332. [CrossRef] [PubMed]
13. Ledgerwood, J.E.; Coates, E.E.; Yamshchikov, G.; Saunders, J.G.; Holman, L.; Enama, M.E.; DeZure, A.; Lynch, R.M.; Gordon, I.; Plummer, S.; et al. Safety, pharmacokinetics and neutralization of the broadly neutralizing HIV-1 human monoclonal antibody VRC01 in healthy adults. *Clin. Exp. Immunol.* **2015**, *182*, 289–301. [CrossRef] [PubMed]
14. Lynch, R.M.; Boritz, E.; Coates, E.E.; DeZure, A.; Madden, P.; Costner, P.; Enama, M.E.; Plummer, S.; Holman, L.; Hendel, C.S.; et al. Virologic effects of broadly neutralizing antibody VRC01 administration during chronic HIV-1 infection. *Sci. Transl. Med.* **2015**, *7*, 319ra206. [CrossRef]
15. Caskey, M.; Schoofs, T.; Gruell, H.; Settler, A.; Karagounis, T.; Kreider, E.F.; Murrell, B.; Pfeifer, N.; Nogueira, L.; Oliveira, T.Y.; et al. Antibody 10-1074 suppresses viremia in HIV-1-infected individuals. *Nat. Med.* **2017**, *23*, 185–191. [CrossRef]

16. First-in-human Study of 10-1074-LS Alone and in Combination with 3BNC117-LS. Available online: https: //clinicaltrials.gov/ct2/show/NCT03554408 (accessed on 28 July 2020).

17. Scheid, J.F.; Horwitz, J.A.; Bar-On, Y.; Kreider, E.F.; Lu, C.L.; Lorenzi, J.C.; Feldmann, A.; Braunschweig, M.; Nogueira, L.; Oliveira, T.; et al. HIV-1 antibody 3BNC117 suppresses viral rebound in humans during treatment interruption. *Nature* **2016**, *535*, 556–560. [CrossRef]

18. 3BNC117-LS First-in-Human Phase 1 Study. Available online: https://clinicaltrials.gov/ct2/show/ NCT03254277 (accessed on 28 July 2020).

19. Evaluating the Safety and Pharmacokinetics of VRC01, VRC01LS, and VRC07-523LS, Potent Anti-HIV Neutralizing Monoclonal Antibodies, in HIV-1-Exposed Infants. Available online: https://clinicaltrials.gov/ ct2/show/NCT02256631 (accessed on 28 July 2020).

20. Safety, PK and Antiviral Activity of PGT121 Monoclonal Antibody in HIV-uninfected and HIV-infected Adults. Available online: https://clinicaltrials.gov/ct2/show/NCT02960581 (accessed on 28 July 2020).

21. A Clinical Trial of PGDM1400 and PGT121 and VRC07-523LS Monoclonal Antibodies in HIV-infected and HIV-uninfected Adults. Available online: https://clinicaltrials.gov/ct2/show/NCT03205917 (accessed on 28 July 2020).

22. Bar-On, Y.; Gruell, H.; Schoofs, T.; Pai, J.A.; Nogueira, L.; Butler, A.L.; Millard, K.; Lehmann, C.; Suarez, I.; Oliveira, T.Y.; et al. Safety and antiviral activity of combination HIV-1 broadly neutralizing antibodies in viremic individuals. *Nat. Med.* **2018**, *24*, 1701–1707. [CrossRef]

23. Mendoza, P.; Gruell, H.; Nogueira, L.; Pai, J.A.; Butler, A.L.; Millard, K.; Lehmann, C.; Suarez, I.; Oliveira, T.Y.; Lorenzi, J.C.C.; et al. Combination therapy with anti-HIV-1 antibodies maintains viral suppression. *Nature* **2018**, *561*, 479–484. [CrossRef]

24. Halper-Stromberg, A.; Nussenzweig, M.C. Towards HIV-1 remission: Potential roles for broadly neutralizing antibodies. *J. Clin. Investig.* **2016**, *126*, 415–423. [CrossRef]

25. Mueller, C.; Altenburger, U.; Mohl, S. Challenges for the pharmaceutical technical development of protein coformulations. *J. Pharm. Pharmacol.* **2018**, *70*, 666–674. [CrossRef]

26. Cao, M.; De Mel, N.; Shannon, A.; Prophet, M.; Wang, C.; Xu, W.; Niu, B.; Kim, J.; Albarghouthi, M.; Liu, D.; et al. Charge variants characterization and release assay development for co-formulated antibodies as a combination therapy. *MAbs* **2019**, *11*, 489–499. [CrossRef] [PubMed]

27. Patel, A.; Gupta, V.; Hickey, J.; Nightlinger, N.S.; Rogers, R.S.; Siska, C.; Joshi, S.B.; Seaman, M.S.; Volkin, D.B.; Kerwin, B.A. Coformulation of Broadly Neutralizing Antibodies 3BNC117 and PGT121: Analytical Challenges During Preformulation Characterization and Storage Stability Studies. *J. Pharm. Sci.* **2018**, *107*, 3032–3046. [CrossRef] [PubMed]

28. Ko, S.Y.; Pegu, A.; Rudicell, R.S.; Yang, Z.Y.; Joyce, M.G.; Chen, X.; Wang, K.; Bao, S.; Kraemer, T.D.; Rath, T.; et al. Enhanced neonatal Fc receptor function improves protection against primate SHIV infection. *Nature* **2014**, *514*, 642–645. [CrossRef] [PubMed]

29. Zalevsky, J.; Chamberlain, A.K.; Horton, H.M.; Karki, S.; Leung, I.W.; Sproule, T.J.; Lazar, G.A.; Roopenian, D.C.; Desjarlais, J.R. Enhanced antibody half-life improves in vivo activity. *Nat. Biotechnol.* **2010**, *28*, 157–159. [CrossRef]

30. Montefiori, D.C. Measuring HIV neutralization in a luciferase reporter gene assay. *Methods Mol. Biol.* **2009**, *485*, 395–405.

31. Sarzotti-Kelsoe, M.; Bailer, R.T.; Turk, E.; Lin, C.L.; Bilska, M.; Greene, K.M.; Gao, H.; Todd, C.A.; Ozaki, D.A.; Seaman, M.S.; et al. Optimization and validation of the TZM-bl assay for standardized assessments of neutralizing antibodies against HIV-1. *J. Immunol. Methods* **2014**, *409*, 131–146. [CrossRef]

32. Fekete, S.; Beck, A.; Fekete, J.; Guillarme, D. Method development for the separation of monoclonal antibody charge variants in cation exchange chromatography, Part II: pH gradient approach. *J. Pharm. Biomed. Anal.* **2015**, *102*, 282–289. [CrossRef]

33. Fekete, S.; Beck, A.; Fekete, J.; Guillarme, D. Method development for the separation of monoclonal antibody charge variants in cation exchange chromatography, Part I: Salt gradient approach. *J. Pharm. Biomed. Anal.* **2015**, *102*, 33–44. [CrossRef]

34. Armbruster, C.; Stiegler, G.M.; Vcelar, B.A.; Jager, W.; Koller, U.; Jilch, R.; Ammann, C.G.; Pruenster, M.; Stoiber, H.; Katinger, H.W. Passive immunization with the anti-HIV-1 human monoclonal antibody (hMAb) 4E10 and the hMAb combination 4E10/2F5/2G12. *J. Antimicrob. Chemother.* **2004**, *54*, 915–920. [CrossRef]

35. Wagh, K.; Bhattacharya, T.; Williamson, C.; Robles, A.; Bayne, M.; Garrity, J.; Rist, M.; Rademeyer, C.; Yoon, H.; Lapedes, A.; et al. Optimal Combinations of Broadly Neutralizing Antibodies for Prevention and Treatment of HIV-1 Clade C Infection. *PLoS Pathog.* **2016**, *12*, e1005520. [CrossRef]

9

Generation and Performance of R132H Mutant IDH1 Rabbit Monoclonal Antibody

Juliet Rashidian, Raul Copaciu †, Qin Su †, Brett Merritt, Claire Johnson, Aril Yahyabeik, Ella French and Kelsea Cummings *

MilliporeSigma, 6600 Sierra College Blvd, Rocklin, CA 95677, USA; jrashidian@sial.com (J.R.); raul.copaciu@sial.com (R.C.); qin.su@sial.com (Q.S.); bmerritt@sial.com (B.M.); claire.johnson@sial.com (C.J.); ayahyabeik@sial.com (A.Y.); ella.french@sial.com (E.F.)
* Correspondence: kcummings@sial.com
† These authors contributed equally to this paper.

Abstract: Isocitrate dehydrogenase 1 (IDH1) gene mutations have been observed in a majority of diffuse astrocytomas, oligodendrogliomas, and secondary glioblastomas, and the mutant IDH1 R132H is detectable in most of these lesions. By specifically targeting the R132H mutation through B-cell cloning, a novel rabbit monoclonal antibody, MRQ-67, was produced that can recognize mutant IDH1 R132H and does not react with the wild type protein as demonstrated by Enzyme-linked immunosorbent assay (ELISA) and Western blotting. Through immunohistochemistry, the antibody is able to highlight neoplastic cells in glioma tissue specimens, and can be used as a tool in glioma subtyping. Immunohistochemistry (IHC) detection of IDH1 mutant protein may also be used to visualize single infiltrating tumor cells in surrounding brain tissue with an otherwise normal appearance.

Keywords: IDH1; R132H; novel rabbit monoclonal antibody; B-cell cloning; immunohistochemistry

1. Introduction

Isocitrate dehydrogenase 1 (IDH1) functions as an enzyme in the Krebs (citric acid) cycle and is biologically active in the cytoplasmic and peroxisomal compartments under normal conditions [1]. Somatic mutations in the gene that encodes IDH1 have been reported to be present in some glioma subtypes in high frequencies. The majority of these particular tumors have been found to harbor heterozygous point mutations in codon 132, with a missense amino acid substitution of arginine to histidine (R132H) being observed to have highest rate of occurrence [2]. The high incidence of glioma-specific IDH1 mutations has implicated them as an early event that occurs during gliomagenesis and provides utility in distinguishing low grade astrocytomas and oligodendrogliomas, as well as secondary glioblastomas from reactive gliosis and primary glioblastomas [3]. The value of this mutant marker is further illustrated by the 2016 World Health Organization (WHO) Classification of Tumors of the Central Nervous System that newly incorporates IDH1 mutation status as a parameter for sub-classifying diffuse astrocytic and oligodendroglial tumors [4]. While genetic testing can be burdensome, a clinically established routine procedure like immunohistochemistry (IHC), using a specific monoclonal antibody directed against IDH1 R132H mutant protein, represents a useful tool for overcoming this diagnostic challenge.

This study describes the generation and performance of a novel rabbit monoclonal IDH1 R132H antibody (MRQ-67) by single B-cell cloning technology, a recently emerging strategy for monoclonal antibody development [5]. The capacity of MRQ-67 to identify mutant IDH1 R132H without reacting with wild type protein is demonstrated through binding specificity assays. The functional utility of the antibody to specifically detect mutant IDH1 protein in astrocytomas, oligodendrogliomas, and glioblastomas is also examined through immunohistochemical analysis.

2. Materials and Methods

2.1. Tissue Specimens

Immunohistochemical evaluation of MRQ-67 performance was assessed using formalin-fixed, paraffin-embedded (FFPE) tissue specimens, which included 18 cases of astrocytoma, 7 cases of oligodendroglioma, 7 cases of glioblastoma, 12 cases of meningioma, and 15 cases of non-neoplastic brain tissue. The FFPE tissue specimens used in this study were procured, qualified, and tested in accordance with the U.S. Food and Drug Administration (FDA) "Guidance on Informed Consent for In Vitro Diagnostic Device Studies Using Leftover Human Specimens that are Not Individually Identifiable". This study exclusively used leftover tissue specimens that are not individually identifiable for conducting IHC testing. More specifically, these are remnants of human specimens collected for routine clinical care or analysis that would have otherwise been discarded and where the identity of the subject is not known to, or may not be readily ascertained by, any individual associated with this study.

2.2. Immunization

New Zealand White Rabbits were immunized with synthetic peptide CKPIIIGHHAYGD coupled to Keyhole limpet hemocyanin (KLH) corresponding the amino acids 126 to 137 of the human IDH1 containing R132H mutation. All of the housing and immunization procedures were performed by Antibodies Incorporated (Antibodies Inc., Davis, CA, USA), according to the approved protocols and guidelines of the Institutional Animal Care and Use Committee (IACUC). The project numbers were 5834 and 5835 under IACUC protocol 0298-9 "Custom Polyclonal Antibody Production in Rabbits", approved on 1 July 2016 (PHS Assurance number A4064-01).

2.3. Isolation and Sorting of Rabbit B-Cells

Peripheral blood mononuclear cells (PBMCs) were isolated from the ethylenediaminetetraacetic acid (EDTA) containing peripheral blood by density-gradient centrifugation with Lympholyte-Mammal (Cedarlane, Burlington, NC, USA), as described in the manual. The isolated PBMCs (10^7 cells) were next washed with RPMI (Life Technologies, Carlsbad, CA, USA) containing DNase I (Roche, Basel, Switzerland) and re-suspended in phosphate-buffered saline (PBS) containing 0.5% bovine serum albumin (BSA). Then, the IgG expressing B-cells were isolated using Anti-Rabbit IgG Microbeads (Miltenyi Biotech, Auburn, CA, USA).

The isolated B-cells were stained for viability, incubated with a cocktail of anti-rabbit IgG and fluorochrome-conjugated specific peptide in the dark for 30 min at 4 °C, and washed with ice-cold PBS. Finally, cells were re-suspended in PBS and subjected to Fluorescence Activated Cell Sorting (FACS) analyses. Sorting was carried out using BD Influx Cell Sorter and BD FACS DIVA software (UC Davis Medical Center, Sacramento, CA, USA). Single B-cells expressing IgG were sorted into a 96-well plate (omitting row H).

2.4. Cloning Antibody Variable Regions

Single-cell reverse transcription polymerase chain reaction (RT-PCR) was performed with reverse transcriptase Superscript III First-Strand Synthesis system (Life Technologies, Carlsbad, CA, USA). Next, the RT-PCR reaction mixtures were used for subsequent polymerase chain reaction (PCR) reactions to amplify variable regions of IgG heavy chain (V_H) and light chain (V_L). The V_H and V_L were separately cloned in pTrans-CMV-MCS expression vectors (CEVEC, Köln, Germany) containing constant region coding sequences for rabbit IgG γ and IgG κ.

2.5. Transfection

Primary human amniocytes CAP-T cells (CEVEC, Köln, Germany) were transiently co-transfected with vectors containing the codon sequences of heavy chain and light chain originating from the same sorted cell using NovaCHOice® transfection kit (MilliporeSigma, Billerica, MA, USA), and the supernatants were harvested after seven days for evaluation by Enzyme-linked immunosorbent assay (ELISA), Western blotting, and IHC.

2.6. ELISA

The concentration of the IgG released by transfected cells was measured using Rabbit IgG ELISA kit (ZeptoMetrix Corp., Franklin, MA, USA). Serial dilutions of a rabbit IgG antibody (60, 30, 15, 7.5, 3.75, and 0 ng/mL), provided by the kit, were used to set up a standard curve. The specificity of the antibody was determined by immobilizing biotinylated synthetic peptides (provided by Antibodies Inc., Davis, CA, USA) KPIIIGHHAYGD (mutant) or KPIIIGRHAYGD (wild type) on a 96-well plate. The plate was coated with 2 µg/mL streptavidin (MilliporeSigma, Billerica, MA, USA) overnight at 4 °C and then the peptides were immobilized at 1 µg/mL for one hour at room temperature. After blocking with 5% skim milk for an hour, the plate was probed with the supernatant of transfected cells or a commercially available mouse monoclonal IDH1 R132H H09 antibody (Dianova, Hamburg, Germany) at different concentrations, starting from 1 µg/mL and lower and incubated for an hour at 37 °C. Next, a peroxidase-conjugated anti-rabbit IgG anibody (Jackson ImmunoResearch Lab, West Grove, PA, USA) (1:1000) was added to the plate and incubated for an hour at room temperature. The enzymatic reaction was conducted with Tetramethylbenzidine (TMB) (MilliporeSigma, Billerica, MA, USA) at room temperature and stopped by 0.25 M Sulfuric acid (MilliporeSigma, Billerica, MA, USA). The optical density was measured at 450 nm. The plate was washed four times after every step with PBS containing 0.05% Tween 20 (MilliporeSigma, Billerica, MA, USA).

2.7. Western Blotting

100 ng of recombinant human IDH1 R132H protein and wild type IDH1 protein (Abcam, Cambridge, MA, USA) were loaded onto 4–12% Bis-Tris mini gels (Life Technologies, Carlsbad, CA, USA) and blotted to PVDF membranes (iBlot™ Transfer Stack, PVDF, Invitrogen, Carlsbad, CA, USA). The Western blot was carried out using WesternBreeze Chromogenic kit (Invitrogen, Carlsbad, CA, USA) and the supernatant of the transfected cells (0.5 µg/mL IgG) or H09 (0.5 µg/mL antibody) were used to probe the membranes.

2.8. Immunohistochemistry

FFPE tissue samples were sectioned at a thickness of 4 µm and were prepared on Superfrost™ Plus microscope slides (Fisherbrand™, Pittsburgh, PA, USA). Prepared slides were stained by routine IHC on a BenchMark ULTRA automated staining instrument (Ventana Medical Systems Inc., Tucson, AZ, USA). Tissue slides were incubated for 64 min at 95 °C using an EDTA-based epitope retrieval solution, followed by a 32 min primary antibody incubation at 36 °C. Staining signal was visualized through a horseradish peroxidase (HRP)-based multimer detection system and 3-3'-Diaminobenzidine (DAB) chromogen. Counterstaining was performed by incubating tissue slides for 4 min with Hematoxylin II, followed by a 4 min incubation with bluing reagent. Stained slides were evaluated using light microscopy for target signal intensity and background signal by a qualified pathologist. Tumor cells exhibiting a strong, diffuse cytoplasmic staining pattern, as well as weaker nuclear labeling, were scored as positive for IDH1 mutant protein. The H09 antibody was used as a reference comparison during performance testing of the antisera from immunized rabbits and optimization of the selected MRQ-67 clone. The H09 clone further served in establishing the IDH1 R132H mutation status of glioma samples that were used in this study. The same automated staining conditions were used for both the MRQ-67 and H09 clones, with optimal antibody titers having been experimentally determined for each clone individually. The MRQ-67 and H09 clones were determined to perform optimally in IHC at concentrations of 2.54 μg/mL and 3.25 μg/mL, respectively.

3. Results

Four rabbits were immunized with the synthetic IDH1 R132H mutant peptide. Sera from immunized rabbits were tested by IHC. The PBMCs from the rabbit with the best immune response were isolated for cloning of V_H and V_L, followed by co-transfection in CAP-T cells.

ELISA analyses of the transfection reactions confirmed the production of rabbit IgG by 73% of the clones (Figure 1a). The positive clones were further screened for specificity of the antibodies and among them, antibody MRQ-67 generated by clone C5 was selected for further evaluations. As shown in Figure 1b, the MRQ-67 antibody specifically reacted with mutant peptide IDH1 R132H in a dose-dependent manner, but not with the wild type peptide IDH1 in ELISA assay, indicating that MRQ-67 specifically recognized IDH1 R132H. This result was consistent with the result obtained using the control antibody, H09 (Figure 1b).

(a)

	1	2	3	4	5	6	7	8	9	10	11	12
A	22.2	16.4	0.0	11.0	22.9	0.0	17.7	18.3	19.2	11.9	1.7	6.5
B	6.5	15.1	11.8	12.2	18.5	0.0	21.1	31.3	20.1	22.7	0.0	16.8
C	29.7	0.0	24.6	15.7	23.3	21.2	36.9	14.8	19.4	0.0	0.0	11.9
D	23.4	18.2	0.0	0.0	17.9	22.9	7.8	30.5	13.8	13.6	22.4	0.0
E	4.0	37.2	5.5	0.0	9.6	0.0	34.6	9.7	21.4	19.2	0.0	18.9
F	18.2	30.6	22.8	34.7	2.9	40.2	10.6	0.0	0.0	0.0	20.1	11.9
G	10.2	0.0	12	0.0	29.6	23.8	0.0	20.5	0.0	0.0	0.0	13
H	EW	EW	EW	EW	EW	EW	EW	EW	EW	EW	EW	EW

Concentration of rabbit IgG (μg/mL)
EW: Empty Well

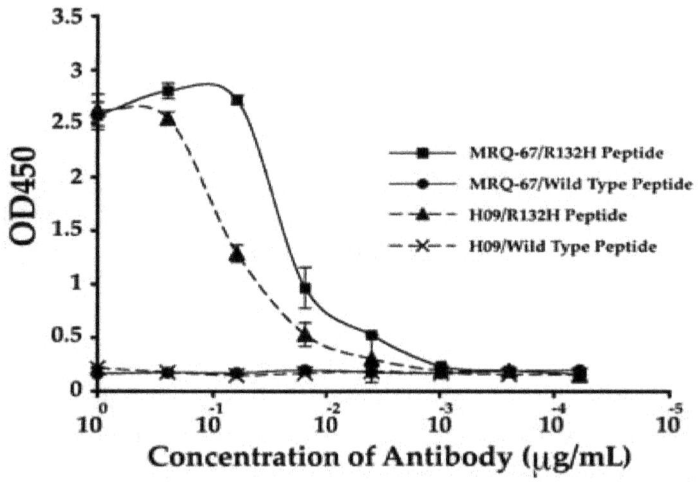

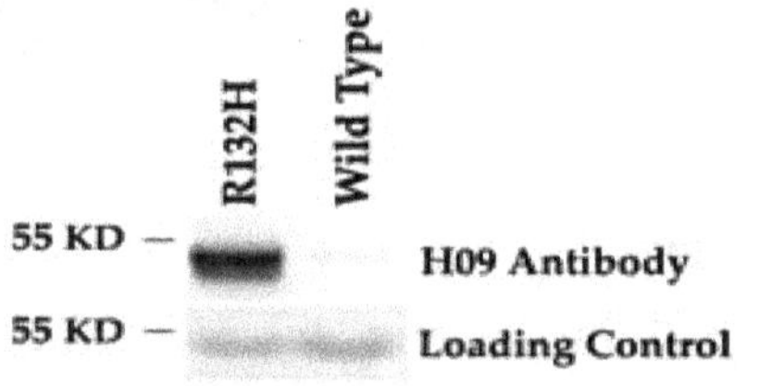

Figure 1. Generation and performance of rabbit monoclonal MRQ-67 antibody against IDH1 R132H and comparing its function with the H09 antibody by Enzyme-linked immunosorbent assay (ELISA) and Western blotting assays: (**a**) The concentration of antibody generated by clones was measured in μg/mL by rabbit IgG ELISA kit; (**b**) Peptide binding ELISA. MRQ-67 antibody specifically recognized only mutant IDH1 R132H peptide and not wild type IDH1 peptide. The ELISA binding assay result for the H09 antibody has been included as a control; (**c**,**d**) Analysis of MRQ-67 and H09 for detecting recombinant human IDH1 R132H and recombinant human IDH1 wild type proteins in Western blotting. MRQ-67 (**c**) and H09 (**d**) antibodies (0.5 μg/mL) were used to probe the membranes. Coomassie blue stainings of the proteins are shown as loading control.

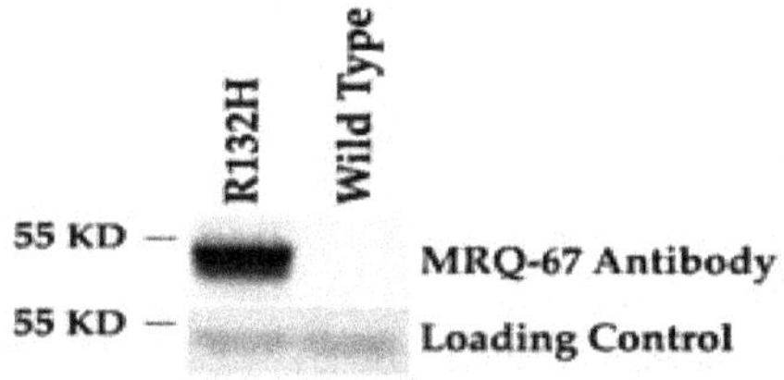

The MRQ-67 antibody's specificity was further analyzed by Western blotting and compared with the specificity of H09 antibody. As shown in Figure 1c,d, MRQ-67 and H09 both detected the recombinant IDH1 R132H protein at a predicted molecular weight of 48 kDa for human IDH1 protein. Notably, while MRQ-67 antibody did not detect any band on the blot with wild type recombinant IDH1 protein (Figure 1c), the H09 antibody showed a weak reaction with this protein (Figure 1d). Overall, this data indicates that MRQ-67 is also useful in detecting not only IDH1 R132H peptide, but also the mutant IDH1 R132H protein.

To further characterize the rabbit IDH1 R132H monoclonal antibody, the capacity of the MRQ-67 antibody to immunohistochemically identify IDH1 mutant protein in FFPE tissues was investigated. The IHC staining results summarized in Table 1 demonstrate equivalent sensitivity and specificity performance of the MRQ-67 clone in comparison to H09 for distinguishing low grade gliomas from glioblastomas, meningiomas, and benign brain samples. The MRQ-67 clone generated strong, diffuse cytoplasmic staining with weaker nuclear reactivity in 50% of the diffuse and anaplastic astrocytomas (Figure 2a) that was equivalent to performance observed with H09 (Figure 2b). Positive tumor staining in 71% of oligodendroglioma samples by MRQ-67 was primarily demonstrated by cytoplasmic reactivity (Figure 3a) and was comparable to observed results from H09 testing (Figure 3b). From the seven high grade glioblastoma cases that were tested, only one reacted positively with MRQ-67 as indicated by weakly diffuse cytoplasmic and nuclear staining (Figure 4a), while no tumor cells were labeled in the rest of the tested cases (Figure 4b).

Table 1. IDH1 R132H immunohistochemistry (IHC) staining data. Summary of IHC staining results comparing the number of cases stained positive out of the total number of cases tested with the MRQ-67 and H09 clones.

Tissue	Cases Stained (MRQ-67)	Cases Stained (H09)
Astrocytoma	9/18 (50%)	9/18 (50%)
Oligodendroglioma	5/7 (71%)	5/7 (71%)
Gliobastoma	1/7 (14%)	1/7 (14%)
Meningioma	0/12	0/12
Non-neoplastic Brain	0/15	0/15

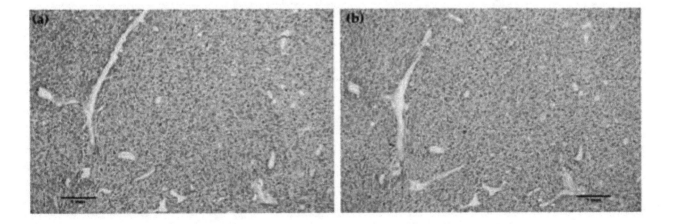

Figure 2. Comparison immunohistochemistry (IHC) staining results with MRQ-67 and H09 in astrocytoma: (**a**) Strong, diffuse cytoplasmic and weak nuclear labeling of tumor cells with MRQ-67 in a case of anaplastic astrocytoma (100×); (**b**) Equivalent cytoplasmic and nuclear staining of tumor cells with H09 in the same case of astrocytoma (100×).

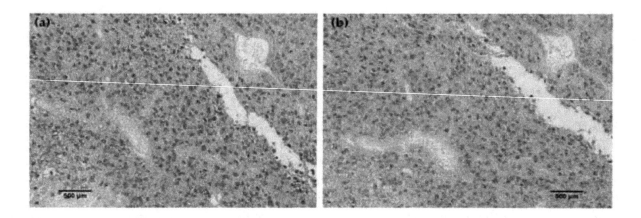

Figure 3. Comparison immunohistochemistry (IHC) staining results with MRQ-67 and H09 in oligodendroglioma: (**a**) Strong cytoplasmic and weak nuclear labeling of tumor cells with MRQ-67 in a case of WHO grade II oligodendroglioma (200×); (**b**) Comparable cytoplasmic and nuclear staining of tumor cells with H09 in the same case of oligodendroglioma (200×).

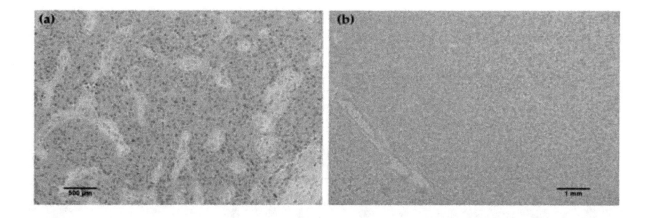

Figure 4. MRQ-67 immunohistochemistry (IHC) staining results in high grade glioblastoma: (**a**) Weak, diffuse cytoplasmic and nuclear labeling of tumor cells in a case of WHO grade IV glioblastoma with anaplastic astrocytoma involvement (200×); (**b**) No observed reactivity in tumor cells in another case of WHO grade IV glioblastoma (100×).

In all cancerous and benign brain samples tested, the MRQ-67 antibody did not react with endothelial cells, lymphocytic cells, or normal glial cells. The 15 cases of benign brain (Figure 5a,b) and 12 cases of meningioma (Figure 6c,d) that were assessed displayed no observable cross-reactivity, with only two cases (16%) of meningioma demonstrating equivocal background staining signal when tested using MRQ-67. However, meningioma samples stained with the H09 clone generated nonspecific background signal in fibrillar and spindle cell components in 11 out of 12 cases (92%), with 4 cases (33%) in particular developing notably strong background staining (Figure 6a,b). One particular case of benign brain was observed to have a small focus of tumor cells that was identified by anti-IDH1 R132H (Figure 7a). Importantly, the surrounding distal nervous tissue was identified to consist of single infiltrative tumor cells that exhibited strong positive reactivity (Figure 7b).

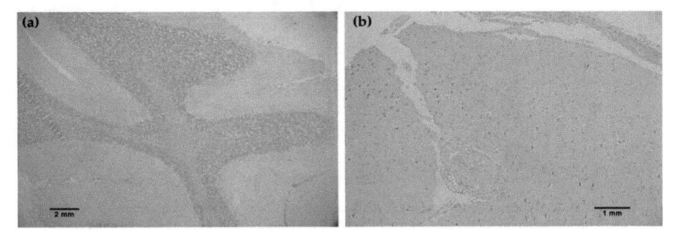

Figure 5. MRQ-67 immunohistochemistry (IHC) staining results in normal brain: (**a**) No observed reactivity in the normal cell types that constitute the gray and white matter in the cerebellar region of the brain (40×); (**b**) No observed reactivity in normal cerebral nervous tissue (100×).

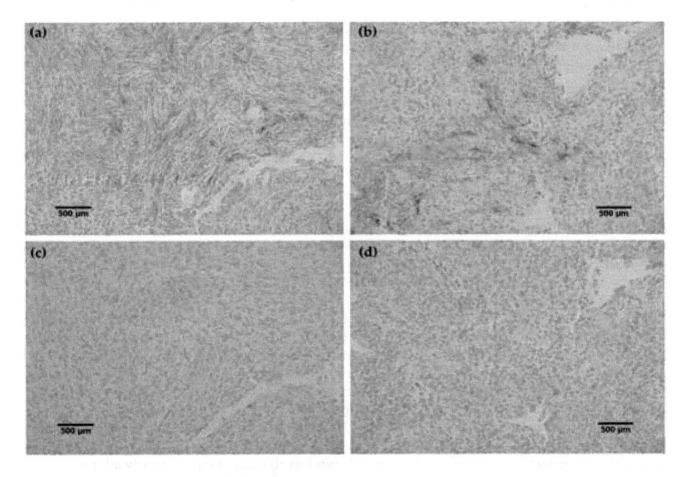

Figure 6. Comparison immunohistochemistry (IHC) staining results of MRQ-67 and H09 in meningioma specimens: (**a**) The H09 clone displayed positive reactivity in spindle cells of a meningioma sample (200×); (**b**) Positive labeling of fine fibrous elements by the H09 clone in another case of meningioma (200×); (**c**) The MRQ-67 clone demonstrated no cross-reactivity with spindle cells in the same meningioma case stained with the H09 clone (200×); (**d**) MRQ-67 also did not generate cross-reaction with fibrous elements as was observed with H09 staining in the same case of meningioma (200×).

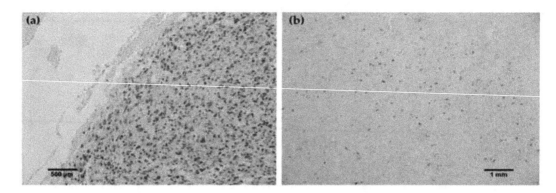

Figure 7. MRQ-67 immunohistochemistry (IHC) staining results in a primarily benign brain sample with a small tumor focus and some scattered tumor cells: (**a**) Cytoplasmic and weak nuclear labeling of cells within a small tumor focus of a benign brain sample (200×); (**b**) Scattered reactivity in single infiltrative tumor cells of the same benign brain case that have dispersed from the focal tumor site (100×).

4. Discussion

In the specific targeting of the IDH1 R132H mutation through B-cell cloning, a novel rabbit monoclonal antibody was produced that promises to be a useful tool for overcoming the diagnostic challenge of differentiating between different subtypes of glioma. The single B-cell cloning technology used to generate MRQ-67 is an attractive method for developing high quality monoclonal antibodies that has several advantages over previously established techniques. This technology is more efficient than cell fusion in hybridoma technique [6], and unlike display methods (e.g., phage display [7] and yeast surface display [8]), both heavy and light chains originate from a single sorted cell. This allows for the natural cognate pairing of the heavy and light chains to be preserved during synthesis and maturation of the antibody [5]. Moreover, culturing of isolated B-cells is not required, which removes a potential source of technical complications from the process.

In ELISA assays and Western blotting analyses, the MRQ-67 rabbit monoclonal antibody reacted with mutant IDH1 R132H, but not with wild type IDH1. This data indicates that MRQ-67 is capable of specifically detecting not only IDH1 R132H peptide, but also the mutant IDH1 R132H protein without cross-reacting with wild type IDH1. The specificity of MRQ-67 to the R132H mutation had not been tested against other less frequent mutations of IDH1 at the time of this report.

Identification of IDH1 mutation status by IHC presents a useful tool for many diagnostic institutions where genetic testing can be burdensome and may be inaccurate, especially regarding tissue samples with low tumor cell content. Detection by IHC provides the opportunity to visualize even single infiltrating tumor cells in otherwise normal appearing brain tissue. The IDH1 status of FFPE tissue samples used in this study had not been determined by sequencing at the time of this report. IDH1 mutation status of these tissues was therefore established through the use of the commercially available mouse monoclonal IDH1 R132H (H09) antibody.

Rabbit monoclonal anti-IDH1 R132H (MRQ-67) labeled each of the same cases as H09, indicating comparable ability to detect IDH1 mutant protein by IHC. However, the H09 clone generated nonspecific background signals in the fibrillar and spindle cell components in nearly all meningioma cases tested, with a few cases in particular developing notably strong background staining. The observed cross-reaction with fibrous elements in meningioma cases has been previously identified as nonspecific binding by anti-IDH1 R132H to extracellular matrix protein or a subtype of collagen fiber [9]. Staining with the MRQ-67 clone demonstrated only two instances of weak, nonspecific background signal in meningioma samples, indicating a particular advantage in specificity compared to the H09 clone. Since no immunoreaction was observed in meningioma tumor cells or normal brain samples, all tumor cells that stained are considered to be IDH1 mutant-positive, including the single infiltrating cells that dispersed from the primary tumor focus as seen in Figure 7.

The presence of IDH1 mutations has been indicated to be much more frequent in secondary glioblastomas compared to primary glioblastomas [10]. Clinical information regarding the progression of the single case of glioblastoma in this study with identified mutant IDH1 staining signal was not available, but histopathological evidence of lower grade glioma involvement was observed. Further, population-based data indicates a considerably greater incidence rate of primary glioblastoma compared to that of secondary glioblastoma [11]. These observations, together with H09 comparison staining data in glioblastoma samples, suggest that MRQ-67 functions as intended for IHC applications.

Overall, the results from ELISA assays, Western blotting, and IHC analyses support the proposed utility of the novel rabbit monoclonal MRQ-67 antibody in the identification of mutated human IDH1 protein. IDH1 (MRQ-67) rabbit monoclonal antibody is a specific marker for immunohistochemical detection of IDH1 mutant protein in glioma subtypes and may have value as a tool in distinguishing between diffuse astrocytomas and oligodendrogliomas from secondary glioblastoma.

Acknowledgments: We would like to acknowledge Maricela Linhares for her support in preparing cell cultures.

Author Contributions: J.R. conceived and designed the experiments; J.R., R.C., B.M., A.Y., and E.F. performed the experiments; J.R., Q.S., and R.C. analyzed the data; J.R., R.C., K.C., and C.J. wrote the paper.

References

1. Guo, C.; Pirozzi, C.J.; Lopez, G.Y.; Yan, H. Isocitrate dehydrogenase mutations in gliomas: Mechanisms, biomarkers and therapeutic target. *Curr. Opin. Neurol.* **2011**, *24*, 648–652. [CrossRef] [PubMed]
2. Balss, J.; Meyer, J.; Mueller, W.; Korshunov, A.; Hartmann, C.; von Deimling, A. Analysis of the IDH1 codon 132 mutation in brain tumors. *Acta Neuropathol.* **2008**, *116*, 597–602. [CrossRef] [PubMed]
3. Watanabe, T.; Nobusawa, S.; Kleihues, P.; Ohgaki, H. IDH1 mutations are early events in the development of astrocytomas and oligodendrogliomas. *Am. J. Pathol.* **2009**, *174*, 1149–1153. [CrossRef] [PubMed]
4. Louis, D.N.; Perry, A.; Reifenberger, G.; von Deimling, A.; Figarella-Branger, D.; Cavenee, W.K.; Ohgaki, H.; Wiestler, O.D.; Kleihues, P.; Ellison, D.W. The 2016 World Health Organization Classification of Tumors of the Central Nervous System: A summary. *Acta Neuropathol.* **2016**, *131*, 803–820. [CrossRef] [PubMed]
5. Zhang, Z.; Liu, H.; Guan, Q.; Wang, L.; Yuan, H. Advances in the Isolation of Specific Monoclonal Rabbit Antibodies. *Front. Immunol.* **2017**, *8*, 494. [CrossRef] [PubMed]
6. Kohler, G.; Milstein, C. Continuous cultures of fused cells secreting antibody of predefined specificity. *Nature* **1975**, *256*, 495–497. [CrossRef] [PubMed]
7. Smith, G.P. Filamentous fusion phage: Novel expression vectors that display cloned antigens on the virion surface. *Science* **1985**, *228*, 1315–1317. [CrossRef] [PubMed]
8. Murai, T.; Ueda, M.; Yamamura, M.; Atomi, H.; Shibasaki, Y.; Kamasawa, N.; Osumi, M.; Amachi, T.; Tanaka, A. Construction of a starch-utilizing yeast by cell surface engineering. *Appl. Environ. Microbiol.* **1997**, *63*, 1362–1366. [PubMed]
9. Capper, D.; Weissert, S.; Balss, J.; Habel, A.; Meyer, J.; Jager, D.; Ackermann, U.; Tessmer, C.; Korshunov, A.; Zentgraf, H.; et al. Characterization of R132H mutation-specific IDH1 antibody binding in brain tumors. *Brain Pathol.* **2010**, *20*, 245–254. [CrossRef] [PubMed]
10. Nobusawa, S.; Watanabe, T.; Kleihues, P.; Ohgaki, H. IDH1 mutations as molecular signature and predictive factor of secondary glioblastomas. *Clin. Cancer Res.* **2009**, *15*, 6002–6007. [CrossRef] [PubMed]
11. Ohgaki, H.; Dessen, P.; Jourde, B.; Horstmann, S.; Nishikawa, T.; Di Patre, P.L.; Burkhard, C.; Schuler, D.; Probst-Hensch, N.M.; Maiorka, P.C.; et al. Genetic pathways to glioblastoma: A population-based study. *Cancer Res.* **2004**, *64*, 6892–6899. [CrossRef] [PubMed]

10

Principles of *N*-Linked Glycosylation Variations of IgG-Based Therapeutics: Pharmacokinetic and Functional Considerations

Souad Boune, Peisheng Hu, Alan L. Epstein and Leslie A. Khawli *☉

Department of Pathology, Keck School of Medicine, University of Southern California, Los Angeles, CA 90089, USA; so3ad86@gmail.com (S.B.); peisheng@usc.edu (P.H.); aepstein@usc.edu (A.L.E.)
* Correspondence: lkhawli@usc.edu

Abstract: The development of recombinant therapeutic proteins has been a major revolution in modern medicine. Therapeutic-based monoclonal antibodies (mAbs) are growing rapidly, providing a potential class of human pharmaceuticals that can improve the management of cancer, autoimmune diseases, and other conditions. Most mAbs are typically of the immunoglobulin G (IgG) subclass, and they are glycosylated at the conserved asparagine position 297 (Asn-297) in the CH2 domain of the Fc region. Post-translational modifications here account for the observed high heterogeneity of glycoforms that may or not impact the stability, pharmacokinetics (PK), efficacy, and immunogenicity of mAbs. These modifications are also critical for the Fc receptor binding, and consequently, key antibody effector functions including antibody-dependent cell-mediated cytotoxicity (ADCC) and complement-dependent cytotoxicity (CDC). Moreover, mAbs produced in non-human cells express oligosaccharides that are not normally found in serum IgGs might lead to immunogenicity issues when administered to patients. This review summarizes our understanding of the terminal sugar residues, such as mannose, sialic acids, fucose, or galactose, which influence therapeutic mAbs either positively or negatively in this regard. This review also discusses mannosylation, which has significant undesirable effects on the PK of glycoproteins, causing a decreased mAbs' half-life. Moreover, terminal galactose residues can enhance CDC activities and Fc–C1q interactions, and core fucose can decrease ADCC and Fc–FcγRs binding. To optimize the therapeutic use of mAbs, glycoengineering strategies are used to reduce glyco-heterogeneity of mAbs, increase their safety profile, and improve the therapeutic efficacy of these important reagents.

Keywords: glycosylation; post-translational modifications; pharmacokinetics; effector functions; antibody-dependent cell-mediated cytotoxicity; complement-dependent cytotoxicity; immunogenicity; pharmacodynamics; glycoengineering; antibody-drug conjugates

1. Introduction

Monoclonal antibody (mAb)-based therapeutics have been increasingly studied and utilized as therapeutic agents for the past 20 years [1]. Even though mAb technology was invented early in 1975 by Milstein and Koehler [2], the potential of these agents was not appreciated originally because of anti-drug antibody (ADA) responses in humans induced by murine antibodies [3]. However, with the rapid growth of biotechnology-derived techniques and the advanced knowledge of the immune system, scientists have realized the roll that mAbs can play in the treatment of many diseases [4]. Today, there are more than 60 products of therapeutic monoclonal antibodies (mAbs) that are approved in the US for human use, about 240 in clinical testing, and around 40 entering clinical trials each year [5,6].

Therapeutic antibodies are generally IgGs. An IgG is a glycoprotein that contains four polypeptide chains: Two identical heavy chains (H) and two identical light chains (L). The light and heavy chains pair by covalent disulfide bonds and noncovalent associations (Figure 1) [4]. Each heavy chain is connected to one light chain by one disulfide bond. Each antibody molecule is made of three globular domain structures forming a "Y" shape, two of which are the fragments that bind to the antigens (Fab) and the other is the fragment crystallizable (Fc) for the activation of Fcγ receptors (FcγRs) on leukocytes and the C1 component of complement [6]. IgG molecules bear N-glycosylation at the conserved asparagine at position 297 (Asn-297) in the heavy chain of the CH2 constant domain of the Fc region [6]. The oligosaccharide is an essential player in Fc effector functions including antibody-dependent cellular cytotoxicity (ADCC) and complement-dependent cytotoxicity (CDC), which are major mechanisms of action of therapeutic antibodies located in the Fc region. Alteration of glycan compositions and structures can impact the effector function by causing conformational changes of the Fc domain, which would affect binding affinity to Fcγ receptors [3,5]. Thus, engineering of Fc glycosylation to develop therapeutic monoclonal antibodies with desired characteristics is a promising strategy to enhance functionality and efficacy of therapeutic IgG antibodies. In this review, Fc N-glycan structure and biosynthesis are briefly reviewed, followed by a discussion of the knowledge acquired recently about the influence of glycosylation of antibodies on therapeutic antibody immunogenicity, pharmacokinetics (PK), and effector functions. Furthermore, current Fc glycoengineering strategies used to produce mAbs with higher homogeneity and effector functions are introduced and discussed. In the following sections we will also discuss those aspects of glycosylation variations which relate to the PK and pharmacodynamic (PD) parameters of currently approved antibody-based therapeutics.

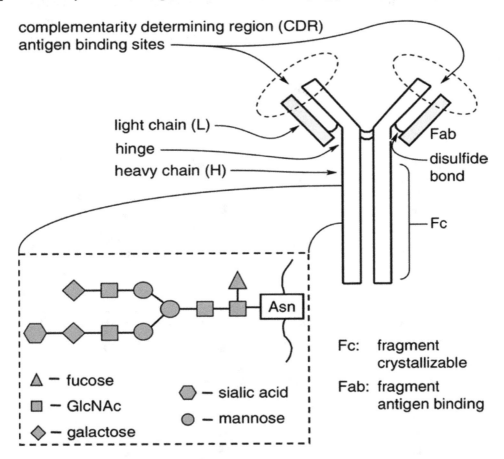

Figure 1. Simplified structure of an immunoglobulin (IgG). Inset shows an example of an IgG Fc diantennary oligosaccharide, which in normal IgG, is attached at an asparagine residue at position 297 (Asn-297). Generally, the oligosaccharide has a core pentasaccharide with varying addition of galactose, fucose, sialic acid, and N-acetylglucosamine (GlcNAc). Reproduced from Bakhtiar, 2012 [4].

2. IgG Glycan Structure and Biosynthesis

Post-translational modification is a biological process that involves the modification of an amino acid side chain, terminal amino, or carboxyl group by means of covalent or enzymatic modifications following IgG biosynthesis. Generally, these modifications may include phosphorylation, acetylation, glycosylation, sialylation of one or more amino acids in the protein, and also may include the formation of S-S bridges between 2 SH groups on amino acids, and proteolysis. Post-translational modifications contribute to the final tertiary (three-dimensional) structure of IgGs and play a key role in the biological activity and interaction with other cellular molecules such as proteins, nucleic acids, lipids, and cofactors. These modifications are not predictable by the sequence of IgG and are often critical in determining the way IgG behaves (e.g., its function and degradation). Therefore, each therapeutic protein will have a unique post-translational modification profile in its natural state, and as discussed further in this review, the post-translational modification profile of an IgG can potentially impact drug stability, safety, and efficacy.

2.1. IgG Glycan Structure

Structurally, the N-linked glycans of human IgGs are typically biantennary complexes. Different residues, such as fucose, bisecting GlcNAc, galactose, and sialic acid, can be added to this core biantennary complex structure (GlcNAc2Man3GlcNAc2), generating heterogeneity of the IgG-Fc glycans of normal polyclonal IgGs [5,7]. The heterogeneous glycans can be classified into three sets (G0, G1, and G2), depending on the number of galactose residues in the outer arms of biantennary glycans. Within each of these sets, there are different species that arise from the presence or absence of core fucose and bisecting GlcNAc (Figure 2) [3].

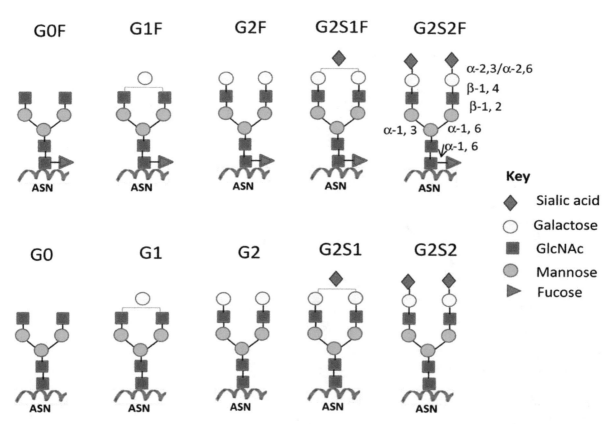

Figure 2. Major N-linked glycoforms of therapeutic monoclonal antibodies (mAbs). Reproduced from Liu, 2015 [3].

2.2. Glycan Biosynthesis in Human Cells

Glycosylation is the most common post-translational modification of proteins. It is a complex process that results in a great diversity of carbohydrate–protein bonds and glycan structures. It is known that it has a great impact on protein structures and functions [8]. Glycosylation of IgG is an enzyme-directed chemical reaction that occurs in the endoplasmic reticulum (ER) and the Golgi apparatus of the cell. Initially, a Glc3Man9GlcNAc2 oligosaccharide is transferred to Asn-297 of the IgG heavy chain via an oligosaccharyltransferase complex in the ER. Subsequently, the N-glycans are subjected to a sequence of consecutive modifications by sets of glycosidases and glycosyltransferases [9]. Polypeptide-associated Glc3Man9GlcNAc2 is trimmed by glucosidases I and II and endo-mannosidase in the lumen of the ER, resulting in the removal of three Glc residues and a mannose residue to produce Man8GlcNAc2 (Figure 3) [5]. In the cis-Golgi, the Man8GlcNAc2 is sequentially subjected to two class I α-mannosidases that act particularly on α-1,2-Man residues to produce the core Man5GlcNAc2 glycan for additional modification in the medial and trans-Golgi, mediated by GlcNAc transferases I, II, and III (GnT I, II, and III), α-1,6-fucosyltransferase (FUT8), galactosyltransferases (GalT), and sialyltransferases (SiaT) [3,5,9].

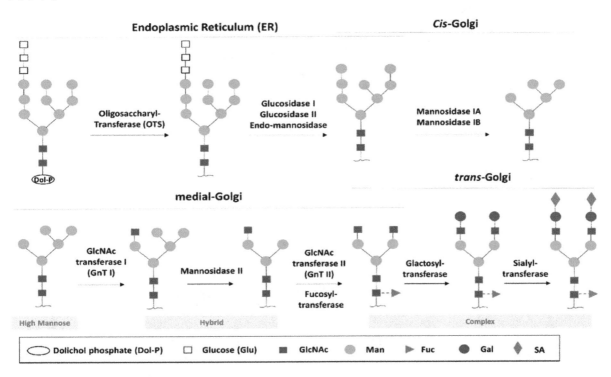

Figure 3. Glycan biosynthesis through the endoplasmic reticulum (ER) and Golgi glycosylation pathways. The biosynthesis begins with the processing of the initial high mannose N-glycan in the ER, followed by transferring into the cis-Golgi to generate the core N-glycan substrate used for further diversification in the trans-Golgi. The potential glycoforms include the high mannose, hybrid, and complex structure. Reprinted from Li et al., 2017 [5] with permission of the copyright owner.

3. N-Glycosylation Impact on mAb Structure and Effector Function

The amount and nature of glycosylation can dramatically affect the behavior of endogenous and recombinant IgGs. The most commonly described roles for glycosylation are related to receptor binding and Fc effector functions. However, the glycosylation profile of an IgG can also substantially affect its PK and distribution. In order to understand the possible manipulations and reasons behind glycosylation and glycoengineering, the reader is also directed to references [3–7,10] for a thorough overview describing the current understanding of glycosylation pattern (and normal variation), normal PK, and effector functions in IgG. As such, Fc glycosylation has great influence on mAbs' efficacy, stability, safety, immunogenicity, PK, and PD.

3.1. Impact of Fc Glycosylation on Structure

It is well established that the glycan structures can directly affect IgG through altering the conformation of the Fc domain [11]. *N*-glycans have essential structural supportive functions. They play a critical role in the stability of CH2 domain of IgGs, which binds to the glycans via extensive non-covalent interactions that reduce the dynamics of CH2 and aid in CH2 folding. Deglycosylation makes mAbs thermally less stable and more prone to unfolding and degradation [10]. Furthermore, removal of sugar residues leads to the generation of a "closed" conformation while the fully galactosylated IgG-Fc correlates with "open" conformation, which may be most favorable for FcγR binding [12] (Figure 4) [6].

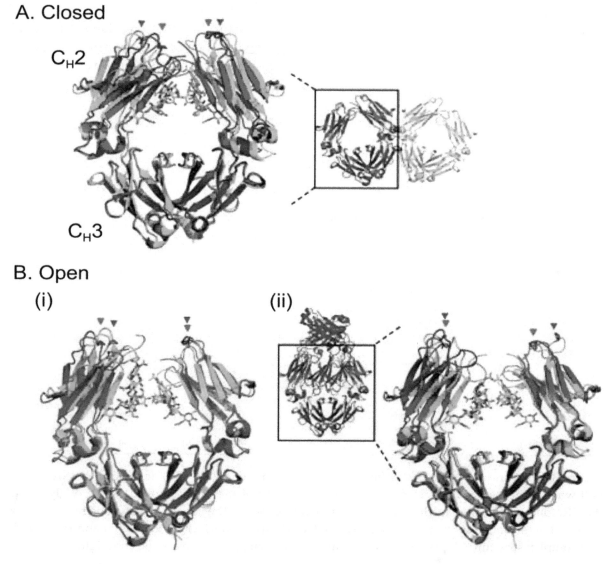

Figure 4. Comparison of non-glycosylated and glycosylated Fc structures. (**A**) Closed conformation of the non-glycosylated Fc. Overall structure of the two aglycosylated Fc molecules is shown in red and green, and the Fc shown in red is superimposed with the glycosylated Fc. (**B**) Open conformation of the non-glycosylated Fc. Overall structure of the two interlocked Fc molecules is shown in pink and blue. The Fc shown in pink is superimposed with the glycosylated Fc. The Fc glycans are shown in green sticks. The Pro329 residues located in the FG loop of the CH2 domains are indicated by red and blue arrowheads for the non-glycosylated and glycosylated CH2 domains, respectively. Reproduced from Mimura et al., 2018 [6].

3.2. Impact of Fc Glycosylation on Immunogenicity

As mentioned above, glycosylated mAbs can alter their safety and immunogenicity. Glycan patterns are highly variable since they depend on the host glycosylation machinery. Thus, different host cells can produce different recombinant antibodies with different glycoforms. Most therapeutic recombinant antibodies are Chinese hamster ovary (CHO)-derived recombinant IgG molecules, and some are made in murine myeloma cell lines NS0 and SP2/0. Recombinant antibodies produced in CHO cells are glycosylated similarly to natural human IgG. On the other hand, recombinant human IgGs derived in murine myeloma cells can have different glycoforms because they add sugars which are not normally found in the human IgG [3,5]. Terminal-sugar residues expressed in non-human glycoforms that are not normally found in endogenous serum IgGs could be highly immunogenic in humans [13]. Immunogenicity of these therapeutic antibodies can lead to reduced efficacy and safety and cause anti-drug Ab responses (ADA) and hypersensitivity reactions. Therefore, the expression system (bacteria, yeast, insect, plant, or mammalian cells) that is used to generate recombinant mAbs is crucial and has tremendous influence on the mAb function in vivo [14].

Glycoproteins that are produced in yeasts, plants, and insect cells usually have high-mannose contents, which can increase immunogenicity of recombinant mAbs [15]. Lam et al. have demonstrated that antigen mannosylation significantly increases protein immunogenicity in mice [16]. Most therapeutic mAbs, however, have very low levels of high-mannose content [17]. Moreover, terminal sialic acids of therapeutic mAbs derived in non-human cells, such as murine myeloma cell lines, have been shown to be a possible factor that cause immunogenicity in patients since they express the N-glycolylneuraminic acid (NGNA) form of sialic acids that are not normally found in human IgGs [18]. The main reason behind this significant immunogenicity could be NGNA-specific antibodies that have been found to be expressed by all humans [19]. More specific investigations by Qian and coworkers have reported that Cetuximab, a murine myeloma cell-derived novel therapeutic monoclonal antibody that contains NGNA, caused immune interaction with NGNA-specific antibodies [20]. Because of these findings, assessment of the immunogenicity of therapeutic Abs is a critical quality attribute that should be considered with respect to the manufacturing of these therapeutic glycoproteins.

3.3. Impact of Fc Glycosylation on Pharmacokinetics

Clearance has a critical impact on the efficacy of therapeutic antibodies. Monoclonal antibodies are high-molecular weight drugs that are large complex proteins (approximately 150 kDa) that are not eliminated through kidney filtration. In addition, they can escape fast degradation in the lysosomes through the neonatal Fc receptor (FcRn) recycling mechanism [21]. The binding of Fc to the neonatal Fc receptor at the CH2–CH3 domain plays a critical role in the PK properties of IgG molecules. Recycling of antibodies results in long half-life of IgGs in the serum (up to 4 weeks) [22]. Roopenian et al. conducted experiments on FcRn knockout mice and they have concluded that FcRn is responsible for protecting IgG from catabolism [22]. Both glycosylated and deglycosylated IgGs bind equally to the (FcRn) receptor [23]. Therefore, the interaction between FcRn and IgG is independent of the Fc glycans due to their protected and buried position within the antibody structure. The significance of Fc glycosylation in the PK of therapeutic mAbs can be examined by comparing the biological activities of glycosylated IgG with either enzymatically deglycosylated IgGs or by preparing aglycosylated IgGs (bearing Asn-297 mutation) using molecular biology techniques. Several studies have compared the biological activity and PK properties of antibodies with different glycoforms in humans and animals [24,25].

Liu et al. confirmed that glycosylation is not required for an IgG antibody's long half-life after they characterized aglycosylated IgGs by chemical modification and genetic engineering [23]. These animal studies demonstrated that the PK profile of an aglycosylated IgG1 mAb with an Asn-297 mutation was almost identical to that of the glycosylated form. Another clinical trial conducted in 2009 by Clarke et al. also demonstrated that aglycosylated mAb ALD518 (clazakizumab), a humanized anti-human IL-6 IgG1 produced in yeast, had a normal PK in humans and animals. In their phase I clinical trial, the circulating half-life for ALD518 was 20–32 days, which is consistent with the half-life of a normal human IgG1 [26]. Moreover, Abuqayyas and colleagues found that 8C2, a mouse IgG mAb, exhibited similar PK and tissue distribution in both FcγR knockout mice and in wild type mice [27]. Similar PK properties of glycosylated and non-glycosylated IgGs confirm that antibody clearance in humans and animals is not significantly affected by Fc glycan removal [10,24,28].

3.4. Effect of Terminal Mannose on Pharmacokinetics

Circulating glycoproteins can be cleared from the blood by receptors that recognize specific glycan forms. Glycan receptors that are involved in the clearance of glycoproteins include the mannose receptor (ManR) and the asialoglycoprotein receptor (ASGPR). The asialoglycoprotein receptors bind to terminal Gal residues and the ManR bind to glycoproteins with terminal Man or GlcNac sugars. Glycan binding to these receptors expressed on tissues was considered to have potential effects on the PK of antibodies bearing these terminal sugars and to cause faster removal from circulation [25]. Consistent with this, Kanda et al. demonstrated that IgG antibodies with high-mannose glycoforms have shorter half-life compared to those with the complex-type glycans in mice [29]. Yu et al. conducted a PK study in mice, and they determined the clearance rate of antibodies bearing Man8/9 and Man5 glycan. They showed that the antibodies bearing the high mannose glycoform were cleared faster compared with antibodies bearing the fucosylated complex glycoform, while the PK properties of antibodies with Man8/9 and Man5 glycoforms appeared similar (Figure 5) [25]. In agreement with previous human studies, Goetze and coworkers observed faster elimination of therapeutic IgGs containing Fc high-mannose glycans from circulation compared to other glycoforms [17]. In addition, differences in high-mannose structural isoform clearance rates in humans were reported by Chen et al., but these investigators suggested that changes in the serum half-life of mAbs bearing high mannose glycoforms were actually due to glycan cleavage [24]. Another investigation done by Millward et al. reached contradictory conclusions. They found no significant difference in serum half-life in mice between high-mannose IgG type and complex IgGs [30]. In summary, high-terminal mannose content appears to be an important point that should be considered as it may affect PK properties and efficacy of therapeutic antibodies. Because of the above findings, most mAbs for clinical use possess relatively low-terminal high-mannose glycan content.

In general, glycans that have a major impact on PK of mAbs include mannose, sialic acids, galactose, and fucose [3,25] (Figure 5). The negatively-charged sialic acids attached to the terminus of glycan chains have been shown to affect half-life for many glycoproteins. It was found that IgGs with exposed terminal Gal (after removal of sialic acid) resulted in a decreased half-life in mice and localization in the liver [3]. To date, the PK properties of different glycan compositions in approved antibody-based therapeutics have not yet been investigated in the clinic.

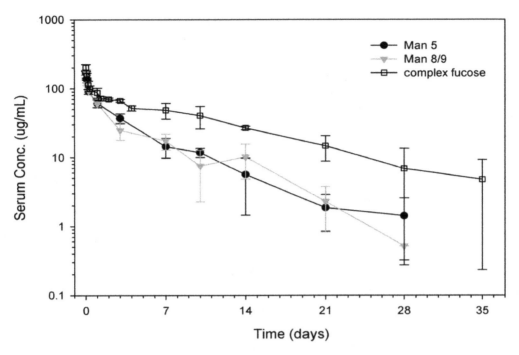

Figure 5.   The influence of high-mannose glycans on the pharmacokinetics (PKs) of mAbs. Pharmacokinetic profiles of mAb variants in athymic nude mice. The two groups conducted in this study were mAb with >99% Man5 (solid black circle) and mAb with >99% Man8/9 (solid gray triangle). The complex-fucosylated profile (open squares) was from a separate study conducted in a similar fashion to the current study. Reproduced from Yu et al., 2012 [25].

4. Impact of Fc Glycosylation on Pharmacodynamics

The oligosaccharides of the IgG-Fc play a critical role in activation of FcγRs and complement C1. FcγR-mediated effector functions result in the killing of the target cell. FcγRs are responsible for ADCC effector function and, while the receptor C1q mediates CDC. Many studies have found that the lack of glycosylation noticeably decreases the binding affinity to FcγRI and eliminates the binding to FcγRII and FcγRIII receptors [31,32].

4.1. Sialic Acid

Sialic acids are present in human serum IgGs as N-acetylneuraminic acid (NANA) attached to a terminal galactose by an α-2,3 or α-2,6 linkage. Recombinant monoclonal antibodies expressed in CHO cell line also have NANA, but it is only attached by α-2,3 linkage [18]. On the other hand, monoclonal antibodies produced in NS0 and SP2/0 cell lines have NGNA, a sialic acid form produced by hydroxylation of NANA utilizing cytidine monophosphate N-acetylneuraminic acid hydroxylase enzyme which is absent in human and CHO cells under normal conditions [33]. Typically, the level of sialic acid in human endogenous IgGs is ~11%–15% [18,34]. Studies to date that explore the effects of sialic acid on Fcγ receptors binding are inconclusive. Scallon and coworkers studied pairs of monoclonal human IgG Abs produced in mouse hybridoma cell lines with different amounts of sialic acid in their Fc glycans [35]. They demonstrated that a higher content of terminal sialylation was correlated with decreased activity in ADCC and lower-affinity binding to FcγRIIIa on natural killer (NK) cells in vitro. Similarly, Kaneko et al. reported that Fc sialylation affects antibody effector functions including reduction of ADCC in both in vitro and in vivo [36].

However, another in vitro study investigated the influence of sialic acid on IgG1 effector functions using different glycosylated forms of a single drug with various levels of sialylation generated by in vitro glycoengineering [37]. They found that terminal sialylation had no impact, neither positive nor negative, on ADCC activity, $Fc\gamma RI$, and RIIIa receptors, but slightly improved affinity to $Fc\gamma RIIa$ was reported [37]. Furthermore, full sialylation of human monoclonal IgG1 was reported to interfere with the induction of CDC in vitro [38].

Recently, Fc sialylation has drawn scientists' attention as it has been attributed to increased anti-inflammatory responses to intravenous Ig (IVIG) for the treatment of autoimmune and inflammatory diseases [36,39]. IVIG suppresses inflammation by binding to inhibitory $Fc\gamma RIIb$. Sialylated IgG initiates anti-inflammatory effects by binding to the murine C-type lectin-like receptor-specific intracellular adhesion molecule-grabbing non-integrin R1 (SIGN-RI) (DCSIGN in humans) expressed by macrophage and dendritic cells. As a result, $Fc\gamma RIIb$ expression will be upregulated and Treg cell populations will expand, leading to significant suppression of inflammatory responses [40,41]. Kaneko et al. approved that sialylated human IgG has elevated anti-inflammatory activity compared to the desialylated IgG utilizing a mouse model of rheumatoid arthritis [36]. However, these findings in mice were contradicted by a study of rheumatoid arthritis during pregnancy [42]. This study showed that remission of rheumatoid arthritis was associated with galactosylation independently of sialylation. In summary, sialylated glycans collectively have both positive and negative influences on IgG effector functions, making it crucial to quantitate the sialylation of mAbs headed for the clinic, especially to treat autoimmune conditions. To date, the functions of different Fc-sialylated glycans in approved antibody-based therapeutics have not yet been investigated in the clinic.

4.2. Terminal Galactose

Recombinant mAbs and the human endogenous IgG Fc region have biantennary complex oligosaccharides with either zero, one, or two terminal galactose moieties, which are the three major glycoforms (G0, G1, or G2) [18,34,43].

The impact of terminal galactose residue on IgG biological functions has been investigated in many studies. Whereas the terminal Gal residue content has shown to play an important role in CDC activity of IgG, the ADCC activity does not seem to be affected by galactosylation of an IgG mAb. Hodoniczky and colleagues have remodeled the Fc N-glycans of recombinant therapeutic monoclonal antibody products, Rituxan and Herceptin, in vitro, yielding degalactosylated mAb and other products varying in content of GlcNAc [44]. By degalactosylation of Rituxan and generating mAbs with various Gal content, they have demonstrated that CDC activities and antibody binding to C1q increase as Gal content increases [8,44] (Figure 6). Lower affinity to C1q is due to hydrophobic and hydrophilic interactions between terminal Gal residue and protein, which alter the conformation of the CH2 domain [12]. They confirmed that ADCC activity is not influenced by terminal Gal residue content [44]. Nevertheless, despite some of these contradictory results, galactosylation can induce a positive impact on the binding affinity of the IgG1 to $Fc\gamma RIIa$ and $Fc\gamma RIIIa$ receptors and ADCC activity [37]. A recent in vitro study also showed that Fc-galactosylation of rituximab enhances CDC activities compared to the degalactosylated glycoform and improvement of C1q binding eventually leads to tumor cell lysis [45]. However, these findings apply to IgG1, but not other subclasses of mAbs. Thus, further detailed, specific investigations of the effects of galactosylation on other IgG subclasses effector functions such as ADCC and CDC are needed.

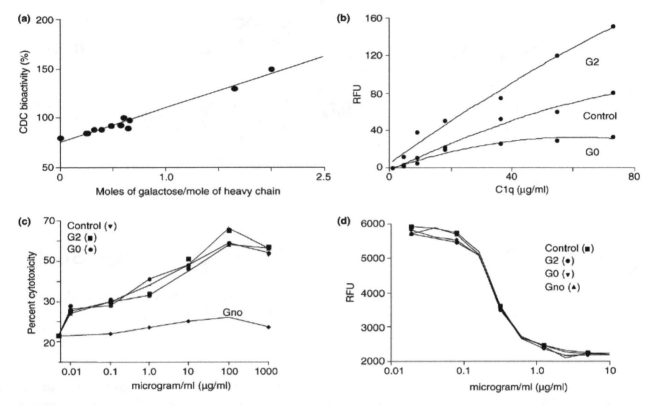

Figure 6. Increase in terminal Gal content increases complement-dependent cytotoxicity (CDC) activity (**a**) and C1q binding (**b**) of rIgGs, but does not affect antibody-dependent cell-mediated cytotoxicity (ADCC) activity (**c**) and antigen binding expressed as relative fluorescence units (RFU) (**d**). G2, G0, and/or Gno (no glycans) glycoforms of Rituxan and/or Herceptin were prepared by in vitro glycosylation methods. These glycoforms, along with control antibody samples (untreated), were subjected to CDC (Rituxan glycoforms), C1q binding (Rituxan glycoforms), ADCC (Herceptin glycoforms), and antigen binding to HER2-ECD (Herceptin glycoforms). Rituxan is a chimeric antibody against CD20 and elicits CDC activity but shows very little ADCC activity. Herceptin is a humanized antibody against HER2-neu antigen and elicits ADCC activity but no CDC activity. Reproduced from Raju 2008 [8].

4.3. Bisecting N-Acetylglucosamine

Approximately 10% of human serum endogenous IgGs glycoforms have bisecting GlcNAc residues. Recombinant antibodies generated in CHO cells do not contain bisecting GlcNAc because of the lack of active *N*-acetylglucosaminyltransferase-III (GnT-III) needed for synthesis of bisecting GlcNAc containing *N*-glycans [8,32,46] (Figure 7). Addition of a bisecting GlcNAc has been reported to enhance the binding affinity to FcγRIIIa, which causes 10–30-fold higher ADCC activities [47,48]. Although Hodoniczky et al. [44] approved that bisecting GlcNAc enhances ADCC activity by approximately 10-fold independently of the lack of core fucosylation of rituximab remodeled in vitro, a study done by Shinkawa et al. [48] has debated these findings. Since loss of core fucosylation is always associated with in vivo addition of bisecting GlcNAc, Shinkawa and colleagues proposed that the presence of bisecting GlcNAc may not be the main cause of an ADCC activity increase. As such, Shinkawa's studies demonstrated that the removal of core fucose rather than bisecting GlcNAc has the biggest impact on ADCC activity of therapeutic antibodies [48]. Similar to Shinkawa's results, Ferrara et al. [49] have reported that antibodies enriched in bisected oligosaccharides have increased ADCC.

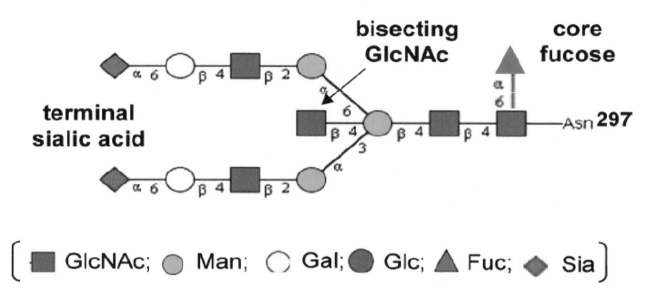

Figure 7. The structure of a full-length biantennary *N*-glycan attached to the Asn-297 in the Fc domain and containing bisecting GlcNAc residue. Reproduced from Huang et al., 2012 [50].

4.4. Fucose

The core fucose residues are added to the core GlcNAc residue which is linked to the protein via α-1,6 linkage. This complex glycoform is dominantly found in both serum IgG (>80%) and recombinant IgG's produced in CHO cells (>90%) [32]. Although absence of core fucose residues in Fc glycans has been shown to dramatically improve antibody binding to FcRIIIa and ADCC activity, many studies have demonstrated that the fucosylation level has slight consequences on binding of antibodies to FcγR1, FcγRII, and C1q [48,51,52]. Shields and coworkers used afucosylated anti-HER2 to demonstrate the significant role played by the absence of core fucose in the enhancement of ADCC activity of IgG [51]. About 100-fold greater ADCC exhibited by afucosylated anti-HER2 compared to fucosylated recombinant IgG has been reported in this study. Furthermore, it has been observed that the binding to FcγRI, C1q, or FcRn was not altered [51]. Using marketed nonfucosylated anti-CD20 IgG1 rituximab, Lida et al. confirmed that nonfucosylated IgG1 mediates very high ADCC at low doses in humans, which enhances the therapeutic potential of the modified mAb [53]. Another study has shown that higher binding affinity of afucosylated IgG to Fcγ RIIIa apply for all IgG subclasses [54]. Inclusively, afucosylation of mAb leads the greatest influence on ADCC enhancement, which mediates the efficacy of potential therapeutic recombinant antibodies. Therefore, many recombinant IgGs modified via glycoengineering strategies to generate low-fucose antibodies are currently under investigation in human clinical trials to improve the clinical efficacy of these therapeutics. A classic example of producing low-fucose content antibodies is the anti-CD20 antibody obinutuzumab, which was approved by the US Food and Drug Administration (FDA) in 2013 for the treatment of non-Hodgkin's lymphoma and chronic lymphocytic leukemia. Obinutuzumab showed significantly increased ADCC activity compared with the prototype antibody (rituximab). The same engineered cell line was used to produce a nonfucosylated anti-CD20 antibody (mogamulizumab) that showed a 100-fold increase in ADCC activity compared with the nonglycoengineered rituximab. As such, mogamulizumab was approved for the treatment of adult T cell leukemia/lymphoma in Japan.

4.5. High Mannose

Typically, high mannose content in Fc glycan of IgG varies from five to nine mannose molecules linked to the core GlcNAc. Although about 0.1% of human serum endogenous IgG's contain Fc glycan with high mannose (mostly Man5GlcNAc2 structure), high mannose glycoforms content varies with cell lines and can represent up to 10% of recombinant IgG [20]. Different studies exploring high mannose type Fc glycans have shown that mannose content can impact antibody effector functions. Zhou and his team have demonstrated that the presence of high mannose structures result in enhanced ADCC activity and increased IgG binding affinity for the FcγRIIIa receptor [55]. However, it is unclear whether enhancement in ADCC activity is due to the absence of fucose, since high mannose type glycans possess no core fucose residues [20]. It has also been shown that the IgG with high mannose structures have a negative impact on CDC activity because of lower binding affinity for C1q [55]. Consistently, Kanda et al. have reported similar results that high mannose structures can lead to reduced C1q binding and complement activation [29]. Nevertheless, it was shown that mAbs with high mannose glycan exhibit higher ADCC in the same study. In conclusion, high mannose type Fc glycans have a positive effect on ADCC activity but a negative impact on CDC activity of IgG molecules.

5. Glycoengineering

Since different glycoforms have positive or negative effects on antibody effector functions, it is necessary to develop Fc glycoengineering strategies to facilitate the generation of therapeutic mAbs with consistent and homogenous glycoforms to improve their therapeutic efficacy. Although much progress in cell glycoengineering has already been achieved and important improvements on glycan quality have been accomplished, it is still very challenging to produce IgGs with highly homogenous glycoforms in host cells. The current Fc glycoengineering strategies include host cell glycoengineering and in vitro chemoenzymatic glycosylation remodeling.

5.1. Cell Glycoengineering

Antibody glycosylation is the result of a multistep process. Host cell-based glycoengineering alters glycoforms by genetically modifying important mediators in the glycan biosynthetic pathways to enhance production of desired glycoforms [56]. This technology has been used recently to generate mAbs with optimized quality and efficacy, and focusing on Fc defucosylation which produces a significant increase in ADCC activity results due to the absence of core fucose [57]. Various approaches have been used to modify host cells in order to enhance the desired or limit the unwanted glycoforms. One approach selects host cell type, environmental factors, and cell culture conditions. Host cells that have low FUT8 activity, such as rat hybridoma cell line YB2/0, allow production of recombinant glycoproteins with low core fucose [58,59]. Recombinant mAbs derived from CHO cells exhibit low sialic acid levels because of the absence of α-2,6-sialyltransferase in these cells [60]. Therefore, this cell type is an attractive alternative for the production of mAbs with low sialic acid content. Moreover, cell culture conditions can be modified to favor antibody glycoforms homogeneity. Crowell et al. have reported that feeding the culture with uridine, manganese chloride, and galactose could result in higher CDC activity of mAb due to increased terminal galactose [61]. Another study used 2-fluorofucose, a fucose analogue, to inhibit fucosylation in vitro and produce fucose-deficient antibodies [62].

Another approach in host cells glycoengeneering uses inhibitors of the enzymes that synthesize N-linked oligosaccharide chains to alter host biosynthesis pathways. Enzyme inhibitors prevent the addition of outer arm sugar residues including fucose [63]. For example, the addition of ER α-mannosidase inhibitors, deoxymannojirimycin and kifunensine, results in the generation of high mannose (Man9GlcNAc2) glycoform. Another example is that ER glucosidases I and II inhibitors include deoxynojirimycin and castanospermine which arrest mAb in Glc3Man9GlcNAc2 glycoform [63].

A third approach is genetic modulation of the host glycan biosynthesis pathway. This strategy can be performed by upregulating or downregulating substrate expression. Sullivan's group succeeded in the generation of defucosylated antibodies by silencing the *GMD* gene responsible for the expression of GDP fucose, the fucose donor [64]. Furthermore, gene editing techniques, such as ZFNs, TALENs, and CRISPR-Cas9, have been widely used to modify N-glycosylation pathways. Chan et al. used these techniques to inactivate the GDP-fucose transporter (SLC35C1) in Chinese hamster ovary (CHO) cells. They concluded that inactivating the *Slc35c1* gene results in production of fucose-free antibodies in CHO cells [65]. Alternatively, small interfering RNis (siRNAs) have been used to knock out multiple genes involved in fucosylation. Finally, inactivation of FUT8 and GDP-mannose 4,6-dehydratase *(GMD)* in CHO cells has led to the production of completely afucosylated IgG with enhanced ADCC [66]. For example, to improve ADCC, a significant improvement through cell-based glycoengineering has been previously reported with the first approved mAbs mogamulizumab and obinutuzumab. Mogamulizumab (POTELIGEO®, KW0761) is a humanized mAb which uses a FUT8 knockout CHO cell line to produce mAbs with nonfucosylated glycan mixtures [66]. Obinutuzumab (Gazyva™, GA-101) is derived from Roche GlycoMAb® technology which overexpresses GnTIII [46,47]. Once the GnT-III adds a bisecting GlcNAc to an oligosaccharide, the core-fucosylation is inhibited. Both technologies produce therapeutic mAbs with enhanced ADCC activity.

5.2. Chemoenzymatic Glycoengineering

Although much successful work in cell glycoengineering has been done to generate therapeutic mAbs with specific glycoforms, it is still very difficult to produce optimized IgGs with homogeneous glycoforms. To accomplish this, chemoenzymatic glycosylation of IgG antibodies provides a new avenue to remodel Fc *N*-glycan from a heterogeneous *N*-glycosylation pattern to a homogeneous one. The Protocol of chemoenzymatic synthesis includes deglycosylation of IgG antibodies using ENG'ase (endo-β-*N*-acetylglucosaminidase) leaving the innermost GlcNAc with or without core fucose at the *N*-glycosylation site. After preparation of glycan oxazolines as donor substrates, a transglycosylation step is used with ENGase-based glycosynthase [66–68] (Figure 8A), and then prepared the glycoengineered mAbs with homogenous *N*-glycans (M3, G0, G2, and A2) via enzymatic reaction (Figure 8B).

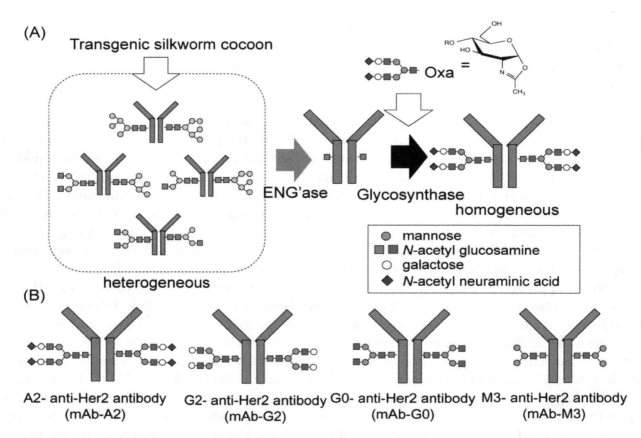

Figure 8. (A) Schematic representation of chemoenzymatic synthesis using ENG'ase and glycosynthase. **(B)** Diagram of the homogeneous glycosylated mAb with M3 (mAb-M3), G0 (mAb-G0), G2 (mAb-G2), and A2 (mAb-A2). Reproduced from Kurogochi et al., 2015 [68].

There are various ENGases mutants (EndoS D233Q, EndoA N171A, EndoA E173Q, EndoMN175A, and EndoM N175Q) that exhibit transglycosylation activity, which have been engineered to have different substrate specificities and limitations [50,69]. As an example, Huang and coworkers [50] generated two glycosynthase mutants (EndoS-D233A and D233Q) to transform rituximab from mixtures of G0F, G1F, and G2F glycoforms to well-defined homogeneous glycoforms. Using EndoS glycosynthase mutants permitted the production of a fully sialylated (S2G2F) glycoform that shows enhanced anti-inflammatory activity of IVIG's Fc glycans, and a nonfucosylated G2 glycoform that favors increased FcγIIIa receptor-bindings and ADCC activity of mAbs [50] (Figure 9).

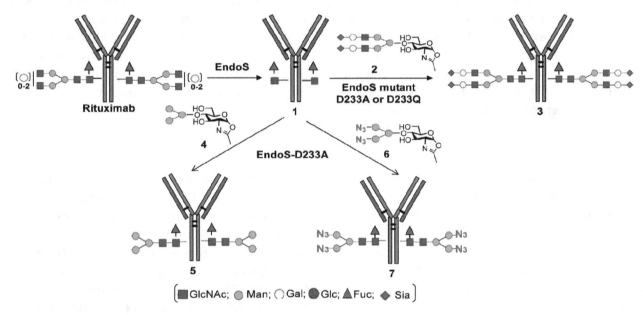

Figure 9. Chemoenzymatic remodeling of rituximab to prepare homogeneous and selectively modified glycoforms. Reproduced from Huang et al., 2012 [50].

While many investigations have demonstrated that Endo-S is limited to action on the complex-type, a more recent study described Endo-S2 glycosynthases (D184M and D184Q) that have relaxed substrate specificity and act on transferring three major types (complex, high-mannose, and hybrid type) of N-glycans [70]. Collectively, chemoenzymatic glycoengineering technology may be used to develop therapeutic monoclonal antibodies that have homogenous glycoforms, which may circumvent all current efficacy and function quality issues.

5.3. Glycoengineering for Site-Specific Antibody-Drug Conjugation

Antibody-drug conjugates or ADCs are emerging as powerful reagents for the selective delivery of highly toxic drugs to target cells. These relatively novel agents combine the ability of mAbs to bind antigen positive tumor cells with the highly potent killing activity of a cytotoxic drug. In one of the several approaches to obtain structurally-defined, homogeneous antibody–drug conjugates, the Fc glycans of the antibody is engineered for site-specific conjugation [71]. As discussed above, IgGs carry a highly conserved N-glycan at the Asn-297 of the Fc domain. Several terminal residues of glycoproteins, including fucose, galactose, and sialic acids that contain vicinal cis diols, can be oxidized selectively with mild periodate (NaIO4) treatment to generate aldehyde groups, which can be further functionalized with other groups, including hydrazides and aminooxy groups for chemoselective conjugation. However, antibody glycosylation is highly heterogeneous, and contains a mixture of galactose and core fucose. As a result, direct oxidation recombinant antibodies usually led to heterogeneous mixtures of the conjugates. For example, to have better control of the homogeneity of ADCs, researchers developed a CHO cell line that could control Fc N-glycosylation at the G0F glycoform, where fucose could be selectively oxidized. Thus, treatment of the G0F antibody with mild NaIO4 selectively oxidized the fucose moiety to provide an aldehyde derivative. In contrast to core fucose, oxidation of sialic acid can take place under relatively different conditions because their cis diols are less hindered and more susceptible to periodate oxidation. The advantage of this site-selective modification at the conserved N-glycan does not change the IgG structure and thus usually will not affect the antibody's inherent affinity for its antigen. A thorough overview on recent approaches behind glycoengineering of antibodies for site-specific antibody–drug conjugation is described in reference [71].

Today, there are 4 antibody-drug conjugates approved by the US FDA, including Genentech/Roche's Kadcyla® (HER2-specific trastuzumab-drug conjugate) used for the treatment of metastatic breast cancer, Seattle Genetics's Adcetris® (CD30-specific brentuximab-drug conjugate) used for treatment of relapsed Hodgkin's lymphoma, Pfizer/Wyeth's Besponsa™ (CD22-specific inotuzumab-drug conjugate) used for relapsed or refractory B cell precursor acute lymphoblastic leukemia, and more recently, Wyeth Pharmaceuticals' Mylotarg™ (CD33-specific gemtuzumab-ozogamicin conjugate) used for the therapy of acute myelogenous leukemia.

6. Conclusions

In summary, therapeutic mAbs are large, complex, and heterogeneous glycoproteins. They are typically glycosylated at amino acid position 297 in the Fc region. The N-glycosylation is crucial for antibody structure and effector functions. The presence or absence of different terminal sugars of Fc glycans can have a significant impact on the PK, PD, and immunogenicity of mAbs (Table 1). Although several studies investigated the correlation between PD and N-glycosylation, the results were often contradictory. Whereas high mannose content was shown to significantly impact PK by decreasing antibody half-life, the impact of other glycans on PK is still not fully understood [72]. Collectively, glycosylation is not essential for IgGs' long half-life, and FcRn is the main factor that maintains IgGs' circulation time. Furthermore, therapeutic IgGs derived from non-human cells can be immunogenic as they may express terminal sugar residues that are not naturally found in human serum IgGs, such as sialic acid NGNA. This immunogenicity can decrease the drug efficacy and cause hypersensitivity reactions. For the effects of glycoform patterns on PD and IgG effector functions, the presence of core fucose can interfere with FcγRIIIa binding and ADCC activity of therapeutic antibody. Therefore, the removal of fucose should be considered to enhance ADCC activity of monoclonal antibody drugs. On the other hand, galactosylation can improve the efficacy and quality of mAbs by increasing antibody binding to C1q and CDC of mAbs. Although progress has occurred, there is still much important work to address the unsolved underlying mechanisms that regulate the relationship between changes in Fc-glycan structures and the efficacy and quality of therapeutic monoclonal antibody functions. Due to the critical role of glycosylation and the great impact of different glycans on therapeutic monoclonal antibodies, the need for developing novel glycoengineering strategies has emerged in the last decade [5]. These strategies offer a new route to produce homogenous IgGs with desired glycoforms in order to enhance efficacy and functionality of therapeutic glycoproteins. Glycoengineering techniques which include glycoengineering of cell lines and chemoenzymatic glycoengineering approaches [50,68] are evolving and offer promising novel avenues to develop stable and safer mAbs, which is ultimately linked to lower risk of immunogenicity and higher therapeutic efficacy in humans [5,73–76]. As such, understanding the ways to control the Fc-glycan heterogeneity is essential to the successful clinical development of antibody-based drugs, which can be used to predict their PK/PD during early clinical development and to ensure faster results. This information can appropriately inform manufacturing process development so that these processes are more finely adjusted to deliver the desired Fc glycosylation [77].

Table 1. Summary of potential effects of the most prevalent Fc-glycans on the pharmacokinetics (PK) and pharmacodynamics (PD) of monoclonal antibodies (mAbs). N-Glycolylneuraminic acid form of sialic acid (NGNA).

Fc-Glycans	Potential Effects	References
Fucose	Absence of core fucose enhances: <ul><li>FcγRIIIa binding</li><li>ADCC activity</li></ul>	[48,51–54]
Galactose	Enhances antibody binding to C1q and CDC	[44,45]
Sialic acid	<ul><li>Anti-inflammatory activity</li><li>NGNA reduces FcγRIIIa binding and ADCC activity</li><li>NGNA may be immunogenic in human</li><li>Removal of sialic acid decreases half-life</li></ul>	[36,39] [35,36] [18–20] [3,25]
High Mannose	<ul><li>Decreases half-life</li><li>Increases FcγRIIIa binding and ADCC activity</li><li>Decreases antibody binding to C1q and CDC</li></ul>	[17,25,29] [55] [29,55]
Bisecting GlcNAc	Increases FcγRIIIa binding and ADCC activity	[44,47–49]

In respect to biosimilar development, site-specific glycosylation is also considered crucial in correlating distinct product attributes with observed in vivo effects [13,78]. In this context, an in-depth method for the characterization and analysis of manufactured biosimilar products is required for the production of optimal and consistent biosimilar therapeutic products. A better understanding of the relationship between glycosylation patterns and clinical performance is also of major importance for biosimilar development, and can be used to develop safe and efficacious antibody-based products on the market. In conclusion, antibody glycosylation is necessary to optimize the stability, safety, functionality, and efficacy of therapeutic IgG antibodies. Furthermore, new methods are being applied to generate the next generation of therapeutic mAbs for the treatment of a wide spectrum of human diseases.

To date, antibody-based products are still presenting academia and the biotechnology industry with novel challenges in terms of glycan characterization, stability, and in vivo behavior. Although many studies have been conducted evaluating the various effects of glycosylation on their physicochemical properties and patterns including their importance to biosimilarity [72], our understanding of how glycosylation translates to potential pharmacologic effects and toxicities is still incomplete. Additional investigations are therefore warranted to obtain a clearer pictu re of its importance to antibodies as a vital and important class of drugs.

Author Contributions: S.B. wrote the first draft of the paper as part of her Master Degree Project. All other authors (L.A.K.; A.L.E.; P.H.) contributed substantially to the final text, tables, figure and references to the paper. All authors have read and agreed to the published version of the manuscript.

Acknowledgments: The authors would like to express their gratitude to Michelle Khawli for her valuable technical editing, language editing, and proofreading. Her willingness to give her time so generously has been very much appreciated.

References

1. Fang, J.; Richardson, J.; Du, Z.; Zhang, Z. Effect of Fc-glycan structure on the conformational stability of IgG revealed by hydrogen/deuterium exchange and limited proteolysis. *Biochemistry* **2016**, *55*, 860–868. [CrossRef] [PubMed]

2.   Kohler, G.; Milstein, C. Continuous cultures of fused cells secreting antibody of predefined specificity. *Nature* **1975**, *256*, 495–497. [CrossRef]

3.   Liu, L. Antibody glycosylation and its impact on the pharmacokinetics and pharmacodynamics of monoclonal antibodies and Fc-fusion proteins. *J. Pharm. Sci.* **2015**, *104*, 1866–1884. [CrossRef]

4.   Bakhtiar, R. Therapeutic recombinant monoclonal antibodies. *J. Chem. Educ.* **2012**, *89*, 1537–1542. [CrossRef]

5.   Li, W.; Zhu, Z.; Chen, W.; Feng, Y.; Dimitrov, D.S. Crystallizable fragment glycoengineering for therapeutic antibodies development. *Front. Immunol.* **2017**, *8*, 1554. [CrossRef] [PubMed]

6.   Mimura, Y.; Katoh, T.; Saldova, R.; O'Flaherty, R.; Izumi, T.; Mimura-Kimura, Y.; Utsunomiya, T.; Mizukami, Y.; Yamamoto, K.; Matsumoto, T.; et al. Glycosylation engineering of therapeutic IgG antibodies: Challenges for the safety, functionality and efficacy. *Protein Cell* **2018**, *9*, 47–62. [CrossRef]

7.   Cymer, F.; Beck, H.; Rohde, A.; Reusch, D. Therapeutic monoclonal antibody N-glycosylation–structure, function and therapeutic potential. *Biologicals* **2018**, *52*, 1–11. [CrossRef] [PubMed]

8.   Raju, T.S. Terminal sugars of Fc glycans influence antibody effector functions of IgGs. *Curr. Opin. Immunol.* **2008**, *20*, 471–478. [CrossRef]

9.   Butters, T.D. Control in the N-linked glycoprotein biosynthesis pathway. *Chem. Biol.* **2002**, *9*, 1266–1268. [CrossRef]

10.   Higel, F.; Seidl, A.; Sörgel, F.; Friess, W. N-glycosylation heterogeneity and the influence on structure, function and pharmacokinetics of monoclonal antibodies and Fc fusion proteins. *Eur. J. Pharm. Biopharm.* **2016**, *100*, 94–100. [CrossRef]

11.   Borrok, M.J.; Jung, S.T.; Kang, T.H.; Monzingo, A.F.; Georgiou, G. Revisiting the role of glycosylation in the structure of human IgG Fc. *ACS Chem. Biol.* **2012**, *7*, 1596–1602. [CrossRef]

12.   Krapp, S.; Mimura, Y.; Jefferis, R.; Huber, R.; Sondermann, P. Structural analysis of human IgG-Fc glycoforms reveals a correlation between glycosylation and structural integrity. *J. Mol. Biol.* **2003**, *325*, 979–989. [CrossRef]

13.   Barbosa, M.D. Immunogenicity of biotherapeutics in the context of developing biosimilars and biobetters. *Drug Discov. Today* **2011**, *16*, 345–353. [CrossRef] [PubMed]

14.   Beck, A.; Wagner-Rousset, E.; Bussat, M.-C.; Lokteff, M.; Klinguer-Hamour, C.; Haeuw, J.-F.; Goetsch, L.; Wurch, T.; Dorsselaer, A.; Corvaia, N. Trends in glycosylation, glycoanalysis and glycoengineering of therapeutic antibodies and Fc-fusion proteins. *Curr. Pharm. Biotechnol.* **2008**, *9*, 482–501. [CrossRef] [PubMed]

15.   Durocher, Y.; Butler, M. Expression systems for therapeutic glycoprotein production. *Curr. Opin. Biotechnol.* **2009**, *20*, 700–707. [CrossRef]

16.   Lam, J.S.; Mansour, M.K.; Specht, C.A.; Levitz, S.M. A model vaccine exploiting fungal mannosylation to increase antigen immunogenicity. *J. Immunol.* **2005**, *175*, 7496–7503. [CrossRef] [PubMed]

17.   Goetze, A.M.; Liu, Y.D.; Zhang, Z.; Shah, B.; Lee, E.; Bondarenko, P.V.; Flynn, G.C. High-mannose glycans on the Fc region of therapeutic IgG antibodies increase serum clearance in humans. *Glycobiology* **2011**, *21*, 949–959. [CrossRef] [PubMed]

18.   Biburger, M.; Lux, A.; Nimmerjahn, F. How immunoglobulin G antibodies kill target cells. *Adv. Immunol.* **2014**, *124*, 67–94. [PubMed]

19.   Tangvoranuntakul, P.; Gagneux, P.; Diaz, S.; Bardor, M.; Varki, N.; Varki, A.; Muchmore, E. Human uptake and incorporation of an immunogenic nonhuman dietary sialic acid. *Proc. Natl. Acad. Sci. USA* **2003**, *100*, 12045–12050. [CrossRef]

20.   Qian, J.; Liu, T.; Yang, L.; Daus, A.; Crowley, R.; Zhou, Q. Structural characterization of N-linked oligosaccharides on monoclonal antibody cetuximab by the combination of orthogonal matrix-assisted laser desorption/ionization hybrid quadrupole–quadrupole time-of-flight tandem mass spectrometry and sequential enzymatic digestion. *Anal. Biochem.* **2007**, *364*, 8–18.

21.   Liu, L. Pharmacokinetics of monoclonal antibodies and Fc-fusion proteins. *Protein Cell* **2018**, *9*, 15–32. [CrossRef] [PubMed]

22.   Roopenian, D.C.; Akilesh, S. FcRn: The neonatal Fc receptor comes of age. *Nat. Rev. Immunol.* **2007**, *7*, 715–725. [CrossRef] [PubMed]

23. Liu, L.; Stadheim, A.; Hamuro, L.; Pittman, T.; Wang, W.; Zha, D.; Hochman, J.; Prueksaritanont, T. Pharmacokinetics of IgG1 monoclonal antibodies produced in humanized Pichia pastoris with specific glycoforms: A comparative study with CHO produced materials. *Biologicals* **2011**, *39*, 205–210. [CrossRef] [PubMed]

24. Chen, X.; Liu, Y.D.; Flynn, G.C. The effect of Fc glycan forms on human IgG2 antibody clearance in humans. *Glycobiology* **2008**, *19*, 240–249. [CrossRef] [PubMed]

25. Yu, M.; Brown, D.; Reed, C.; Chung, S.; Lutman, J.; Stefanich, E.; Wong, A.; Stephan, J.-P.; Bayer, R. Production, characterization and pharmacokinetic properties of antibodies with N-linked Mannose-5 glycans. *MABS* **2012**, *4*, 475–487. [CrossRef]

26. Clarke, S.; Gebbie, C.; Sweeney, C.; Olszewksi, N.; Smith, J. A phase I, pharmacokinetic (PK) and preliminary efficacy assessment of ALD518, a humanized anti-IL-6 antibody, in patients with advanced cancer (Abstract). *J. Clin. Oncol.* **2009**, *27*, 3025.

27. Abuqayyas, L.; Zhang, X.; Balthasar, J.P. Application of knockout mouse models to investigate the influence of FcγR on the pharmacokinetics and anti-platelet effects of MWReg30, a monoclonal anti-GPIIb antibody. *Int. J. Pharm.* **2013**, *444*, 185–192. [CrossRef]

28. Batra, J.; Rathore, A.S. Glycosylation of monoclonal antibody products: Current status and future. *Biotechnol. Prog.* **2016**, *32*, 1091–1102. [CrossRef]

29. Kanda, Y.; Yamada, T.; Mori, K.; Okazaki, A.; Inoue, M.; Kitajima-Miyama, K.; Kuni-Kamochi, R.; Nakano, R.; Yano, K.; Kakita, S.; et al. Comparison of biological activity among nonfucosylated therapeutic IgG1 antibodies with three different N-linked Fc oligosaccharides: The high mannose, hybrid, and complex types. *Glycobiology* **2006**, *17*, 104–118. [CrossRef]

30. Millward, T.A.; Heitzmann, M.; Bill, K.; Längle, U.; Schumacher, P.; Forrer, K. Effect of constant and variable domain glycosylation on pharmacokinetics of therapeutic antibodies in mice. *Biologicals* **2008**, *36*, 41–47. [CrossRef]

31. Sazinsky, S.L.; Ott, R.G.; Silver, N.W.; Tidor, B.; Ravetch, J.V.; Wittrup, K.D. Aglycosylated immunoglobulin G1 variants productively engage activating Fc receptors. *Proc. Natl. Acad. Sci. USA* **2008**, *105*, 20167–20172. [CrossRef] [PubMed]

32. Raju, T.; Briggs, J.B.; Borge, S.M.; Jones, A.J.S. Species-specific variation in glycosylation of IgG: Evidence for the species-specific sialylation and branch-specific galactosylation and importance for engineering recombinant glycoprotein therapeutics. *Glycobiology* **2000**, *10*, 477–486. [CrossRef] [PubMed]

33. Ambrogelly, A.; Gozo, S.; Katiyar, A.; Dellatore, S.; Kune, Y.; Bhat, R.; Sun, J.; Li, N.; Wang, D.; Nowak, C.; et al. Analytical comparability study of recombinant monoclonal antibody therapeutics. *MABS* **2018**, *10*, 513–538. [CrossRef] [PubMed]

34. Flynn, G.C.; Chen, X.; Liu, Y.D.; Shah, B.; Zhang, Z. Naturally occurring glycan forms of human immunoglobulins G1 and G2. *Mol. Immunol.* **2010**, *47*, 2074–2082. [CrossRef]

35. Scallon, B.J.; Tam, S.H.; McCarthy, S.G.; Cai, A.N.; Raju, T.S. Higher levels of sialylated Fc glycans in immunoglobulin G molecules can adversely impact functionality. *Mol. Immunol.* **2007**, *44*, 1524–1534. [CrossRef]

36. Kaneko, Y.; Nimmerjahn, F.; Ravetch, J.V. Anti-Inflammatory activity of immunoglobulin G resulting from Fc sialylation. *Science* **2006**, *313*, 670–673. [CrossRef]

37. Thomann, M.; Schlothauer, T.; Dashivets, T.; Malik, S.; Avenal, C.; Bulau, P.; Rüger, P.; Reusch, D. In vitro glycoengineering of IgG1 and its effect on Fc receptor binding and ADCC activity. *PLoS ONE* **2015**, *10*, e0134949. [CrossRef]

38. Quast, I.; Keller, C.W.; Maurer, M.A.; Giddens, J.P.; Tackenberg, B.; Wang, L.-X.; Münz, C.; Nimmerjahn, F.; Dalakas, M.C.; Lünemann, J.D. Sialylation of IgG Fc domain impairs complement-dependent cytotoxicity. *J. Clin. Investig.* **2015**, *125*, 4160–4170. [CrossRef]

39. Nimmerjahn, F.; Ravetch, J.V. Anti-Inflammatory actions of intravenous immunoglobulin. *Ann. Rev. Immunol.* **2008**, *26*, 513–533. [CrossRef]

40. Anthony, R.M.; Ravetch, J.V. A novel role for the IgG Fc glycan: The anti-inflammatory activity of sialylated IgG Fcs. *J. Clin. Immunol.* **2010**, *30*, 9–14. [CrossRef]

41. Anthony, R.M.; Nimmerjahn, F.; Ashline, D.J.; Reinhold, V.N.; Paulson, J.C.; Ravetch, J.V. Recapitulation of IVIG anti-inflammatory activity with a recombinant IgG Fc. *Science* **2008**, *320*, 373–376. [CrossRef]

42. Bondt, A.; Selman, M.H.J.; Deelder, A.M.; Hazes, J.M.; Willemsen, S.P.; Wuhrer, M.; Dolhain, R.J.E.M. Association between galactosylation of immunoglobulin G and improvement of rheumatoid arthritis during pregnancy is independent of sialylation. *J. Proteome Res.* **2013**, *12*, 4522–4531. [CrossRef] [PubMed]

43. Raju, T.S.; Jordan, R.E. Galactosylation variations in marketed therapeutic antibodies. *MABS* **2012**, *4*, 385–391. [CrossRef] [PubMed]

44. Hodoniczky, J.; Zheng, Y.; James, D. Control of recombinant monoclonal antibody effector functions by Fc N-glycan remodeling in vitro. *Biotechnol. Prog.* **2005**, *21*, 1644–1652. [CrossRef] [PubMed]

45. Peschke, B.; Keller, C.W.; Weber, P.; Quast, I.; Lünemann, J.D. Fc-galactosylation of human immunoglobulin gamma isotypes improves C1q binding and enhances complement-dependent cytotoxicity. *Front. Immunol.* **2017**, *8*, 646. [CrossRef] [PubMed]

46. Patnaik, S.K.; Stanley, P. Lectin-resistant CHO glycosylation mutants. *Meth. Enzymol.* **2006**, *416*, 159–182.

47. Davies, J.; Jiang, L.; Pan, L.-Z.; Labarre, M.J.; Anderson, D.; Reff, M. Expression of GnTIII in a recombinant anti-CD20 CHO production cell line: Expression of antibodies with altered glycoforms leads to an increase in ADCC through higher affinity for FCγRIII. *Biotechnol. Bioeng.* **2001**, *74*, 288–294. [CrossRef]

48. Shinkawa, T.; Nakamura, K.; Yamane, N.; Shoji-Hosaka, E.; Kanda, Y.; Sakurada, M.; Uchida, K.; Anazawa, H.; Satoh, M.; Yamasaki, M.; et al. The absence of fucose but not the presence of galactose or bisecting N-acetylglucosamine of human IgG1 complex-type oligosaccharides shows the critical role of enhancing antibody-dependent cellular cytotoxicity. *J. Biol. Chem.* **2003**, *278*, 3466–3473. [CrossRef]

49. Ferrara, C.; Brünker, P.; Suter, T.; Moser, S.; Püntener, U.; Umaña, P. Modulation of therapeutic antibody effector functions by glycosylation engineering: Influence of Golgi enzyme localization domain and co-expression of heterologous β1, 4-N-acetylglucosaminyltransferase III and Golgi α-mannosidase II. *Biotechnol. Bioeng.* **2006**, *93*, 851–861. [CrossRef]

50. Huang, W.; Giddens, J.; Fan, S.-Q.; Toonstra, C.; Wang, L.-X. Chemoenzymatic glycoengineering of intact IgG antibodies for gain of functions. *J. Am. Chem. Soc.* **2012**, *134*, 12308–12318. [CrossRef]

51. Shields, R.L.; Lai, J.; Keck, R.; Oconnell, L.Y.; Hong, K.; Meng, Y.G.; Weikert, S.H.A.; Presta, L.G. Lack of fucose on human IgG1 N-linked oligosaccharide improves binding to human FcγRIII and antibody-dependent cellular toxicity. *J. Biol. Chem.* **2002**, *277*, 26733–26740. [CrossRef] [PubMed]

52. Niwa, R.; Hatanaka, S.; Shoji-Hosaka, E.; Sakurada, M.; Kobayashi, Y.; Uehara, A.; Yokoi, H.; Nakamura, K.; Shitara, K. Enhancement of the antibody-dependent cellular. *Clin. Cancer Res.* **2004**, *10*, 6248–6255. [CrossRef] [PubMed]

53. Iida, S.; Misaka, H.; Inoue, M.; Shibata, M.; Nakano, R.; Yamane-Ohnuki, N.; Wakitani, M.; Yano, K.; Shitara, K.; Satoh, M. Nonfucosylated therapeutic IgG1 antibody can evade the inhibitory effect of serum immunoglobulin G on antibody-dependent cellular cytotoxicity through its high binding to Fc RIIIa. *Clin. Cancer Res.* **2006**, *12*, 2879–2887. [CrossRef]

54. Niwa, R.; Natsume, A.; Uehara, A.; Wakitani, M.; Iida, S.; Uchida, K.; Satoh, M.; Shitara, K. IgG subclass-independent improvement of antibody-dependent cellular cytotoxicity by fucose removal from Asn297-linked oligosaccharides. *J. Immunol. Meth.* **2005**, *306*, 151–160. [CrossRef] [PubMed]

55. Zhou, Q.; Shankara, S.; Roy, A.; Qiu, H.; Estes, S.; Mcvie-Wylie, A.; Culm-Merdek, K.; Park, A.; Pan, C.; Edmunds, T. Development of a simple and rapid method for producing non-fucosylated oligomannose containing antibodies with increased effector function. *Biotechnol. Bioeng.* **2007**, *99*, 652–665. [CrossRef]

56. Butler, M.; Spearman, M. The choice of mammalian cell host and possibilities for glycosylation engineering. *Curr. Opin. Biotechnol.* **2014**, *30*, 107–112. [CrossRef]

57. Suzuki, E.; Niwa, R.; Saji, S.; Muta, M.; Hirose, M.; Lida, S.; Shiotsu, Y.; Satoh, M.; Shitara, K.; Kondo, M.; et al. A nonfucosylated anti-HER2 antibody augments antibody-dependent cellular cytotoxicity in breast cancer patients. *Clin. Cancer Res.* **2007**, *13*, 1875–1882. [CrossRef]

58. Yamane-Ohnuki, N.; Satoh, M. Production of therapeutic antibodies with controlled fucosylation. *MABS* **2009**, *1*, 230–236. [CrossRef]

59. Urbain, R.; Teillaud, J.L.; Prost, J.F. EMABling antibodies: From feto-maternal allo-immunisation prophylaxis to chronic lymphocytic leukaemia therapy. *Med. Sci.* **2009**, *25*, 1141–1144.

60. Dicker, M.; Strasser, R. Using glyco-engineering to produce therapeutic proteins. *Expert Opin. Biol. Ther.* **2015**, *15*, 1501–1516. [CrossRef]

61. Crowell, C.K.; Grampp, G.E.; Rogers, G.N.; Miller, J.; Scheinman, R.I. Amino acid and manganese supplementation modulates the glycosylation state of erythropoietin in a CHO culture system. *Biotechnol. Bioeng.* **2006**, *96*, 538–549. [CrossRef]

62. Okeley, N.M.; Alley, S.C.; Anderson, M.E.; Boursalian, T.E.; Burke, P.J.; Emmerton, K.M.; Jeffrey, S.C.; Klussman, K.; Law, C.-L.; Sussman, D.; et al. Development of orally active inhibitors of protein and cellular fucosylation. *Proc. Natl. Acad. Sci. USA* **2013**, *110*, 5404–5409. [CrossRef] [PubMed]

63. Powell, L.D. Inhibition of N-Linked Glycosylation. *Curr. Protoc. Mol. Biol.* **1995**, *32*, 17101–17109. [CrossRef]

64. Sullivan, F.X.; Kumar, R.; Kriz, R.; Stahl, M.; Xu, G.-Y.; Rouse, J.; Chang, X.-J.; Boodhoo, A.; Potvin, B.; Cumming, D.A. Molecular cloning of human GDP-mannose 4,6-dehydratase and reconstitution of GDP-fucose biosynthesis in vitro. *J. Biol. Chem.* **1998**, *273*, 8193–8202. [CrossRef]

65. Chan, K.F.; Shahreel, W.; Wan, C.; Teo, G.; Hayati, N.; Tay, S.J.; Tong, W.H.; Yang, Y.; Rudd, P.M.; Zhang, P.; et al. Inactivation of GDP-fucose transporter gene (Slc35c1) in CHO cells by ZFNs, TALENs and CRISPR-Cas9 for production of fucose-free antibodies. *Biotechnol. J.* **2015**, *11*, 399–414. [CrossRef] [PubMed]

66. Imai-Nishiya, H.; Mori, K.; Inoue, M.; Wakitani, M.; Lida, S.; Shitara, K.; Satoh, M. Double knockdown of alpha 1,6-fucosyltransferase (FUT8) and GDP-mannose 4,6-dehydratase (GMD) in antibody-producing cells: A new strategy for generating fully non-fucosylated therapeutic antibodies with enhanced ADCC. *BMC Biotechnol.* **2007**, *7*, 84. [CrossRef] [PubMed]

67. Giddens, J.P.; Wang, L.-X. Chemoenzymatic Glyco-engineering of monoclonal antibodies. *Methods Mol. Biol.* **2015**, *1321*, 375–387. [PubMed]

68. Kurogochi, M.; Mori, M.; Osumi, K.; Tojino, M.; Sugawara, S.-I.; Takashima, S.; Hirose, Y.; Tsukimura, W.; Mizuno, M.; Amano, J.; et al. Glycoengineered monoclonal antibodies with homogeneous glycan (M3, G0, G2, and A2) using a chemoenzymatic approach have different affinities for FcγRIIIa and variable antibody-dependent cellular cytotoxicity activities. *PLoS ONE* **2015**, *10*, e0132848. [CrossRef]

69. Umekawa, M.; Huang, W.; Li, B.; Fujita, K.; Ashida, H.; Wang, L.-X.; Yamamoto, K. Mutants of mucor hiemalis endo-β-N-acetylglucosaminidase show enhanced transglycosylation and glycosynthase-like activities. *J. Biol. Chem.* **2007**, *283*, 4469–4479. [CrossRef]

70. Li, T.; Tong, X.; Yang, Q.; Giddens, J.P.; Wang, L.-X. Glycosynthase mutants of endoglycosidase S2 show potent transglycosylation activity and remarkably relaxed substrate specificity for antibody glycosylation remodeling. *J. Biol. Chem.* **2016**, *291*, 16508–16518. [CrossRef]

71. Wang, L.-X.; Tong, X.; Li, C.; Giddens, J.P.; Li, T. Glycoengineering of Antibodies for Modulating Functions. *Annu. Rev. Biochem.* **2019**, *88*, 433–459. [CrossRef]

72. Bumbaca, D.; Boswell, C.A.; Fielder, P.J.; Khawli, L.A. Physiochemical and biochemical factors influencing the pharmacokinetics of antibody therapeutics. *AAPS J.* **2012**, *14*, 554–558. [CrossRef] [PubMed]

73. Jefferis, R. Glycosylation as a strategy to improve antibody based therapeutics. *Nat. Rev. Drug Discov.* **2009**, *8*, 226–234. [CrossRef] [PubMed]

74. Smith, A.; Manoli, H.; Jaw, S.; Frutoz, K.; Epstein, A.L.; Theil, F.P.; Khawli, L.A. Unraveling the effect of immunogenicity response on the PK/PD, efficacy, and safety of biologics. *J. Immunol. Res.* **2016**, *2016*, 9. [CrossRef] [PubMed]

75. Lu, Y.; Khawli, L.A.; Purushothama, S.; Theil, F.P.; Partridge, M. Recent advances in assessing immunogenicity of therapeutic proteins: Impact on biotherapeutic development. *J. Immunol. Res.* **2016**, *2016*, 1–2. [CrossRef] [PubMed]

76. Beck, A.; Liu, H. Macro-and micro-heterogeneity of natural and recombinant IgG antibodies. *Antibodies* **2019**, *8*, 18. [CrossRef] [PubMed]

77. Reusch, D.; Tejada, M.L. Fc glycans of therapeutic antibodies as critical quality attributes. *Glycobiology* **2015**, *25*, 1325–1334. [CrossRef] [PubMed]

78. Duivelshof, B.L.; Jiskoot, W.; Beck, A.; Veuthey, J.-L.; Guillarme, D.; D'Atri, V. Glycosylation of biosimilars: Recent advances in analytical characterization and clinical implications. *Anal. Chim. Acta* **2019**, *1089*, 1–18. [CrossRef]

11

Antibody Fragments as Tools for Elucidating Structure-Toxicity Relationships and for Diagnostic/Therapeutic Targeting of Neurotoxic Amyloid Oligomers

André L. B. Bitencourt [1,†], Raquel M. Campos [1,†], Erika N. Cline [2], William L. Klein [2] and Adriano Sebollela [1,*]

[1]   Department of Biochemistry and Immunology, Ribeirao Preto Medical School, University of São Paulo, Ribeirão Preto, SP 14049-900, Brazil; brandaobqi@hotmail.com (A.L.B.B.); raquelmariacampos@usp.br (R.M.C.)
[2]   Department of Neurobiology, Northwestern University, Evanston, IL 60208-3520, USA; erika.cline@northwestern.edu (E.N.C.); wklein@northwestern.edu (W.L.K.)
*   Correspondence: sebollela@fmrp.usp.br
†   These authors contributed equally to this work.

Abstract: The accumulation of amyloid protein aggregates in tissues is the basis for the onset of diseases known as amyloidoses. Intriguingly, many amyloidoses impact the central nervous system (CNS) and usually are devastating diseases. It is increasingly apparent that neurotoxic soluble oligomers formed by amyloidogenic proteins are the primary molecular drivers of these diseases, making them lucrative diagnostic and therapeutic targets. One promising diagnostic/therapeutic strategy has been the development of antibody fragments against amyloid oligomers. Antibody fragments, such as fragment antigen-binding (Fab), scFv (single chain variable fragments), and VHH (heavy chain variable domain or single-domain antibodies) are an alternative to full-length IgGs as diagnostics and therapeutics for a variety of diseases, mainly because of their increased tissue penetration (lower MW compared to IgG), decreased inflammatory potential (lack of Fc domain), and facile production (low structural complexity). Furthermore, through the use of in vitro-based ligand selection, it has been possible to identify antibody fragments presenting marked conformational selectivity. In this review, we summarize significant reports on antibody fragments selective for oligomers associated with prevalent CNS amyloidoses. We discuss promising results obtained using antibody fragments as both diagnostic and therapeutic agents against these diseases. In addition, the use of antibody fragments, particularly scFv and VHH, in the isolation of unique oligomeric assemblies is discussed as a strategy to unravel conformational moieties responsible for neurotoxicity. We envision that advances in this field may lead to the development of novel oligomer-selective antibody fragments with superior selectivity and, hopefully, good clinical outcomes.

Keywords: antibody fragments; single chain; amyloid; oligomer; neurotoxicity; NUsc1

1. Toxic Protein Oligomers in Central Nervous System Diseases

In living systems, proteins must assume and maintain a three-dimensional conformation, which dictates their biological functions. Under certain conditions, however, monomeric protein units may self-associate to form oligomeric structures that display both loss of biological, and gain of toxic, function [1]. Ultimately, these oligomers have the potential to aggregate into insoluble amyloid fibrils, highly stable non-branched insoluble structures rich in β-sheet content [2–4]. Although this property is inherent to all proteins [5–7], a number of amyloidogenic proteins accumulate in tissues, causing diseases known as amyloidoses, which can be systemic but commonly impact the central nervous system (CNS) [1,8–11].

It is now evident that soluble oligomers are the most toxic form of amyloidogenic proteins, more so than their monomeric or fibrillar forms, disrupting, e.g., synaptic function, membrane permeability, calcium homeostasis, gene transcription, mitochondrial activity, autophagy, and/or endosomal transport in an array of disease models [12–15]. The first reports on the brain accumulation of toxic soluble oligomers were in Alzheimer's disease (AD); the associated oligomers mainly composed of the 4.5 kDa amyloid β (Aβ) peptide [16–18]. Since then, toxic soluble oligomers of other proteins have been implicated in the onset and progression of several debilitating CNS diseases, e.g., tau, α-synuclein, the prion protein (PrP^c), and huntingtin protein (htt) in Alzheimer's, Parkinson's, prion, and Huntington's diseases, respectively [19–24]. In fact, many of these protein oligomers are found together in multiple diseases [25,26].

Amyloidogenic oligomers have been frequently implicated as promising diagnostic and therapeutic targets for CNS amyloidoses [12,14,27–33]. Despite their disease relevance, the structural hallmarks of such soluble oligomers remain elusive due to their metastability and heterogeneity, hampering our ability to target them therapeutically and diagnostically [12,34–36]. One promising strategy in the structural analysis of amyloidogenic oligomers is the utilization of antibody fragments, which can achieve high conformational selectivity, enabling the isolation and stabilization of different oligomeric species. Furthermore, the structural properties of the antibody fragments themselves make them promising diagnostic/therapeutic tools. In this review, we discuss their application as tools for structural research and diagnostic/therapeutic targeting of oligomers acting in brain amyloidoses.

2. Antibody Fragments

Monoclonal antibodies (mAbs) are currently the largest, and most rapidly growing, class of biopharmaceuticals on the market to treat a variety of diseases [37,38]. However, only four mAbs have been approved to treat a neurodegenerative disease (multiple sclerosis), and these antibodies are thought to work primarily in the periphery [37]. There are a number of challenges in utilizing monoclonal antibodies for the diagnosis or treatment of brain diseases. For one, their large molecular mass hinders their ability to cross the blood–brain barrier [38,39]. Moreover, the crystallizable fraction (Fc) of mAbs can mediate deleterious inflammatory responses resulting in, e.g., meningoencephalitis, vasogenic edema, cerebral microhemorragies, and even death [40–47]. Regarding diagnostics, poor contrast of mAbs in imaging applications due to a long serum half-life has been reported as a drawback [48].

During the past 20 years, antibody fragments have been developed as an alternative to full-length IgGs for the diagnosis and treatment of a variety of diseases, including brain disorders [13,38,39,47,49–52]. These molecules are simple protein motifs of large diversity that include the IgG antigen-binding domain(s) but lack the inflammatory Fc domain, retaining the total (fragment antigen-binding: Fab and single-chain variable fragment: scFv) or partial (VH) antigen specificity of intact IgGs [38,39,52].

Compared to full-length IgGs, antibody fragments have advantages and disadvantages as therapeutics. An important advantage is their smaller size (12–50 kDa), thought to potentiate the blood–brain barrier crossing and tissue penetration and enable access to challenging, cryptic epitopes [38,39,52]. Furthermore, their fast blood clearance makes them ideal imaging agents [39]. On the other hand, their smaller size leads to a shorter half-life in vivo, in part due to rapid kidney clearance, which limits the chance of target engagement without the addition of half-life extension moieties (e.g., PEG and albumin-binding fragments) [38,44]. Another advantage of antibody fragments, is their lack of the inflammatory Fc domain (see discussion above). On the other hand, it is noteworthy that the lack of Fc-dependent activation of immune cells may reduce the efficiency of an immunotherapy when a robust inflammatory response is required [53,54], as in cancer immunotherapy, which requires T cell recruiting [55].

Another advantage of antibody fragments, is their excellent manufacturability and low cost of production [38,39]. They can be efficiently selected from in vitro display libraries (phage or yeast) and cloned and expressed in heterologous expression systems (e.g., bacteria); this facilitates the production of large quantities in an easy and affordable way. Importantly, the in vitro approach eliminates animal immunization, which may be key when the conformation of the immunogen plays a role in antibody specificity [46,56]. Finally, engineered antibody fragments yielding multimers (diabodies, triabodies, and tetrabodies) have been shown to present higher avidity and lower blood clearance than their monomeric counterparts without compromising tissue penetration abilities [38,48,54].

The main types of antibody fragments under development are Fab, scFv (single chain variable fragments), and heavy chain variable domain VH/VHH (single-domain antibodies) fragments [38,39,49,52,57]. The potential of isolated light chain variable domain (VL) chains has not been significantly investigated due to their low stability [56]. An overview of the structures of these molecules is presented in Figure 1. The first artificial antibody fragments reported in the literature were initially obtained by removing the Fc domain through proteolysis [44]. Later advances have enabled the further reduction of antibody structure to scFv and VH/VHH (also called minibodies or nanobodies) [38,39,52–54,57]. These fragment types are described in more detail below.

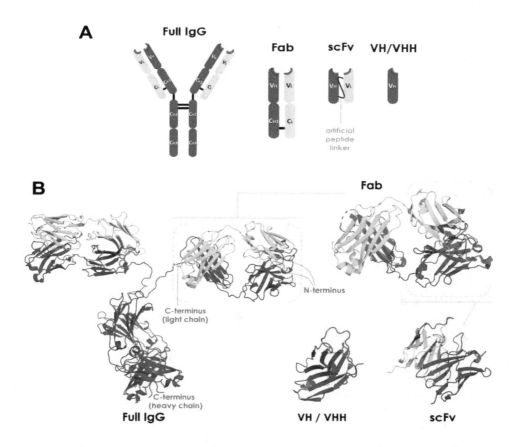

Figure 1. Overview of the structure of antibody fragments. (**A**) General schematic of domain framework and (**B**) ribbon diagrams of full-length IgG and fragment molecules. Structures were obtained from the Protein Data Bank (http://www.rcsb.org/pdb/). CH, CL, VH, and VL stand for constant heavy, constant light, variable heavy, and variable light domains, respectively. Heavy or light chains are depicted in dark blue or cyan, respectively. Complementarity-determining region (CDR) segments are highlighted in red. PDB codes: 1IGT (full length IgG), 5VH3 (Fab), 4NKO (scFv), and 3R0M (VHH) [58]. Fab: fragment antigen-binding; scFv: single chain variable fragments; VH/VHH: heavy chain variable domain fragment.

Fab fragments are independent structural units of ~50 kDa containing two antigen-binding sites, with the heavy chain variable domain (VH) linked to the heavy constant domain 1 (CH1) and the light chain variable domain (VL) linked to the light constant domain (CL) [44]. These domains interact through a large interface between the chains (VH/VL and CH1/CL) and a small one between the variable and the constant domains (VH/CH1 and VL/CL) of each chain [59]. The packing between the variable domains creates the antigen binding site [56]. The CH1 and CL domains are also covalently connected by a disulfide bond between Cys residues at their carboxyl terminal region [60,61]. Each Ig domain presents two layers of β-sheet structures, with three to five β-sheets per layer. The variable Ig domains (cyan; Figure 1B) are slightly longer than the constant domains (dark blue; Figure 1B), as they contain two more β-sheets per layer. The β-sheets are connected through loops, and the β-sheet layers of constant domains are attached through a disulfide bond. All amino terminal variable domain loops pack together in a β-sheet motif arranged as an antiparallel barrel-like structure, forming the complete complementarity-determining region (CDR), which is ultimately responsible for the antibody specificity (highlighted in red in Figure 1B) [44,59]. Each Ig domain contains three amino terminal loops encoding different CDR segments. Since the sequence variation associated with the specificity of immunoglobulins is found in CDRs, these regions are also referred to as hypervariable regions [59]. The hypervariable regions assemble into the antigen binding site and interact directly with the epitope. The framework regions, those comprising the variable domain sequences besides CDRs, fold into β-sheet motif structures and provide the scaffold for antibody-antigen interactions [62].

Single-chain variable fragments (scFvs), the smallest antibody fragments containing a complete antigen binding site, are recombinant molecules of ~30 kDa in which the variable domains of both VL and VH chains are engineered into a single polypeptide chain connected by a flexible peptide linker and/or a disulfide bond [20,43,45,46]. Their hypervariable segments (amino terminal loops) are approximately 10 amino acid residues long and, as in full length IgGs, form the antigen binding site [59]. The length and amino acid composition of the linker are crucial in maintaining the correct fold of these proteins [54]. The linker is typically about 3.5 nm in length and must contain small, hydrophilic residues (typically Gly and Ser) for enhanced solubility and flexibility [44,54].

VH/VHH fragments (~15–20 kDa) are N-terminal Ig domains derived only from the heavy chain, thus retaining antigen binding specificity within a single polypeptide domain [53,59,63]. Similar to VH fragments (Figure 1), VHHs (high affinity variable domains naturally found in camelids) contain three CDRs forming the antigen binding site [59,62]. Human VH domains and camelid VHH framework regions show a high sequence homology [61]. VHH fragments are naturally occurring [38,39,49,52] and especially stable.

3. Antibody Fragments Assisting the Study, and Diagnostic/Therapeutic Targeting, of Neurotoxic Amyloid Oligomers in CNS Amyloidoses

In the last two decades, several studies using antibody fragments to study the role of protein oligomers in CNS amyloidoses have been published (Table 1). Considering the discussion in the first two sections above, a major motivation for the use of antibody fragments as research and diagnostic/therapeutic tools for this disease class is the augmented chance of obtaining high affinity, conformation-sensitive antibodies over the typical animal immunization approach. Antibody fragments that display high selectivity for toxic oligomeric conformations are likely to be capable of neutralizing these neurotoxic aggregates without interfering with the physiological function of their monomeric counterparts, therefore presenting as preferred candidates for immunotherapies to treat amyloidogenic diseases. In the following sections, we review studies describing conformational antibody fragments capable of recognizing soluble oligomeric species formed by distinct proteins linked to prevalent CNS amyloidosis that currently lack a cure. We also highlight reports that, in our view, should provide guidance for the development of improved antibody fragments targeting neurotoxic oligomers.

Table 1. Conformation-sensitive antibody fragments directed to oligomeric species of proteins implicated in central nervous system (CNS) amyloidoses.

Antibody	Fragment Type	CNS Amyloidosis	Target		Ref.
			High Affinity *	Low Affinity	
NUsc1	scFv	AD	Aβ42 Oligomers (>50 kDa) ¶	not reported	[64,65]
MO6	scFv	AD	Aβ42 Oligomers and Immature fibrils (18–37 kDa #)	not reported	[66]
AS	scFv	AD	Aβ42 Oligomers and Immature Protofibrils (25–55 kDa #)	not reported	[67]
HT6	scFv	AD	Aβ42 Oligomers (18–45 kDa #)	not reported	[68]
11A5	scFv	AD	Aβ42 Oligomers (34 kDa #)	not reported	[69]
A4	scFv	AD	Aβ42 Oligomers	Aβ42 Monomers and Fibrils	[70]
E1	scFv	AD	Aβ42 Oligomers	not reported	[71]
scFv59	scFv	AD	Aβ42 Oligomers and Plaques	not reported	[72]
scFv235	scFv	AD	phosphoTau Oligomers (50–70 kDa) #	Tau monomers	[73]
F9T, D11C, H2A	scFv	AD	Tau Oligomers (Trimers) ¶	not reported	[74]
RN2N	scFv	AD	Tau Oligomers	not reported	[75]
D5	scFv	PD	α-Synuclein Oligomers	not reported	[76]
10H	scFv	PD	α-Synuclein Oligomers (Trimers and Hexamers) ¶	α-Synuclein Monomers	[77]
VH14, NbSyn87	VH	PD	α-Synuclein Oligomers	not reported	[78]
D5-apoB	scFv	PD	α-Synuclein Oligomers (28–80 kDa) #	not reported	[79]
W20	scFv	Various diseases	Oligomers of Aβ40 and Aβ42, PrP^C, α-Syn, amylin, insulin, lysozyme	not reported	[80]

* MW/size of targeted oligomers is presented when available. It is also indicated whether MW/size have been determined under non-denaturing ¶ or denaturing # conditions. AD: Alzheimer's Disease; PD: Parkinson's Disease; PrP^c: cellular prion protein.

3.1. Alzheimer's Disease

3.1.1. Amyloid β

The increasing collection of antibody fragments against toxic aggregates associated with Alzheimer's Disease (AD) has enabled the elucidation of important information related to the biochemical nature of these toxic aggregates and their contribution to AD pathogenesis. As discussed above, a major challenge for all amyloidogenic proteins, but perhaps especially for the AD toxins Aβ oligomers (AβOs), has been to identify the most toxic aggregated species. This difficulty in characterization is due to the heterogeneous distribution of metastable species (including non-toxic or differentially toxic species) formed during the aggregation process [81]. Although robust evidence suggests that soluble AβOs and protofibrils play a prominent role in AD progression [12,82], the precise structural features of these soluble aggregates that contribute to AD pathogenesis remain elusive [1,12,81]. However, recent advances in this area have been made possible with the use of conformation-selective fragment antibodies [64–72,82,83]. One of those is the scFv antibody NUsc1, selected from a phage-display library by our group [64,65]. NUsc1 presents a marked selectivity for soluble AβOs compared to monomers or fibrils (Figure 2A) and, importantly, provides neuroprotection against AβO toxicity in cell cultures, blocking AβO binding and reducing AβO-induced oxidative stress and Tau hyperphosphorylation [64,65]. NUsc1 is of particular interest since it recognizes a unique conformational epitope displayed on oligomers of Aβ but not those formed by other proteins (such as Tau or Lysozyme); other anti-AβO scFvs have been shown to recognize a common epitope present on oligomers formed by different proteins [73,81,84]. Moreover, NUsc1 exhibits a marked oligomer size-dependent selectivity, preferentially targeting neurotoxic AβO species larger than 50 kDa, as analyzed under non-denaturing conditions by size-exclusion chromatography (Figure 2B).

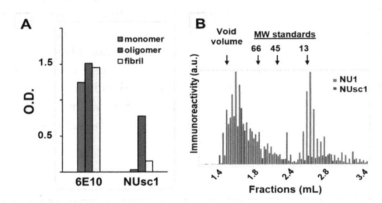

Figure 2. The scFv antibody NUsc1 is highly selective to high molecular weight Aβ oligomers (AβO). (**A**) NUsc1 shows high selectivity for Aβ oligomers over monomers and fibrils as determined via ELISA. The anti-pan Aβ IgG 6E10 is shown for comparison. Adapted with permission from (Velasco et al., ACS Chem. Neurosci. 2012 [64]). Copyright (2020) American Chemical Society. (**B**) Within a synthetic AβO population, NUsc1 selectively targets a high molecular weight subset, showing little binding to a lower molecular weight subset that is readily bound by the anti-AβO IgG NU1. Reactivity of both antibodies to AβO fractions separated by size-exclusion chromatography under non-denaturing conditions was determined by dot immunoblotting. Reprinted with permission from (Sebollela et al., Journal of Neurochem. 2017 [65]).

Other anti-AβO scFvs have been reported that are promising tools for the study of AβO structure–toxicity relationships as well as their diagnostic and therapeutic targeting. The scFv MO6 was found to target AβO species (18–37 kDa) that are on-pathway to fibril formation and toxic to SH-SY5Y cells [66]. Important to its diagnostic/therapeutic potential, MO6 was demonstrated to cross the blood–brain barrier (BBB) in an in vitro BBB model with a delivery efficiency of 66% 60 min post-administration. Another study reported the scFv b4.4, which recognized an epitope in the central region of Aβ42 (comprising residues H^{13}, K^{16} V^{18}, F^{19}) and was able to neutralize the toxicity of either AβOs or fibrillar Aβ to SH-SY5Y cells [83]. The scFv AS was found to recognize cytotoxic medium-sized AβO species (25–55 kDa) and protofibrils [67]. While scFvs are commonly identified via phage display, AS was identified from a library constructed from the immune repertoire of AD patients. The scFv HT6 also was found to bind efficiently to an N-terminal epitope present in cytotoxic medium-sized AβOs (mainly 18–45 kDa) in vitro [68]. Significantly, the anti-AβO scFv 11A5, selected by phage display and found to target a 34 kDa assembly, has been reported to ameliorate cognitive decline in rats induced by injection of AβOs [69]. It is important to consider that in all of these studies, AβO size has been evaluated by denaturing SDS-PAGE/Western immunoblotting, and therefore may not accurately reflect the AβO size in the physiological milieu. Additionally, an interesting approach has been developed wherein atomic force microscopy is utilized to biopan for conformation-selective antibodies by phage display. Following this approach, two scFvs were identified, named A4 and E1, that targeted distinct oligomeric species presenting either high [70] or low [71] cytotoxicity potentials. Further studies with these conformer-selective scFvs, and others like them, promise to shed additional light on the AβO structural properties contributing to AD pathogenesis.

The scFvs highlighted above were all identified by their unique selectivities from antibody libraries. One promising strategy for the rational engineering of scFvs with even further improved selectivity for oligomeric species of interest, is complementarity-determining region (CDR) mapping (i.e., determination of the complementarity-determining region (CDR) amino acid sequences, the regions responsible for antibody specificity) of existing scFvs. So far, CDR mapping has only been reported for non-conformational anti-Aβ scFvs. In one of these reports, Tiller and colleagues (2017) used a series of mutations in the CDR sequences of scFvs to identify the contribution of arginine residues to the affinity and selectivity for Aβ monomers [85]. Other recent studies have contributed to the identification and importance of particular amino acids within CDRs, e.g., tyrosine, glycine, serine, and especially arginine, in the binding to different Aβ aggregated species [86,87]. If similar studies are conducted with anti-AβO scFvs in the future, comparison to these data obtained with non-conformational anti-Aβ scFvs may indicate the key interactions underlying conformational preference for oligomeric over monomeric and fibrillar species. From a therapeutic perspective, the ectopic expression of neurotoxic-selective fragment antibodies by using brain-optimized viral vectors is emerging as an exciting path to be exploited. For instance, recent data in AD-mouse models indicate a cognitive benefit provided by the brain expression of the scFv NUsc1, which was discussed above (unpublished data [88]).

3.1.2. Tau

Another AD-relevant amyloidogenic protein is the microtubule-associated protein Tau. Upon abnormal hyperphosphorylation or co-factor binding, this protein forms oligomers and larger aggregates that contribute to neuronal dysfunction and death in AD and other tauopathies (reviewed in [89,90]). Since Tau oligomers have been linked to neurodegeneration, structural studies aimed to unravel the conformation of soluble Tau aggregates have been the focus of recent investigations [91]. As with AβOs, antibody fragments are emerging as promising tools for these studies [74,75,92]. For instance, Tian et al. (2015) reported the selection of three conformation-selective anti-Tau scFvs (F9T, D11C, H2A) capable of binding trimeric but not monomeric or fibrillar Tau [74]. These scFvs distinguished AD from cognitively normal post-mortem human brains and are capable of detecting oligomeric Tau at earlier ages, compared to typical ages in which neurofibrillary tangles can be detected. In terms of therapy, these oligomer-selective scFv antibodies represent an advantage over non-conformational antibodies as they do not block the physiological functions carried out by monomeric Tau.

3.2. Parkinson's Disease

Parkinson's disease (PD) is a neurodegenerative disorder associated with the abnormal aggregation of the neuronal membrane protein alpha synuclein (α-syn) (reviewed in Shulz-Schaeffer [93]). It has been shown that, besides the formation of insoluble aggregates that deposit inside neurons as inclusion bodies, termed Lewy bodies, α-syn also forms neurotoxic soluble oligomers/protofibrils [94,95]. As with Aβ and Tau, antibody fragments are beginning to emerge in the literature with selectivity for oligomeric over monomeric or fibrillar forms of α-syn. Emadi and colleagues have identified two scFv antibodies of particular use in elucidating α-syn oligomer structure–function relationships. The scFv D5 was found to be selective for oligomers more abundant in initial stages of α-syn aggregation and to block further aggregation of these oligomers and their toxicity in SH-SY5Y cells [76]. D5 was also seen to interact with oligomers formed by the Huntington's disease-associated protein htt51Q [96], in line with the notion that many antibodies raised against amyloid oligomers cross-react with structurally similar oligomers formed by non-related proteins [97]. In contrast, 10H, an scFv that targets oligomers more abundant in later stages of α-syn aggregation, appears to be selective for oligomers of α-syn [77]. Both scFvs D5 and 10H provided neuroprotection in an α-syn overexpressing transgenic mouse model when fused to penetratin (a cell-penetrating peptide), raising a potential immunotherapeutic benefit of these scFvs in PD [98]. Although in principle antibodies targeting pan-amyloid aggregates such as scFv D5 may represent a promising therapeutic strategy, it is also important to consider that cross-reactivity may be harmful in some cases. For instance, Kvam et al. (2009) showed that the anti-fibrillar α-syn scFv-6E, which also binds mutant huntingtin and ataxin-3, increased the aggregation of these polyglutamine-rich proteins in striatal cells, aggravating intracellular dysfunction and cell death [99].

Although few antibody fragments selective for oligomeric α-syn conformations have been reported in the literature, studies utilizing antibody fragments selective for linear α-syn sequences (i.e., non-conformational antibodies) have increased our understanding of α-syn aggregation and toxicity. Zhou et al. (2004) reported the scFv antibody D10, which presented nanomolar affinity for α-syn monomers and inhibited aggregation to oligomeric and protofibrillar forms. The authors localized the D10 epitope within the C-terminus of α-syn, suggesting that perturbation in this region interferes with the aggregation process. In the same study, it was also shown that co-expression of D10 in HEK293 cells engineered to overexpresses α-syn reduced the formation of high-molecular weight α-syn aggregates, thus suggesting a positive action of D10 as an intrabody [100] (i.e., a fragment antibody engineered to accumulate within its producing cell). The VHH single domain antibodies NbSyn2 and NbSyn87 have been used to identify the role of different C-terminal regions of α-syn in fibril formation [101–103]. NbSyn2, which recognizes an epitope between residues 136–140, did not affect fibril formation [78,102,103]. In contrast, NbSyn87, which recognizes an epitope comprised by residues 118–128, induced conformational changes on both secondary and tertiary structures of α-syn, consequentially reducing the half-time of fibril formation [78,101].

scFvs targeting the α-syn nonamyloid component (NAC) have also shown therapeutic promise in pre-clinical studies. The NAC presents a high tendency to adopt β-pleated sheet structures and is known to play a key role in the aggregation and toxicity of α-syn in vitro and in vivo [104]. In 2008, Lynch and colleagues showed a novel NAC-selective scFv named NAC32 capable of reducing the aggregation and neurotoxicity of α-syn aggregates [105]. Other single domain antibodies targeting the NAC, NAC1 and VH14, acted similarly to NAC32 in preventing a-syn aggregation [106].

Although considerable advances towards the understanding of α-syn aggregation and toxicity have been attained by the use of fragment antibodies, few reports have been published so far evaluating the consequences of the in vivo expression/administration of these antibody fragments. Although few, these reports do demonstrate therapeutic promise. In one of these studies, the single-domain antibodies VH14 and NbSyn87 were expressed in fusion with the proteasome-targeting PEST motif, resulting in increased cytoplasmic solubility and enhanced degradation of α-syn in neuronal cell lines [78]. In another interesting piece of work, Spencer et al. (2014) induced the expression of a scFv directed to α-syn oligomers in fusion with the low-density lipoprotein receptor-binding domain from apolipoprotein B (LDL ApoB) in vivo [79]. This construction increased the penetration of the scFv into the brain via the endosomal sorting complex required for transport (ESCRT) pathway, consequently leading to lysosomal degradation of α-syn aggregates [79]. These exciting reports suggest the feasibility of in vivo expression of engineered anti-oligomeric scFvs as a therapeutic alternative for PD.

3.3. Huntington's Disease

Huntingtin (HTT) is a ubiquitously expressed large protein (3144 amino acids) involved in the pathogenesis of Huntington's disease (HD) [107]. Although the diverse physiological roles of HTT are not yet fully understood, it is well known that its aggregation and neurotoxicity are dependent on the presence of an aberrant polyglutamine (polyQ) stretch encoded in exon 1 of the htt gene (corresponding to the N-terminus in the protein) [108–110]. In mutant-disease-associated HTT, this polyQ stretch is longer than in wild type HTT, reaching 40 or more glutamine residues (as opposed to normally 20 on average) [110]. Interestingly, this increment is enough to impact the stability of the whole molecule, driving its aggregation into both soluble oligomers and insoluble aggregates [111].

Since HTT aggregates are exclusively intraneuronal, intrabodies have been the antibody fragment type preferentially applied to their structure-function study and their therapeutic targeting. One of the first scFv-type intrabodies directed to huntingtin was reported by Lecerf et al. (2001). Named C4, this scFv binds to residues 1–17 of HTT, a sequence N-terminal to the polyQ repeat in HTT exon 1, stabilizing an alpha helix-rich oligomeric complex and preventing amyloid formation [112,113]. When co-expressed with HTT exon 1 in non-neuronal cells, C4 was capable of reducing the amount of HTT aggregates and redirecting the subcellular localization of HTT exon 1. Moreover, C4 efficiently reduced cell death in malonate-treated brain slice cultures expressing mutant HTT [114]. Additionally of importance, expression of C4 in the HD disease mouse model B6.HDR6/1, via AAV2/1 vector, led to delayed HTT aggregation in both early and late disease stages [115]. The authors also generated scFv-C4 in fusion with the PEST domain to increase proteasomal degradation of the antigen–antibody complex [115].

A piece of pioneering work by Khoshnan et al. (2002) reported three scFvs (MW1, MW2, and MW7) produced by cloning the antigen-binding domains of monoclonal IgGs targeting either polyQ or an adjacent domain in HTT exon 1 rich in proline residues (named PRD) into scFv scaffolds [116]. The scFv MW7, selective for PRD, inhibited cell death induced by mutant HTT in co-transfected HEK293 cells [116]. Surprisingly MW1 and MW2, both selective for polyQ, accelerated aggregation and cell death in the same culture model. Possible explanations for this unexpected result are that MW1 and MW2 either stabilized a toxic aggregated conformation of HTT or interfered with the binding of HTT to other molecules mediating HTT toxicity [116]. These findings highlight the complexity and importance of identifying fragment antibodies that indeed target toxic oligomeric species, which are expected to show promise as therapeutics and/or diagnostics.

In another piece of work, multiple intrabodies targeting HTT PRD domains (scFv MW7; VL Happ1; VL Happ3) or the HTT N-terminus (VL 12.3) were used to investigate the role of these domains in HTT aggregation and toxicity [117]. VL 12.3 had been previously shown to reduce toxicity in a neuronal culture model of HD [118]. All of these intrabodies reduced mutant HTT exon 1 aggregation and toxicity in both cell culture and brain slice models of HD, although the mechanisms of protection were different. While the N-terminus-targeting intrabody altered HTT subcellular localization, the PRD-targeting intrabodies were seen to increase the turnover rate of HTT [119]. These results reinforce the notion of a strong correlation between the structural domains targeted by each intrabody and their mechanism of neuroprotection. Fragment antibodies VL 12.3 and Haap1 were also employed to investigate the contribution of N-terminus and PRD domains to HD pathology in vivo using five different HD mouse models. While VL 12.3 showed no significant effects on one model, and increased mortality in another, Haap1 alleviated HD neuropathology in all the five animal models tested, including prolonged lifespan in one model [120].

Finally, the scFv-EM48, which targets the C-terminus of human mutant HTT exon 1, also showed promising results in an HD mouse model, as decreased formation of neuropil aggregates and cognitive HD-like symptoms [114]. In conjunction with data obtained with antibody fragments targeting the N-terminus, the polyQ domain, and the PRD domain, these data indicate that all domains within HTT exon 1 play a role in mutant HTT aggregation and toxicity. When used as an intrabody, scFv-EM48 also suppressed the toxicity of mutant HTT in HEK293 cells. The ability of this antibody fragment to increase the ubiquitination and consequent degradation of cytoplasmatic HTT suggests that scFv-EM48 acts by promoting the cytoplasmic clearance of mutant HTT thereby preventing its accumulation.

3.4. Prion Diseases

Prion diseases are characterized by the brain accumulation of aggregated and neurotoxic forms of the prion protein (PrP). Under physiological conditions, PrP presents as a ~24 kDa transmembrane protein that exerts a number of functions, such as metal ion hemostasis and cell adhesion [121]. On the other hand, in diseased brains, it converts into a beta-sheet-rich confirmation named PrP^{sc} (i.e., the scrapie isoform), which forms both soluble oligomers and amyloid fibrils [122–124]. Importantly, PrP^{sc} is known to catalyze the conversion of harmless PrP molecules into the aggregation-prone conformation PrP^{sc}, thus conferring to Prion diseases their unique infectious nature [123]. Finding molecules capable of inhibiting either the formation or the toxicity of PrP^{sc} aggregates, including soluble oligomers, has been a major goal in the prion diseases field, as a way to provide a disease-modifying therapy for patients. In this regard, some fragment antibodies have been selected that display promising inhibitory activity on PrP^{sc} oligomerization and fibrillization both in vitro and in cellular models [125,126].

In 2001, Peretz et al. reported the Fab antibody fragment D18, which binds to an epitope within residues 132–156 in helix 1 of the Prion protein in its native conformation, a region thought to contribute to PrP^{sc} assembly and prion elongation. Although the aggregation states targeted by D18 have not yet been identified experimentally, D18 was found to inhibit prion elongation in cultured mouse neuroblastoma cells infected with PrP^{sc} [126]. Subsequently, Campana et al. (2009) engineered scFv-D18 from Fab-D18 and used in silico tools to create a structural model of scFv-D18 bound to PrP. In that model, PrP residue Arg151 was seen to be key in the interaction with the antibody fragment, by anchoring PrP to the cavity formed on antigen binding site of the scFv [127].

More recently, Fujita et al. (2011) cloned the variable region of mAb 3S9—previously shown to inhibit PrP^{sc} accumulation in cell lines infected with mouse-adapted scrapie strains [128,129]—into the scaffold of a scFv antibody. The resulting antibody, named scFv-3S9, recognized an epitope containing Tyr154 in the helix 1 of PrP. When injected into mice brains, Prion-infected cells expressing scFv-3S9 presented less Prion pathology than infected cells not expressing this scFv [128].

Lastly, Sonati and coworkers (2013) used a panel composed of full-length antibodies and antibody fragments (Fab and scFv) directed to either the globular domain or the flexible tail on PrP, to investigate the role of these regions in oligomerization and neurotoxicity. Results generated on cerebellar organotypic cultured slices showed that both domains are required for toxicity, as the flexible tail acquires oxidative stress-mediated toxicity upon undergoing a conformational change originated from the globular domain [130]. This comprehensive work reinforced the notion that antibody-based therapeutic developments against Prion diseases must include a detailed analysis of the targeted structural epitope of each antibody candidate as well as the molecular and clinical outcomes of targeting these epitopes.

4. Concluding Remarks

Increased knowledge about the aggregation pathways and conformations of the toxic aggregate species relevant to CNS amyloidoses has been obtained with the use of fragment antibodies, in particular Fab, scFv, and VHH (Table 1). As technologies for engineering fragment antibodies are constantly improving, the perspective for the generation of novel fragment antibodies with high selectivity for toxic oligomeric conformations as diagnostic and/or therapeutic candidates for CNS amyloidoses, is also rising.

Methodologies for rational Aβ-targeting antibody design have been reviewed (e.g., Plotkin and Cashman, 2020 [131]). For example, just as our group has successfully generated full-length IgGs with selectivity for AβOs over monomers and fibrils [132], rational immunization with specific toxic AβO species can be employed, followed by conversion of the resulting anti-AβO IgG to an antibody fragment. Alternatively, specific toxic AβO species can be utilized in rational bio-panning of antibody fragment libraries. These specific AβO species can be generated by size-based separation methods (reviewed in [12]) or by utilizing specific Aβ monomeric proteoforms ([133,134]) and can be stabilized by various methods. For example, chemical crosslinking via DFDNB (1,5-difluoro-2,4-dinitrobenzene) has been shown to stabilize high molecular weight AβOs that exhibit toxicity in cell cultures and in vivo [135]. Alternatively, computational prediction of regions present on the surface of toxic oligomeric species is emerging as an additional strategy for rational identification of target species [136].

We envision that the use of fragment antibodies in structural studies aimed to unravel the molecular mechanisms of protein aggregation and related toxicity has a strong potential to make unique contributions to the field. In conjunction with CDR mapping and the detailed analysis of the assembly selectivity of each fragment antibody described, this approach may significantly improve our knowledge regarding key atomic contacts between antibodies and toxic oligomers, and as a consequence, the structural moieties that confer toxicity to amyloid oligomers. These advances could enhance the field's capability of engineering antibody fragments able to selectively target neurotoxic aggregates amongst a multitude of oligomeric assemblies co-existing in diseased human tissue. Even in a likely case in which different oligomeric species contribute to neurotoxicity, and thus a single, highly specific antibody would not able to fully neutralize the pathogenic cascade, a therapeutic strategy based on the combination of multiple oligomer-selective antibody fragments directed against different species could be employed to circumvent this issue.

The cognitive benefit and lowering of multiple AD markers reported in AD patients treated with the antibody aducanumab (Biogen)—a monoclonal IgG that preferentially targets aggregated Aβ [137,138]—has brought hope, reinforcing the notion that selectively targeting neurotoxic aggregates would guide the field toward disease-modifying treatments against brain amyloidosis. Indeed, the FDA has recently granted aducanumab priority review [139]. However, there is still room for improvement in the field as the therapeutic benefits of aducanumab were only apparent following a re-analysis of the phase three trials that were initially halted due to a lack of efficacy [138]. In our view, this improvement will stem from the development of antibodies even more selective to neurotoxic oligomeric assemblies. In this context, detailed structural information on these toxic oligomers will be invaluable to the targeted design of new oligomer-selective fragment antibodies with improved specificity and clinical outcomes.

Author Contributions: All authors have read and agree to the published version of the manuscript. Conceptualization, A.L.B.B., R.M.C. and A.S.; data curation, A.L.B.B., R.M.C. and E.N.C.; writing—original draft preparation, A.L.B.B., R.M.C. and A.S.; writing—review and editing, E.N.C., W.L.K. and A.S.; supervision, A.S. All authors have read and agreed to the published version of the manuscript.

Abbreviations

AD   Alzheimer's Disease
Aβ   Amyloid-β
AβOs   Amyloid-β Peptide Oligomers
CDR   Complementary-determining Region
CNS   Central Nervous System
Fab   Fragment Antigen-Binding
Fc   Fragment Crystallizable
HD   Huntington's Disease
HTT   Huntingtin Protein
IgG   Immunoglobulin G
mAbs   Monoclonal Antibodies
NAC   Nonamyloid Component
PD   Parkinson's Disease
PrP^c Cellular Prion Protein
PrP^{sc} Scrapie Prion Protein
scFv   Single-chain Variable Fragment

References

1. Chiti, F.; Dobson, C.M. Protein Misfolding, Amyloid Formation, and Human Disease: A Summary of Progress Over the Last Decade. *Annu. Rev. Biochem.* **2017**, *86*, 27–68. [CrossRef]

2. Bleiholder, C.; Dupuis, N.F.; Wyttenbach, T.; Bowers, M.T. Ion mobilityg-mass spectrometry reveals a conformational conversion from random assembly to β-sheet in amyloid fibril formation. *Nat. Chem.* **2011**, *3*, 172–177. [CrossRef]

3. Lomont, J.P.; Rich, K.L.; Maj, M.; Ho, J.-J.; Ostrander, J.S.; Zanni, M.T. Spectroscopic Signature for Stable β-Amyloid Fibrils versus β-Sheet-Rich Oligomers. *J. Phys. Chem. B* **2018**, *122*, 144–153. [CrossRef]

4. Lu, J.-X.; Qiang, W.; Yau, W.-M.; Schwieters, C.D.; Meredith, S.C.; Tycko, R. Molecular structure of β-amyloid fibrils in Alzheimer's disease brain tissue. *Cell* **2013**, *154*, 1257–1268. [CrossRef]

5. Kayed, R.; Head, E.; Thompson, J.L.; McIntire, T.M.; Milton, S.C.; Cotman, C.W.; Glabel, C.G. Common structure of soluble amyloid oligomers implies common mechanism of pathogenesis. *Science* **2003**, *300*, 486–489. [CrossRef]

6. Chiti, F.; Webster, P.; Taddei, N.; Clark, A.; Stefani, M.; Ramponi, G.; Dobson, C.M. Designing conditions for in vitro formation of amyloid protofilaments and fibrils. *Proc. Natl. Acad. Sci. USA* **1999**, *96*, 3590–3594. [CrossRef]

7. Bucciantini, M.; Giannoni, E.; Chiti, F.; Baroni, F.; Taddei, N.; Ramponi, G.; Dobson, C.M.; Stefani, M. Inherent toxicity of aggregates implies a common mechanism for protein misfolding diseases. *Nature* **2002**, *416*, 507–511. [CrossRef]

8. Dobson, C.M. The structural basis of protein folding and its links with human disease. *Proc. Philos. Trans. R. Soc. B Biol. Sci.* **2001**, *356*, 133–145. [CrossRef]

9. Kelly, J.W. The alternative conformations of amyloidogenic proteins and their multi-step assembly pathways. *Curr. Opin. Struct. Biol.* **1998**, *8*, 101–106. [CrossRef]

10. Hardy, J.A.; Higgins, G.A. Alzheimer's disease: The amyloid cascade hypothesis. *Science* **1992**, *256*, 184–185. [CrossRef]

11. Vieira, M.N.N.; Forny-Germano, L.; Saraiva, L.M.; Sebollela, A.; Martinez, A.M.B.; Houzel, J.C.; De Felice, F.G.; Ferreira, S.T. Soluble oligomers from a non-disease related protein mimic Aβ-induced tau hyperphosphorylation and neurodegeneration. *J. Neurochem.* **2007**, *103*, 736–748. [CrossRef]

12. Cline, E.N.; Bicca, M.A.; Viola, K.L.; Klein, W.L. The Amyloid-β Oligomer Hypothesis: Beginning of the Third Decade. *J. Alzheimer's Dis.* **2018**, *64*, S567–S610. [CrossRef]

13. Valera, E.; Spencer, B.; Masliah, E. Immunotherapeutic Approaches Targeting Amyloid-β, α-Synuclein, and Tau for the Treatment of Neurodegenerative Disorders. *Neurotherapeutics* **2016**, *13*, 179–189. [CrossRef]

14. Bittar, A.; Bhatt, N.; Kayed, R. Advances and considerations in AD tau-targeted immunotherapy. *Neurobiol. Dis.* **2020**, *134*, 104707. [CrossRef]

15. Choi, M.L.; Gandhi, S. Crucial role of protein oligomerization in the pathogenesis of Alzheimer's and Parkinson's diseases. *FEBS J.* **2018**, *285*, 3631–3644. [CrossRef]

16. Gong, Y.; Chang, L.; Viola, K.L.; Lacor, P.N.; Lambert, M.P.; Finch, C.E.; Krafft, G.A.; Klein, W.L. Alzheimer's disease-affected brain: Presence of oligomeric A ligands (ADDLs) suggests a molecular basis for reversible memory loss. *Proc. Natl. Acad. Sci. USA* **2003**, *100*, 10417–10422. [CrossRef]

17. Shankar, G.M.; Li, S.; Mehta, T.H.; Garcia-Munoz, A.; Shepardson, N.E.; Smith, I.; Brett, F.M.; Farrell, M.A.; Rowan, M.J.; Lemere, C.A.; et al. Amyloid-β protein dimers isolated directly from Alzheimer's brains impair synaptic plasticity and memory. *Nat. Med.* **2008**, *14*, 837–842. [CrossRef]

18. Lambert, M.P.; Barlow, A.K.; Chromy, B.A.; Edwards, C.; Freed, R.; Liosatos, M.; Morgan, T.E.; Rozovsky, I.; Trommer, B.; Viola, K.L.; et al. Diffusible, nonfibrillar ligands derived from A 1-42 are potent central nervous system neurotoxins. *Proc. Natl. Acad. Sci. USA* **1998**, *95*, 6448–6453. [CrossRef]

19. Theillet, F.X.; Binolfi, A.; Bekei, B.; Martorana, A.; Rose, H.M.; Stuiver, M.; Verzini, S.; Lorenz, D.; Van Rossum, M.; Goldfarb, D.; et al. Structural disorder of monomeric α-synuclein persists in mammalian cells. *Nature* **2016**. [CrossRef]

20. Spillantini, M.G.; Schmidt, M.L.; Lee, V.M.Y.; Trojanowski, J.Q.; Jakes, R.; Goedert, M. Alpha-synuclein in Lewy bodies. *Nature* **1997**, *388*, 839–840. [CrossRef]

21. Hatters, D.M. Protein misfolding inside cells: The case of Huntingtin and Huntington's disease. *IUBMB Life* **2008**, *60*, 724–728. [CrossRef]

22. Imarisio, S.; Carmichael, J.; Korolchuk, V.; Chen, C.W.; Saiki, S.; Rose, C.; Krishna, G.; Davies, J.E.; Ttofi, E.; Underwood, B.R.; et al. Huntington's disease: From pathology and genetics to potential therapies. *Biochem. J.* **2008**, *412*, 191–209. [CrossRef]

23. Grassmann, A.; Wolf, H.; Hofmann, J.; Graham, J.; Vorberg, I. Cellular aspects of prion replication in vitro. *Viruses* **2012**, *5*, 374–405. [CrossRef]

24. Soto, C.; Satani, N. The intricate mechanisms of neurodegeneration in prion diseases. *Trends Mol. Med.* **2011**, *17*, 14–24. [CrossRef]

25. Rabinovici, G.D.; Carrillo, M.C.; Forman, M.; DeSanti, S.; Miller, D.S.; Kozauer, N.; Petersen, R.C.; Randolph, C.; Knopman, D.S.; Smith, E.E.; et al. Multiple comorbid neuropathologies in the setting of Alzheimer's disease neuropathology and implications for drug development. *Alzheimer's Dement. Transl. Res. Clin. Interv.* **2017**, *3*, 83–91. [CrossRef]

26. Visanji, N.P.; Lang, A.E.; Kovacs, G.G. Beyond the synucleinopathies: Alpha synuclein as a driving force in neurodegenerative comorbidities. *Transl. Neurodegener.* **2019**, *8*, 28. [CrossRef]

27. Goure, W.F.; Krafft, G.A.; Jerecic, J.; Hefti, F. Targeting the proper amyloid-beta neuronal toxins: A path forward for Alzheimer's disease immunotherapeutics. *Alzheimer's Res. Ther.* **2014**, *6*, 42. [CrossRef]

28. Sengupta, U.; Nilson, A.N.; Kayed, R. The Role of Amyloid-β Oligomers in Toxicity, Propagation, and Immunotherapy. *EBioMedicine* **2016**, *6*, 42–49. [CrossRef]

29. Oertel, W.H. Recent advances in treating Parkinson's disease. *F1000Research* **2017**, *6*, 260. [CrossRef]

30. Masnata, M.; Cicchetti, F. The evidence for the spread and seeding capacities of the mutant huntingtin protein in in vitro systems and their therapeutic implications. *Front. Neurosci.* **2017**, *11*, 647. [CrossRef]

31. Jankovic, J.; Rousseaux, M.W.C.; Shulman, J.M. Progress toward an integrated understanding of Parkinson's disease. *F1000Research* **2017**, *6*, 1121.

32. Velayudhan, L.; Ffytche, D.; Ballard, C.; Aarsland, D. New Therapeutic Strategies for Lewy Body Dementias. *Curr. Neurol. Neurosci. Rep.* **2017**, *17*, 68. [CrossRef]

33. Zella, S.M.A.; Metzdorf, J.; Ciftci, E.; Ostendorf, F.; Muhlack, S.; Gold, R.; Tönges, L. Emerging Immunotherapies for Parkinson Disease. *Neurol. Ther.* **2019**, *8*, 29–44. [CrossRef]

34. De Genst, E.; Messer, A.; Dobson, C.M. Antibodies and protein misfolding: From structural research tools to therapeutic strategies. *Biochim. Biophys. Acta* **2014**, *8*, 29–44. [CrossRef]

35. Villar-Piqué, A.; Lopes da Fonseca, T.; Outeiro, T.F. Structure, function and toxicity of alpha-synuclein: the Bermuda triangle in synucleinopathies. *J. Neurochem.* **2016**, *139*, 240–255. [CrossRef]

36. Hoffner, G.; Djian, P. Polyglutamine Aggregation in Huntington Disease: Does Structure Determine Toxicity? *Mol. Neurobiol.* **2015**, *52*, 1297–1314. [CrossRef]

37. Carter, L.; Kim, S.J.; Schneidman-Duhovny, D.; Stöhr, J.; Poncet-Montange, G.; Weiss, T.M.; Tsuruta, H.; Prusiner, S.B.; Sali, A. Prion Protein—Antibody Complexes Characterized by Chromatography-Coupled Small-Angle X-Ray Scattering. *Biophys. J.* **2015**, *109*, 793–805. [CrossRef]

38. Bates, A.; Power, C.A. David vs. Goliath: The Structure, Function, and Clinical Prospects of Antibody Fragments. *Antibodies* **2019**, *8*, 28. [CrossRef]

39. Bélanger, K.; Iqbal, U.; Tanha, J.; MacKenzie, R.; Moreno, M.; Stanimirovic, D. Single-Domain Antibodies as Therapeutic and Imaging Agents for the Treatment of CNS Diseases. *Antibodies* **2019**, *8*, 27. [CrossRef]

40. Nicoll, J.A.; Wilkinson, D.; Holmes, C.; Steart, P.; Markham, H.; Weller, R.O. Neuropathology of human Alzheimer disease after immunization with amyloid-beta peptide: a case report. *Nat Med* **2003**, *9*, 448–452. [CrossRef]

41. Ferrer, I.; Rovira, M.B.; Guerra, M.L.S.; Rey, M.J.; Costa-Jussá, F. Neuropathology and Pathogenesis of Encephalitis following Amyloid β Immunization in Alzheimer's Disease. *Brain Pathol.* **2004**, *14*, 11–20. [CrossRef]

42. Gilman, S.; Koller, M.; Black, R.S.; Jenkins, L.; Griffith, S.G.; Fox, N.C.; Eisner, L.; Kirby, L.; Boada Rovira, M.; Forette, F.; et al. Clinical effects of Aβ immunization (AN1792) in patients with AD in an interrupted trial. *Neurology* **2005**, *64*, 1553–1562. [CrossRef]

43. Lee, M.; Bard, F.; Johnson-Wood, K.; Lee, C.; Hu, K.; Griffith, S.G.; Black, R.S.; Schenk, D.; Seubert, P. Aβ42 immunization in Alzheimer's disease generates Aβ N-terminal antibodies. *Ann. Neurol.* **2005**, *28*, 430–435. [CrossRef]

44. Strohl, W.R.; Strohl, L.M. *Therapeutic Antibody Engineering: Current and Future Advances Driving the Strongest Growth Area in the Pharmaceutical Industry*; Woodhead Publishing: Cambridge, UK, 2012; ISBN 9781907568374.

45. Meyer-Luehmann, M.; Spires-Jones, T.L.; Prada, C.; Garcia-Alloza, M.; De Calignon, A.; Rozkalne, A.; Koenigsknecht-Talboo, J.; Holtzman, D.M.; Bacskai, B.J.; Hyman, B.T. Rapid appearance and local toxicity of amyloid-β plaques in a mouse model of Alzheimer's disease. *Nature* **2008**, *451*, 720–724. [CrossRef]

46. Esquerda-Canals, G.; Martí-Clúa, J.; Villegas, S. Pharmacokinetic parameters and mechanism of action of an efficient anti-Aβ single chain antibody fragment. *PLoS One* **2019**, *14*, e0217793. [CrossRef]

47. Manoutcharian, K.; Perez-Garmendia, R.; Gevorkian, G. Recombinant Antibody Fragments for Neurodegenerative Diseases. *Curr. Neuropharmacol.* **2016**, *5*, 779–788. [CrossRef]

48. Holliger, P.; Hudson, P.J. Engineered antibody fragments and the rise of single domains. *Nat. Biotechnol.* **2005**, *23*, 1126–1136. [CrossRef]

49. Pain, C.; Dumont, J.; Dumoulin, M. Camelid single-domain antibody fragments: Uses and prospects to investigate protein misfolding and aggregation, and to treat diseases associated with these phenomena. *Biochimie* **2015**, *111*, 82–106. [CrossRef]

50. Chia, K.Y.; Ng, K.Y.; Koh, R.Y.; Chye, S.M. Single-chain Fv Antibodies for Targeting Neurodegenerative Diseases. *CNS Neurol. Disord.* **2018**, *17*, 671–679. [CrossRef]

51. Chatterjee, D.; Kordower, J.H. Immunotherapy in Parkinson's disease: Current status and future directions. *Neurobiol. Dis.* **2019**, *132*, 104587. [CrossRef]

52. Messer, A.; Butler, D.C. Optimizing intracellular antibodies (intrabodies/nanobodies) to treat neurodegenerative disorders. *Neurobiol. Dis.* **2020**, *134*, 104619. [CrossRef]

53. Nelson, A.L.; Reichert, J.M. Development trends for therapeutic antibody fragments. *Nat. Biotechnol.* **2009**, *27*, 331–337. [CrossRef]

54. Monnier, P.; Vigouroux, R.; Tassew, N. In Vivo Applications of Single Chain Fv (Variable Domain) (scFv) Fragments. *Antibodies* **2013**, *2*, 193–208. [CrossRef]

55. Alspach, E.; Lussier, D.M.; Miceli, A.P.; Kizhvatov, I.; DuPage, M.; Luoma, A.M.; Meng, W.; Lichti, C.F.; Esaulova, E.; Vomund, A.N.; et al. MHC-II neoantigens shape tumour immunity and response to immunotherapy. *Nature* **2019**, *574*, 696–701. [CrossRef]

56. Ewert, S.; Huber, T.; Honegger, A.; Plückthun, A. Biophysical properties of human antibody variable domains. *J. Mol. Biol.* **2003**, *325*, 531–553. [CrossRef]

57. Nelson, A.L. Antibody fragments: Hope and hype. *MAbs* **2010**, *2*, 77–83. [CrossRef]

58. Rose, A.S.; Hildebrand, P.W. NGL Viewer: A web application for molecular visualization. *Nucleic Acids Res.* **2015**, *43*, W576–W579. [CrossRef]

59. Abbas, A.K.; Lichtman, A.H. *Cellular and Molecular Immunology*; Saunders: Philadelphia, PA, USA, 2014; ISBN 9780323315937.

60. Wörn, A.; Plückthun, A. Stability engineering of antibody single-chain Fv fragments. *J. Mol. Biol.* **2001**, *305*, 989–1010. [CrossRef]

61. Harmsen, M.M.; De Haard, H.J. Properties, production, and applications of camelid single-domain antibody fragments. *Appl. Microbiol. Biotechnol.* **2007**, *77*, 13–22. [CrossRef]

62. Paul, W.E. *Fundamental Immunology*; LWW: Philadelphia, PA, USA, 2012; ISBN 9781451117837.

63. Mitchell, L.S.; Colwell, L.J. Comparative analysis of nanobody sequence and structure data. *Proteins Struct. Funct. Bioinforma.* **2018**, *86*, 697–706. [CrossRef]

64. Velasco, P.T.; Heffern, M.C.; Sebollela, A.; Popova, I.A.; Lacor, P.N.; Lee, K.B.; Sun, X.; Tiano, B.N.; Viola, K.L.; Eckermann, A.L.; et al. Synapse-binding subpopulations of Abeta oligomers sensitive to peptide assembly blockers and scFv antibodies. *ACS Chem Neurosci* **2012**, *3*, 972–981. [CrossRef]

65. Sebollela, A.; Cline, E.N.; Popova, I.; Luo, K.; Sun, X.; Ahn, J.; Barcelos, M.A.; Bezerra, V.N.; Lyra e Silva, N.M.; Patel, J.; et al. A human scFv antibody that targets and neutralizes high molecular weight pathogenic amyloid-β oligomers. *J. Neurochem.* **2017**, *142*, 934–947. [CrossRef]

66. Zhang, Y.; Chen, X.; Liu, J.; Zhang, Y. The protective effects and underlying mechanism of an anti-oligomeric Aβ42 single-chain variable fragment antibody. *Neuropharmacology* **2015**, *99*, 387–395. [CrossRef]

67. Zhang, Y.; Sun, Y.; Huai, Y.; Zhang, Y.J. Functional Characteristics and Molecular Mechanism of a New scFv Antibody Against Aβ42 Oligomers and Immature Protofibrils. *Mol. Neurobiol.* **2015**, *52*, 1269–1281. [CrossRef]

68. Zhang, X.; Huai, Y.; Cai, J.; Song, C.; Zhang, Y. Novel antibody against oligomeric amyloid-β: Insight into factors for effectively reducing the aggregation and cytotoxicity of amyloid-β aggregates. *Int. Immunopharmacol.* **2019**, *67*, 176–185. [CrossRef]

69. Wang, J.; Wang, J.; Li, N.; Ma, J.; Gu, Z.; Yu, L.; Fu, X.; Liu, X. Effects of an amyloid-beta 1-42 oligomers antibody screened from a phage display library in APP/PS1 transgenic mice. *Brain Res.* **2016**, *1635*, 169–179. [CrossRef]
70. Zameer, A.; Kasturirangan, S.; Emadi, S.; Nimmagadda, S. V.; Sierks, M.R. Anti-oligomeric Aβ Single-chain Variable Domain Antibody Blocks Aβ-induced Toxicity Against Human Neuroblastoma Cells. *J. Mol. Biol.* **2008**, *384*, 917–928. [CrossRef]
71. Kasturirangan, S.; Li, L.; Emadi, S.; Boddapati, S.; Schulz, P.; Sierks, M.R. Nanobody specific for oligomeric beta-amyloid stabilizes nontoxic form. *Neurobiol. Aging* **2012**, *33*, 1320–1328. [CrossRef]
72. Yang, J.; Pattanayak, A.; Song, M.; Kou, J.; Taguchi, H.; Paul, S.; Ponnazhagan, S.; Lalonde, R.; Fukuchi, K.I. Muscle-directed anti-Aβ Single-Chain Antibody Delivery Via AAV1 reduces cerebral Aβ load in an Alzheimer's disease mouse model. *J. Mol. Neurosci.* **2013**, *49*, 277–288. [CrossRef]
73. Krishnaswamy, S.; Lin, Y.; Rajamohamedsait, W.J.; Rajamohamedsait, H.B.; Krishnamurthy, P.; Sigurdsson, E.M. Antibody-derived in Vivo imaging of tau pathology. *J. Neurosci.* **2014**, *34*, 16835–16850. [CrossRef]
74. Tian, H.; Davidowitz, E.; Lopez, P.; He, P.; Schulz, P.; Moe, J.; Sierks, M.R. Isolation and characterization of antibody fragments selective for toxic oligomeric tau. *Neurobiol. Aging* **2015**, *36*, 1342–1355. [CrossRef]
75. Nisbet, R.M.; Van Der Jeugd, A.; Leinenga, G.; Evans, H.T.; Janowicz, P.W.; Götz, J. Combined effects of scanning ultrasound and a tau-specific single chain antibody in a tau transgenic mouse model. *Brain* **2017**, *140*, 1220–1230. [CrossRef]
76. Emadi, S.; Barkhordarian, H.; Wang, M.S.; Schulz, P.; Sierks, M.R. Isolation of a Human Single Chain Antibody Fragment Against Oligomeric α-Synuclein that Inhibits Aggregation and Prevents α-Synuclein-induced Toxicity. *J. Mol. Biol.* **2007**, *368*, 1132–1144. [CrossRef]
77. Emadi, S.; Kasturirangan, S.; Wang, M.S.; Schulz, P.; Sierks, M.R. Detecting morphologically distinct oligomeric forms of α-synuclein. *J. Biol. Chem.* **2009**, *284*, 11048–11058. [CrossRef]
78. Butler, D.C.; Joshi, S.N.; De Genst, E.; Baghel, A.S.; Dobson, C.M.; Messer, A. Bifunctional anti-non-amyloid component α-Synuclein nanobodies are protective in situ. *PLoS ONE* **2016**, *11*, e0165964. [CrossRef]
79. Spencer, B.; Emadi, S.; Desplats, P.; Eleuteri, S.; Michael, S.; Kosberg, K.; Shen, J.; Rockenstein, E.; Patrick, C.; Adame, A.; et al. ESCRT-mediated uptake and degradation of brain-targeted α-synuclein single chain antibody attenuates neuronal degeneration in vivo. *Mol. Ther.* **2014**, *22*, 1753–1767. [CrossRef]
80. Zhang, X.; Sun, X.X.; Xue, D.; Liu, D.G.; Hu, X.Y.; Zhao, M.; Yang, S.G.; Yang, Y.; Xia, Y.J.; Wang, Y.; et al. Conformation-dependent scFv antibodies specifically recognize the oligomers assembled from various amyloids and show colocalization of amyloid fibrils with oligomers in patients with amyloidoses. *Biochim. Biophys. Acta* **2011**, *1814*, 1703–1712. [CrossRef]
81. Benilova, I.; Karran, E.; De Strooper, B. The toxic Aβ oligomer and Alzheimer's disease: An emperor in need of clothes. *Nat. Neurosci.* **2012**, *15*, 349–357. [CrossRef]
82. Haass, C.; Selkoe, D.J. Soluble protein oligomers in neurodegeneration: Lessons from the Alzheimer's amyloid β-peptide. *Nat. Rev. Mol. Cell Biol.* **2007**, *8*, 101–112. [CrossRef]
83. Solórzano-Vargas, R.S.; Vasilevko, V.; Acero, G.; Ugen, K.E.; Martinez, R.; Govezensky, T.; Vazquez-Ramirez, R.; Kubli-Garfias, C.; Cribbs, D.H.; Manoutcharian, K.; et al. Epitope mapping and neuroprotective properties of a human single chain FV antibody that binds an internal epitope of amyloid-beta 1-42. *Mol. Immunol.* **2008**. [CrossRef]
84. Williams, S.M.; Schulz, P.; Sierks, M.R. Oligomeric α-synuclein and β-amyloid variants as potential biomarkers for Parkinson's and Alzheimer's diseases. *Eur. J. Neurosci.* **2016**. [CrossRef]
85. Tiller, K.E.; Li, L.; Kumar, S.; Julian, M.C.; Garde, S.; Tessier, P.M. Arginine mutations in antibody complementarity-determining regions display context-dependent affinity/specificity trade-offs. *J. Biol. Chem.* **2017**, *45*, 881–886. [CrossRef]
86. Das, U.; Hariprasad, G.; Ethayathulla, A.S.; Manral, P.; Das, T.K.; Pasha, S.; Mann, A.; Ganguli, M.; Verma, A.K.; Bhat, R.; et al. Inhibition of protein aggregation: Supramolecular assemblies of Arginine hold the key. *PLoS ONE* **2007**, *2*, e1176. [CrossRef]
87. Kawasaki, T.; Onodera, K.; Kamijo, S. Selection of peptide inhibitors of soluble Aβ1-42 oligomer formation by phage display. *Biosci. Biotechnol. Biochem.* **2010**, *74*, 2214–2219. [CrossRef]
88. Sellés, M.C.; Fortuna, J.; Cercato, M.; Bitencourt, A.; Souza, A.; Prado, V.; Prado, M.; Sebollela, A.; Arancio, O.; Klein, W.; et al. Neuronal expression of NUsc1, a single-chain variable fragment antibody against Ab oligomers, protects synapses and rescues memory in Alzheimer's disease models. *IBRO Rep.* **2019**, *6*, S497. [CrossRef]

89. Castellani, R.J.; Perry, G.; Tabaton, M. Tau biology, tauopathy, traumatic brain injury, and diagnostic challenges. *J. Alzheimer's Dis.* **2019**, *67*, 447–467. [CrossRef]

90. Buée, L.; Bussière, T.; Buée-Scherrer, V.; Delacourte, A.; Hof, P.R. Tau protein isoforms, phosphorylation and role in neurodegenerative disorders. *Brain Res. Rev.* **2000**, *33*, 95–130. [CrossRef]

91. Kundel, F.; Hong, L.; Falcon, B.; McEwan, W.A.; Michaels, T.C.T.; Meisl, G.; Esteras, N.; Abramov, A.Y.; Knowles, T.J.P.; Goedert, M.; et al. Measurement of Tau Filament Fragmentation Provides Insights into Prion-like Spreading. *ACS Chem. Neurosci.* **2018**, *9*, 1276–1282. [CrossRef]

92. Ising, C.; Gallardo, G.; Leyns, C.E.G.; Wong, C.H.; Jiang, H.; Stewart, F.; Koscal, L.J.; Roh, J.; Robinson, G.O.; Serrano, J.R.; et al. AAV-mediated expression of anti-tau scFvs decreases tau accumulation in a mouse model of tauopathy. *J. Exp. Med.* **2017**, *214*, 1227–1238. [CrossRef]

93. Schulz-Schaeffer, W.J. The synaptic pathology of α-synuclein aggregation in dementia with Lewy bodies, Parkinson's disease and Parkinson's disease dementia. *Acta Neuropathol.* **2010**, *12*, 131–143. [CrossRef]

94. Langston, J.W.; Sastry, S.; Chan, P.; Forno, L.S.; Bolin, L.M.; Di Monte, D.A. Novel α-synuclein-immunoreactive proteins in brain samples from the Contursi kindred, Parkinson's, and Alzheimer's disease. *Exp. Neurol.* **1998**, *154*, 684–690. [CrossRef]

95. Conway, K.A.; Harper, J.D.; Lansbury, P.T. Fibrils formed in vitro from α-synuclein and two mutant forms linked to Parkinson's disease are typical amyloid. *Biochemistry* **2000**, *39*, 2552–2563. [CrossRef]

96. Nannenga, B.L.; Zameer, A.; Sierks, M.R. Anti-oligomeric single chain variable domain antibody differentially affects huntingtin and α-synuclein aggregates. *FEBS Lett.* **2008**, *582*, 517–522. [CrossRef]

97. Kayed, R.; Head, E.; Sarsoza, F.; Saing, T.; Cotman, C.W.; Necula, M.; Margol, L.; Wu, J.; Breydo, L.; Thompson, J.L.; et al. Fibril specific, conformation dependent antibodies recognize a generic epitope common to amyloid fibrils and fibrillar oligomers that is absent in prefibrillar oligomers. *Mol. Neurodegener.* **2007**, *2*, 18. [CrossRef]

98. Spencer, B.; Williams, S.; Rockenstein, E.; Valera, E.; Xin, W.; Mante, M.; Florio, J.; Adame, A.; Masliah, E.; Sierks, M.R. α-synuclein conformational antibodies fused to penetratin are effective in models of Lewy body disease. *Ann. Clin. Transl. Neurol.* **2016**, *3*, 588–606. [CrossRef]

99. Kvam, E.; Nannenga, B.L.; Wang, M.S.; Jia, Z.; Sierks, M.R.; Messer, A. Conformational targeting of fibrillar polyglutamine proteins in live cells escalates aggregation and cytotoxicity. *PLoS One* **2009**, *4*, e5727. [CrossRef]

100. Zhou, C.; Emadi, S.; Sierks, M.R.; Messer, A. A human single-chain Fv intrabody blocks aberrant cellular effects of overexpressed α-synuclein. *Mol. Ther.* **2004**, *10*, 1023–1031. [CrossRef]

101. De Genst, E.J.; Guilliams, T.; Wellens, J.; Day, E.M.; Waudby, C.A.; Meehan, S.; Dumoulin, M.; Hsu, S.T.D.; Cremades, N.; Verschueren, K.H.G.; et al. Structure and properties of a complex of α-synuclein and a single-domain camelid antibody. *J. Mol. Biol.* **2010**, *402*, 326–343. [CrossRef]

102. Vuchelen, A.; O'Day, E.; De Genst, E.; Pardon, E.; Wyns, L.; Dumoulin, M.; Dobson, C.M.; Christodoulou, J.; Hsu, S.T.D. 1H, 13C and 15N assignments of a camelid nanobody directed against human α-synuclein. *Biomol. NMR Assign.* **2009**, *3*, 231–233. [CrossRef]

103. El-Turk, F.; Newby, F.N.; De Genst, E.; Guilliams, T.; Sprules, T.; Mittermaier, A.; Dobson, C.M.; Vendruscolo, M. Structural Effects of Two Camelid Nanobodies Directed to Distinct C-Terminal Epitopes on α-Synuclein. *Biochemistry* **2016**, *55*, 3116–3122. [CrossRef]

104. Emamzadeh, F.N. Alpha-synuclein structure, functions, and interactions. *J. Res. Med. Sci.* **2016**, *9*, 21–29. [CrossRef]

105. Lynch, S.M.; Zhou, C.; Messer, A. An scFv Intrabody against the Nonamyloid Component of α-Synuclein Reduces Intracellular Aggregation and Toxicity. *J. Mol. Biol.* **2008**, *377*, 136–147. [CrossRef]

106. Guilliams, T.; El-Turk, F.; Buell, A.K.; O'Day, E.M.; Aprile, F.A.; Esbjörner, E.K.; Vendruscolo, M.; Cremades, N.; Pardon, E.; Wyns, L.; et al. Nanobodies raised against monomeric α-synuclein distinguish between fibrils at different maturation stages. *J. Mol. Biol.* **2013**, *425*, 2397–2411. [CrossRef]

107. Ross, C.A.; Tabrizi, S.J. Huntington's disease: From molecular pathogenesis to clinical treatment. *Lancet Neurol.* **2011**, *10*, 83–98. [CrossRef]

108. Davies, S.W.; Turmaine, M.; Cozens, B.A.; DiFiglia, M.; Sharp, A.H.; Ross, C.A.; Scherzinger, E.; Wanker, E.E.; Mangiarini, L.; Bates, G.P. Formation of neuronal intranuclear inclusions underlies the neurological dysfunction in mice transgenic for the HD mutation. *Cell* **1997**, *90*, 537–548. [CrossRef]

109. Lecerf, J.M.; Shirley, T.L.; Zhu, Q.; Kazantsev, A.; Amersdorfer, P.; Housman, D.E.; Messer, A.; Huston, J.S. Human single-chain Fv intrabodies counteract in situ huntingtin aggregation in cellular models of Huntington's disease. *Proc. Natl. Acad. Sci. USA* **2001**, *98*, 4764–4769. [CrossRef]

110. Saudou, F.; Humbert, S. The Biology of Huntingtin. *Neuron* **2016**, *89*, 910–926. [CrossRef]

111. Koyuncu, S.; Fatima, A.; Gutierrez-Garcia, R.; Vilchez, D. Proteostasis of huntingtin in health and disease. *Int. J. Mol. Sci.* **2017**, *18*, 1568. [CrossRef]

112. De Genst, E.; Chirgadze, D.Y.; Klein, F.A.C.; Butler, D.C.; Matak-Vinković, D.; Trottier, Y.; Huston, J.S.; Messer, A.; Dobson, C.M. Structure of a single-chain Fv bound to the 17 N-terminal residues of huntingtin provides insights into pathogenic amyloid formation and suppression. *J. Mol. Biol.* **2015**, *427*, 2166–2178. [CrossRef]

113. Murphy, R.C.; Messer, A. A single-chain Fv intrabody provides functional protection against the effects of mutant protein in an organotypic slice culture model of Huntington's disease. *Mol. Brain Res.* **2004**, *121*, 141–145. [CrossRef]

114. Butler, D.C.; Messer, A. Bifunctional anti-huntingtin proteasome-directed intrabodies mediate efficient degradation of mutant huntingtin exon 1 protein fragments. *PLoS One* **2011**, *6*, e29199. [CrossRef]

115. Snyder-Keller, A.; McLear, J.A.; Hathorn, T.; Messer, A. Early or late-stage anti-N-terminal huntingtin intrabody gene therapy reduces pathological features in B6.HDR6/1 mice. *J. Neuropathol. Exp. Neurol.* **2010**, *69*, 1078–1085. [CrossRef]

116. Khoshnan, A.; Ko, J.; Patterson, P.H. Effects of intracellular expression of anti-huntingtin antibodies of various specificities on mutant huntingtin aggregation and toxicity. *Proc. Natl. Acad. Sci. USA* **2002**, *99*, 1002–1007. [CrossRef]

117. Southwell, A.L.; Khoshnan, A.; Dunn, D.E.; Bugg, C.W.; Lo, D.C.; Patterson, P.H. Intrabodies binding the proline-rich domains of mutant Huntingtin increase its turnover and reduce neurotoxicity. *J. Neurosci.* **2008**, *28*, 9013–9020. [CrossRef]

118. Shimizu, Y.; Kaku-Ushiki, Y.; Iwamaru, Y.; Muramoto, T.; Kitamoto, T.; Yokoyama, T.; Mohri, S.; Tagawa, Y. A novel anti-prion protein monoclonal antibody and its single-chain fragment variable derivative with ability to inhibit abnormal prion protein accumulation in cultured cells. *Microbiol. Immunol.* **2010**, *54*, 112–121. [CrossRef]

119. Wang, C.E.; Zhou, H.; McGuire, J.R.; Cerullo, V.; Lee, B.; Li, S.H.; Li, X.J. Suppression of neuropil aggregates and neurological symptoms by an intracellular antibody implicates the cytoplasmic toxicity of mutant huntingtin. *J. Cell Biol.* **2008**, *181*, 803–816. [CrossRef]

120. Southwell, A.L.; Ko, J.; Patterson, P.H. Intrabody gene therapy ameliorates motor, cognitive, and neuropathological symptoms in multiple mouse models of Huntington's disease. *J. Neurosci.* **2009**, *29*, 13589–13602. [CrossRef]

121. Biasini, E.; Turnbaugh, J.A.; Unterberger, U.; Harris, D.A. Prion protein at the crossroads of physiology and disease. *Trends Neurosci.* **2012**, *35*, 92–103. [CrossRef]

122. Martins, S.M.; Frosoni, D.J.; Martinez, A.M.B.; De Felice, F.G.; Ferreira, S.T. Formation of soluble oligomers and amyloid fibrils with physical properties of the scrapie isoform of the prion protein from the C-terminal domain of recombinant murine prion protein mPrP-(121-231). *J. Biol. Chem.* **2006**, *281*, 26121–26128. [CrossRef]

123. Aguzzi, A.; Lakkaraju, A.K.K. Cell Biology of Prions and Prionoids: A Status Report. *Trends Cell Biol.* **2016**, *26*, 40–51. [CrossRef]

124. Pan, K.M.; Baldwin, M.; Nguyen, J.; Gasset, M.; Serban, A.; Groth, D.; Mehlhorn, I.; Huang, Z.; Fletterick, R.J.; Cohen, F.E.; et al. Conversion of α-helices into β-sheets features in the formation of the scrapie prion proteins. *Proc. Natl. Acad. Sci. USA* **1993**. [CrossRef]

125. Donofrio, G.; Heppner, F.L.; Polymenidou, M.; Musahl, C.; Aguzzi, A. Paracrine Inhibition of Prion Propagation by Anti-PrP Single-Chain Fv Miniantibodies. *J. Virol.* **2005**. [CrossRef]

126. Peretz, D.; Williamson, R.A.; Kaneko, K.; Vergara, J.; Leclerc, E.; Schmitt-Ulms, G.; Mehlhorn, I.R.; Legname, G.; Wormald, M.R.; Rudd, P.M.; et al. Antibodies inhibit prion propagation and clear cell cultures of prion infectivity. *Nature* **2001**, *412*, 739–743. [CrossRef]

127. Campana, V.; Zentilin, L.; Mirabile, I.; Kranjc, A.; Casanova, P.; Giacca, M.; Prusiner, S.B.; Legname, G.; Zurzolo, C. Development of antibody fragments for immunotherapy of prion diseases. *Biochem. J.* **2009**, *418*, 507–515. [CrossRef]

128. Fujita, K.; Yamaguchi, Y.; Mori, T.; Muramatsu, N.; Miyamoto, T.; Yano, M.; Miyata, H.; Ootsuyama, A.; Sawada, M.; Matsuda, H.; et al. Effects of a brain-engraftable microglial cell line expressing anti-prion scFv antibodies on survival times of mice infected with scrapie prions. *Cell. Mol. Neurobiol.* **2011**, *31*, 999–1008. [CrossRef]

129. Miyamoto, K.; Nakamura, N.; Aosasa, M.; Nishida, N.; Yokoyama, T.; Horiuchi, H.; Furusawa, S.; Matsuda, H. Inhibition of prion propagation in scrapie-infected mouse neuroblastoma cell lines using mouse monoclonal antibodies against prion protein. *Biochem. Biophys. Res. Commun.* **2005**, *335*, 197–204. [CrossRef]

130. Sonati, T.; Reimann, R.R.; Falsig, J.; Baral, P.K.; O'Connor, T.; Hornemann, S.; Yaganoglu, S.; Li, B.; Herrmann, U.S.; Wieland, B.; et al. The toxicity of antiprion antibodies is mediated by the flexible tail of the prion protein. *Nature* **2013**, *501*, 102–106. [CrossRef]

131. Plotkin, S.S.; Cashman, N.R. Passive immunotherapies targeting Aβ and tau in Alzheimer's disease. *Neurobiol. Dis.* **2020**, *144*, 26. [CrossRef]

132. Lambert, M.P.; Velasco, P.T.; Chang, L.; Viola, K.L.; Fernandez, S.; Lacor, P.N.; Khuon, D.; Gong, Y.; Bigio, E.H.; Shaw, P.; et al. Monoclonal antibodies that target pathological assemblies of Aβ. *J. Neurochem.* **2007**, *100*, 23–35. [CrossRef]

133. Wildburger, N.C.; Esparza, T.J.; Leduc, R.D.; Fellers, R.T.; Thomas, P.M.; Cairns, N.J.; Kelleher, N.L.; Bateman, R.J.; Brody, D.L. Diversity of Amyloid-beta Proteoforms in the Alzheimer's Disease Brain. *Sci. Rep.* **2017**, *7*, 9520. [CrossRef]

134. Condello, C.; Stöehr, J. Aβ propagation and strains: Implications for the phenotypic diversity in Alzheimer's disease. *Neurobiol. Dis.* **2018**, *109*, 191–200. [CrossRef]

135. Cline, E.N.; Das, A.; Bicca, M.A.; Mohammad, S.N.; Schachner, L.F.; Kamel, J.M.; DiNunno, N.; Weng, A.; Paschall, J.D.; Bu, R. Lo; et al. A novel crosslinking protocol stabilizes amyloid β oligomers capable of inducing Alzheimer's-associated pathologies. *J. Neurochem.* **2019**, *148*, 822–836. [CrossRef]

136. Gibbs, E.; Silverman, J.M.; Zhao, B.; Peng, X.; Wang, J.; Wellington, C.L.; Mackenzie, I.R.; Plotkin, S.S.; Kaplan, J.M.; Cashman, N.R. A Rationally Designed Humanized Antibody Selective for Amyloid Beta Oligomers in Alzheimer's Disease. *Sci. Rep.* **2019**, *9*, 9870. [CrossRef]

137. Sevigny, J.; Chiao, P.; Bussière, T.; Weinreb, P.H.; Williams, L.; Maier, M.; Dunstan, R.; Salloway, S.; Chen, T.; Ling, Y.; et al. The antibody aducanumab reduces Aβ plaques in Alzheimer's disease. *Nature* **2016**, *537*, 50–56. [CrossRef]

138. Rogers, M.B. Exposure, Exposure, Exposure? At CTAD, Aducanumab Scientists Make a Case. Available online: https://www.alzforum.org/news/conference-coverage/exposure-exposure-exposure-ctad-aducanumab-scientists-make-case#comment-34176 (accessed on 29 September 2020).

139. Biogen. FDA Accepts Biogen's Aducanumab Biologics License Application for Alzheimer's Disease with Priority Review|Biogen. Available online: https://investors.biogen.com/news-releases/news-release-details/fda-accepts-biogens-aducanumab-biologics-license-application (accessed on 29 September 2020).

12

Host Cell Proteins in Biologics Manufacturing: The Good, the Bad, and the Ugly

Martin Kornecki [1], **Fabian Mestmäcker** [1], **Steffen Zobel-Roos** [1], **Laura Heikaus de Figueiredo** [2], **Hartmut Schlüter** [2] and **Jochen Strube** [1,*]

[1]   Institute for Separation and Process Technology, Clausthal University of Technology, Leibnizstr. 15, 38678 Clausthal-Zellerfeld, Germany; kornecki@itv.tu-clausthal.de (M.K.); mestmaecker@itv.tu-clausthal.de (F.M.); zobel-roos@itv.tu-clausthal.de (S.Z.-R.)

[2]   Institute of Clinical Chemistry, Department for Mass Spectrometric Proteomics, University Medical Center Hamburg-Eppendorf, Martinistr. 52, 20246 Hamburg, Germany; l.heikaus@uke.de (L.H.d.F.); hschluet@uke.de (H.S.)

*   Correspondence: strube@itv.tu-clausthal.de

Abstract: Significant progress in the manufacturing of biopharmaceuticals has been made by increasing the overall titers in the USP (upstream processing) titers without raising the cost of the USP. In addition, the development of platform processes led to a higher process robustness. Despite or even due to those achievements, novel challenges are in sight. The higher upstream titers created more complex impurity profiles, both in mass and composition, demanding higher separation capacities and selectivity in downstream processing (DSP). This creates a major shift of costs from USP to DSP. In order to solve this issue, USP and DSP integration approaches can be developed and used for overall process optimization. This study focuses on the characterization and classification of host cell proteins (HCPs) in each unit operation of the DSP (i.e., aqueous two-phase extraction, integrated countercurrent chromatography). The results create a data-driven feedback to the USP, which will serve for media and process optimizations in order to reduce, or even eliminate nascent critical HCPs. This will improve separation efficiency and may lead to a quantitative process understanding. Different HCP species were classified by stringent criteria with regard to DSP separation parameters into "The Good, the Bad, and the Ugly" in terms of pI and MW using 2D-PAGE analysis depending on their positions on the gels. Those spots were identified using LC-MS/MS analysis. HCPs, which are especially difficult to remove and persistent throughout the DSP (i.e., "Bad" or "Ugly"), have to be evaluated by their ability to be separated. In this approach, HCPs, considered "Ugly," represent proteins with a MW larger than 15 kDa and a pI between 7.30 and 9.30. "Bad" HCPs can likewise be classified using MW (>15 kDa) and pI (4.75–7.30 and 9.30–10.00). HCPs with a MW smaller than 15 kDa and a pI lower than 4.75 and higher than 10.00 are classified as "Good" since their physicochemical properties differ significantly from the product. In order to evaluate this classification scheme, it is of utmost importance to use orthogonal analytical methods such as IEX, HIC, and SEC.

Keywords: upstream; downstream; host cell protein; CHO; ATPE; iCCC

1. Introduction

The amounts of biotechnology products produced worldwide, prescription as well as over-the-counter drugs, are estimated to account for around 50% of the most successful pharmaceutical products by the year 2020 [1]. Oncology constitutes the biggest therapeutic sector, with an annual growth rate of around 12.5% and sales of approximately $83.2 billion in 2015. Among the five top-selling oncological products, three will be monoclonal antibodies by the year 2020 [2]. The manufacturing process of biopharmaceuticals such as monoclonal antibodies (e.g., IgG, immunoglobulin G) is divided into upstream (USP) and downstream processing (DSP) [3–8]. The production of the monoclonal antibody in bioreactors (BR) using mammalian cells as an expression host and the separation of the liquid phase from the cells using centrifuges or filters is defined as USP [9]. The subsequent DSP is designed to separate side components like host cell proteins (HCP) or host cell DNA (hDNA) from the main component [6,7,10]. The most common unit operations used in the DSP are typically chromatography and filtration.

The commercial success of monoclonal antibodies of course led to significantly increased demand in their production scale [11]. Coping with these demands without significantly changing the approved manufacturing facilities almost forced companies to follow the route of increasing titers within the existing facilities.

Hence, compared to earlier yields of a couple of grams per liter, today antibody concentrations of up to 25 g/L can be achieved using a modified perfusion process [12,13]. Routinely, antibody concentrations of between three and five grams per liter can be generated in fed-batch processes [3,14,15]. However, increasing product titers at constant volumes due to higher cell concentrations will lead to capacity limitations in the DSP, which has to be compensated for by longer process times, higher material consumption, and corresponding costs [4]. This will significantly shift the cost of goods from the USP to the DSP [5]. Therefore, DSP technologies are required that circumvent this upcoming "downstream bottleneck," handling high titer volumes [4,16,17].

Optimizations in the USP concepts have led to increasing product titers. Along with this, raised impurity profiles have been observed [8,9]. Various compositions of the cultivation broth present challenges in the DSP of biotechnologically produced proteins. Considering the generic platform production process for antibodies, unit operations like centrifugation, micro- and ultrafiltration, protein A affinity chromatography, two orthogonal virus inactivation steps, ion-exchange (IEX), and hydrophobic interaction chromatography (HIC) are being used [5]. For the characterization of protein purification stages, key performance parameters can be used. These are typically resolution, speed, recovery, and capacity, as seen in Figure 1.

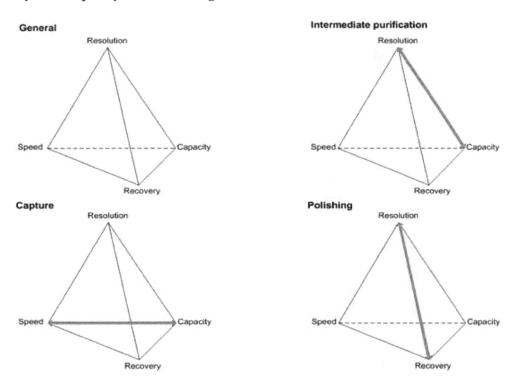

Figure 1. Key performance parameters of the capture, intermediate purification, and polishing step for protein purifications according to [18].

The objectives vary depending on the purification stage in focus, and therefore generate different challenges that have to be addressed during process optimization [18]. For example, the protein A affinity chromatography, used as a capture step, will reach its capacity limitation due to increasing product titers. This can be problematic since this criterion characterizes the capture step and is one of its two objectives. Moving downstream, selectivity challenges occurring during the intermediate purification and polishing step will prevent each step from reaching one of its objectives. Selectivity challenges are going to affect the resolution in IEX and HIC separation operations when HCP resemble the product in terms of pI and hydrophobicity, respectively [12,18].

Impurities like HCPs, which resemble the desired product only in one characteristic (e.g., pI), may challenge the IEX but can probably be easily separated from the product by an additional chromatographic step (e.g., HIC). Impurities similar to the product in more than one characteristic (e.g., pI and hydrophobicity) will be troublesome during purification and polishing. Therefore, the pI and hydrophobic distribution of the impurity spectrum can negatively affect IEX and HIC separations, respectively.

Critical performance parameters regarding the separation efficiency during the capture of monoclonal antibodies using affinity chromatography are capacity limitations as well as (un-)specific HCP co-elution [19]. Consequently, new approaches and technology are needed in order to circumvent future bottlenecks and separation challenges [4].

Furthermore, the existing challenges in process engineering have worsened since regulatory agencies demand higher product quality, an advanced understanding of the process and product, as well as batch-independent product quality [20–22]. Bioprocess engineering will probably focus in regulated industries on quality by design and process analytical technology mechanisms, in order to design, analyze, and control manufacturing processes [23]. This shall lead to improved process control by knowledge-based and statistical methods, which ultimately guarantees the process' robustness.

For example, monoclonal antibodies and fragments represent an interesting group of biopharmaceuticals due to their broad field of application (e.g., analysis or diagnostic). Those glycoproteins are structurally complex and differ in various formats, as can be seen in Figure 2. IgG is the most common format as a biopharmaceutical drug [2].

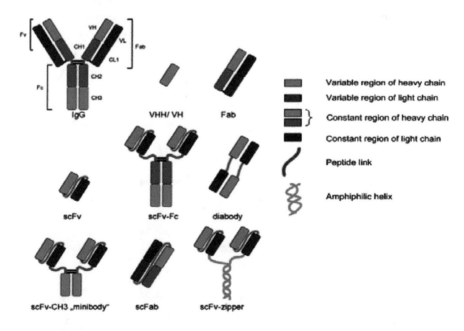

Figure 2. Various formats of recombinant antibodies [24].

The post-translational modifications, especially glycosylations, of these proteins are of utmost importance for their correct function [20]. The immense diversity of glycosylation patterns impacts the functionality, immunogenicity, and pharmacokinetics of the antibody [24,25]. Due to this, posttranslational modifications should be considered critical quality attributes (CQA) and verified throughout the manufacturing of monoclonal antibodies [26–30]. Antibody N-glycans can be quantitatively determined by normal phase chromatography after N-glycosidase digestion and glycan labeling, for example [31]. The most prevalent N-linked glycosylation patterns at the Cγ2 domain of the heavy chain (Fc) of an immunoglobulin G (IgG) are depicted in Figure 3, where the most common glycosylation of IgG is shown in section D.

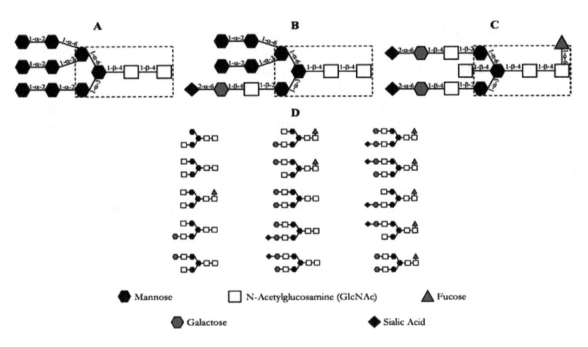

Figure 3. Common glycosylation patterns of an IgG. (**A**) high mannose content; (**B**) hybrid; (**C**) complex biantennary oligosaccharide with core fucosylation; (**D**) most prevalent oligosaccharide structures of IgG [20].

Besides critical process parameters (CPP) like pH, pO_2 and pCO_2, more often impurities play an important role in affecting CQA of the biopharmaceutical product. For example, extracellular proteases and glycosidases accumulating during the cultivation negatively influence the CQA of monoclonal antibodies [14,32–35]. The impurity spectrum consists of a multiplicity of different substances (HCP, hDNA, virus, cells, and cell debris). In this integration approach, HCPs are considered as the primary impurity based on their broad composition and range of isoelectric point (pI), molecular weight (MW), and hydrophobicity, as can be seen in Table 1 [36–40]. They exhibit no constant level, composition, or property distribution. HCPs caused by secretion or cell lysis can range in pI (2–11), MW (10–200 kDa), and variable hydrophobicity, and are therefore difficult to separate if their physicochemical properties resemble the product of interest.

Table 1. Physicochemical properties of the main impurities during the production of biopharmaceuticals, according to [38].

Class	pI	MW (kDa)	Hydrophobicity	Origin	Cause
HCP	2–11	10–200	Variable	Host cells	Secretion, lysis
hDNA	2–3	90–1000	Low	Host cells	Lysis
Insulin	5.3–5.5	5.8	Low	Media	Supplement
Virus	4–7.5	200–7200	Variable	Host cells, media	Contamination
Endotoxins	1–4	3–40	Variable	Media, contamination	Contamination

Primary recovery and purification steps for a biopharmaceutical DSP are based on physicochemical properties in order to efficiently purify the product. However, especially in the case of increasing product titers, a sub-population of impurities (i.e., HCP), which negatively affect the product quality, may remain with the desired protein and represent a certain risk [40]. Therefore, it is of critical importance to validate qualitatively and quantitatively the separation efficiency of each unit operation in the DSP.

This assessment will lead to an expanded understanding of each unit operation by classifying the impurities into "The Good, the Bad, and the Ugly":

- Impurities, which can be separated easily from the main component, are considered "the Good." They possess physicochemical properties significantly different from the protein of interest (i.e., pI, MW, hydrophobicity). As a result, they may be separated by only one unit operation in an efficient way (ion exchange in terms of charge differences).

- Side components showing more similarity to the product are more difficult to separate or are persistent throughout (i.e., not separable from the product) and thus are considered as "the Bad" or "the Ugly."

By characterizing the HCP criteria for an efficient DSP, it is possible to gain a deeper understanding of the process and preserve the quality of the product. This categorization can be used for an USP DSP integration approach towards an efficient production process by circumventing the generation or accumulation of "Bad" and "Ugly" impurities (Figure 4).

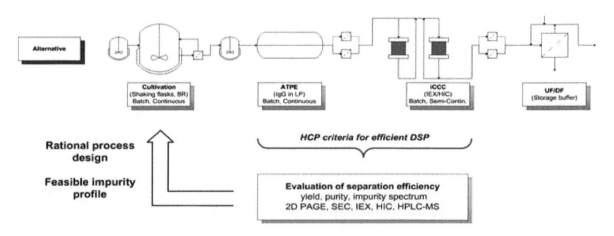

Figure 4. USP DSP integration approach for a systematic development of a bioprocess.

The considered process for the production of monoclonal antibodies utilizes mammalian cell cultivations. Afterwards, the aqueous two-phase extraction (ATPE) is used as a cell harvesting or capture step, depending on the system composition used [41–45]. Following the ATPE, the integrated counter current chromatography (iCCC), which is a combination of an IEX and HIC, is employed as a purification and polishing step. This combination of chromatographic columns leads to a highly purified product [46].

The integration approach begins with a data-driven characterization of HCP occurring in the broth and in each unit operation. The separation efficiency is determined by analytical methods (i.e., 2D SDS-PAGE, SEC, IEX, HIC, and HPLC-MS/MS). The SEC chromatograms qualitatively describe the impurity spectrum and can be used for a determination of impurities in the molecular weight range of the considered product (150 kDa). The IEX and HIC are used for characterizing the charge and hydrophobicity of the HCPs. 2D SDS-PAGE analysis, combined with HPLC-MS/MS measurements, is used for the identification and, of utmost importance, classification of "The Good, the Bad, and the Ugly" HCPs. This classification is done by evaluating the molecular weight, isoelectric point, and hydrophobicity of the HCPs, as seen in Table 2.

Afterwards, these findings are used in rational process design in order to minimize or even eliminate "Ugly" HCPs, which cannot be easily separated from the product (Figure 4).

Table 2. Analytical methods used for the characterization of HCP.

Characteristic	Method	Orthogonal Method
Isoelectric point	2D-SDS PAGE	IEX; HPLC-MS/MS
Molecular weight	SEC	2D-SDS PAGE; HPLC-MS/MS
Hydrophobicity	HIC	-

One possible process design optimization procedure is the improvement of media components. Media optimization is capable of changing the broth's HCP composition towards a population that is easier to separate or at least exhibits a lower HCP concentration. In addition, an optimized medium not only shifts the HCP profile but also improves the cell growth and product titer, which is depicted in Table 3 [47].

Table 3. Improved parameters by using an optimized medium according to [47].

Parameter	Optimized medium
Titer increase	Factor 2.5
Cell growth	Factor 2–2.3
IgG/HCP	65%
HCP profile	Shift

The shifted HCP profile can be seen in the 2D-SDS PAGE comparison in Figure 5.

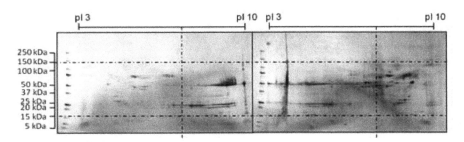

Figure 5. Comparison of 2D-SDS PAGE of a reference (**right**) and optimized medium (**left**) during a CHO cultivation according to [47]. Media was improved by a three-level DoE design.

In this work, the results of the characterization of the HCP profile from a mAb production process are presented. Process-related data as well as analysis-related data are used for the characterization of the process and for the classification of HCPs. The results of each analytical method are critically evaluated in order to determine a process flow being suitable for USP DSP integration and process optimization. Analytical methods such as SEC, 2D-PAGE, IEX, HIC as well as HPLC-MS/MS were used in order to identify critical HCP in the cell-free broth and during each unit operation (i.e., ATPE, IEX, and HIC).

2. Results and Discussion

A schematic overview of the considered alternative process as well as process- and analysis-related data are shown in Figure 6.

The HCP criteria for an efficient DSP have to be evaluated for each unit operation, according to Figure 4. Here, the classification of HCP focuses on the broth, the broth after diafiltration and on a side component fraction after HIC separation. Process-related data such as titer, yield, and purity of each unit operation are shown in Table 4.

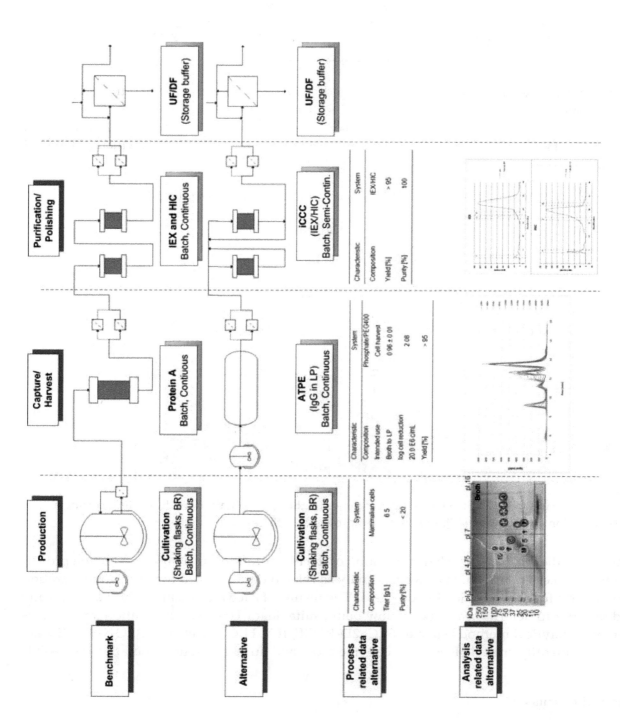

Figure 6. Schematic overview of the considered alternative process in comparison of the benchmark manufacturing route. In addition, process and analysis related data are shown and discussed in the text.

This analytical procedure focuses on the classification and characterization of HCPs. Therefore, each unit operation of the DSP has to be evaluated by its separation efficiency, using analytical methods such as 2D-SDS PAGE, IEX, HIC, and SEC to determine HCP criteria for an efficient DSP, as seen in Figure 3. Protein A and size-exclusion chromatography are used to determine yield and purity, respectively. Each unit operation was loaded with the native broth in order to determine their separation efficiency.

Table 4. Process related data of the cultivation, ATPE, and iCCC. Yield and purity were determined using protein A chromatography and SEC, respectively.

	Cultivation	ATPE	iCCC
System	Mammalian cells	PEG400/40 wt% PO$_4$	IEX/HIC combination
Titer/yield	6.5 g/L	>95%	>95%
Log cell reduction 20.0 E6 cells/mL	-	2.08	-
Purity	<20%	up to 80% *	100%

* Protein-based according to SEC.

The fraction number five occurring on the HIC was chosen due to the high side component content near the target product, as seen in Figure 7. In the following, the classification of the HCPs will be performed by 2D-PAGE gels, as depicted in Figure 8.

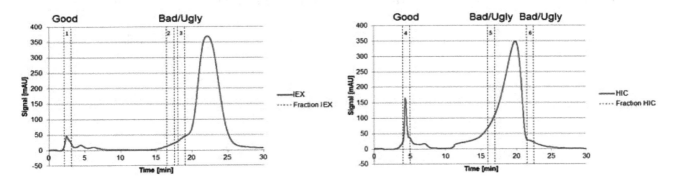

Figure 7. Chromatograms of an analytical IEX (**left**) and HIC (**right**) measurement of the diafiltrated cell-free CHO supernatant. The vertical sections represent the number of fractions taken, representing "Good", "Bad," and "Ugly" impurities.

The classification criterion of the considered HCP was selected by comparing their pI and molecular weight to the target product, as seen in Table 5.

Table 5. Classification of the "Good, Bad, and Ugly" HCP in comparison to the physicochemical properties of the monoclonal antibody (mAb). MW, molecular weight; pI, isoelectric point.

Characteristic	mAb	Good	Bad	Ugly
MW [kDa]	144.2	<15	>15	>15
pI [−]	8.30	<4.75 >10.00	4.75–7.30 9.30–10.00	7.30–9.30

While considering the 2D-PAGE gels, proteins with a MW lower than 15 kDa can be considered "Good" since they can be separated by using diafiltration subsequent to an ATPE with a suitable MW cutoff. Therefore, this filtration step is coupled to a buffer change, which is necessary for the use of the iCCC, since the specific light phase contains PEG400, resulting in a more viscous solution, which would make the chromatographic steps more difficult to handle.

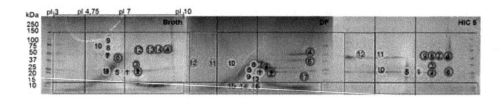

Figure 8. 2D SDS-PAGE of the broth, diafiltrated broth (DF) and HIC fraction. Green circles represent "Good", yellow circles "Bad," and red circles "Ugly" HCP.

Proteins larger than 15 kDa have to be separated by another unit operation, which is based on other physicochemical properties (i.e., pI, hydrophobicity). Therefore, "Bad" and "Ugly" proteins possess a MW larger than 15 kDa. The horizontal line at 150 kDa represents the target protein in its functional condition. The vertical lines depict the isoelectric point at 4.75 and 7.0. Impurities with a pI of 4.75 can be subjected to a possible precipitation step using hydrochloric acid, which significantly reduces their concentration [42]. Those impurities exhibit a different pI than the target protein and can efficiently be separated by an IEX and are therefore classified as "Good." Experimental IEX data show a distinctly different interaction with the stationary phase due to their surface charge distribution, as seen in Figure 9, which resemble the "Good" HCP. They elute near the void volume and can be easily separated. A similar train of thought can be conducted while characterizing the HIC chromatogram. As can be seen in Figure 9, the target product gets concentrated by each cycle in the iCCC mode.

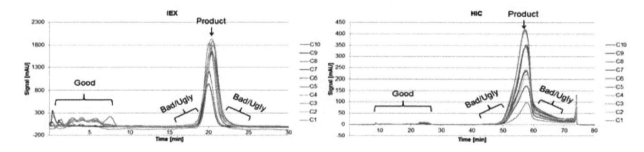

Figure 9. Chromatograms of the IEX (**left**) and HIC (**right**) after various cycles in the iCCC mode.

Impurities with a pI range close to the target protein (i.e., 7.30–9.30) are more difficult to separate via an IEX and are therefore considered "Ugly." However, since the separation efficiency of the IEX will depend on the column, buffer solution, and process parameters, this range can vary depending on the system used. Impurities with characteristics in between those of "Good" and "Ugly" are defined as "Bad." They possess a pI of 4.75–7.30 and 9.30–10.00 and can be difficult to separate when other physicochemical properties (i.e., hydrophobicity) resemble the target product. This dependency can of course also occur with "Ugly" HCP but since they are already classified as difficult to separate, they will not be characterized differently. Regarding the "Good" HCP, this dependency will not occur even if other physicochemical properties show close similarity to the product, since at least one physicochemical attribute is significantly different from the target product. The pI is restricted to 10 due to the pH gradient used in the IEF prior to 2D gel electrophoresis.

The 2D-PAGE analysis seen in Figure 8 is suitable for the visualization of the side component spectrum. However, the sample preparation requires reducing agents such as DTT, which destroys the protein's structure by reducing the disulfide bonds. This preparation procedure results in spots on the gel, which do not resemble their native structure in the supernatant. Following the aforementioned classification and separation system, proteins with a MW lower than 15 kDa but with an isoelectric point near the target product will sometimes be classified as "Good" since they can be separated by filtration. Hence, the native protein can be "Ugly" even if it appears as "Good" in the gel (assuming no change in surface charge). Thus, it is of the utmost importance to use orthogonal analytical methods to validate the classification. In terms of MW, SEC analysis can be conducted in order to determine the size distribution of side components, as seen in Figure 10. The advantage of using SEC analysis is the determination of the side component's native MW distribution as well as their qualitative mass in proportion to the product's signal. The disadvantage is the less sensitive detection of low mass content side components as well as proteins resulting in a signal overlap with the mAb.

In order to identify proteins present in the 2D-PAGE gel spots, their tryptic peptides were identified via analysis with liquid chromatography (LC) coupled to tandem mass spectrometry (MS/MS) and a database search. The numbers in the gels in Figure 8 indicate the spots that were analyzed using LC-MS/MS. The first five spots occurred in every gel. The subsequent spots were unique in each gel. The identified peptides and their corresponding proteins of each spot in these gels are presented in the appendix (Tables A1–A3). The identified proteins of the first recurrent spots are listed alongside with their MW and pI in Table 6.

As can be seen in Table 6, the MW and pI of the spots analyzed with 2D-PAGE do not correspond to the value in the protein database. This is a result of proteins existing in different species due to posttranslational modifications and proteolytic processing (proteolytic degradation and sample preparation, respectively). In contrast, the theoretically calculated pI values obtained by the ExPASy computation tool (http://web.expasy.org/compute_pi/) represent the unmodified full length amino acid sequence of a defined protein. SEC analysis, for example, is a non-invasive analytical method for the determination of MW distribution of side components, if the salt concentration used in aqueous eluents allows for separation based on molecular size exclusion alone due to the hydrodynamic radius [48]. Nevertheless, for a systematic integration approach, the classification of HCPs based on their physicochemical properties can lead to an enhanced process understanding, especially in the DSP.

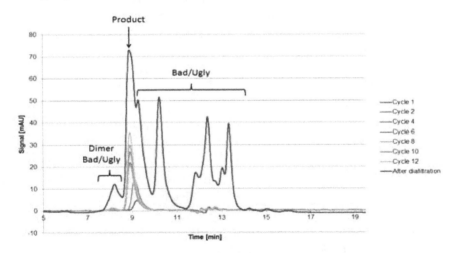

Figure 10. SEC chromatograms after various cycles as well as the broth after diafiltration.

Table 6. Classification of CHO proteins identified via LC-MS/MS analysis and characterized by 2D-PAGE gel. Comparison of theoretical (UniProt; pI calculated according to the amino acid sequences) and observed MW and pI with respect to the spot position on the 2D-PAGE gel.

Spot Gel	MW Gel	pI Gel	Class Gel	MW [1]	pI [2]	Class MS	Protein	UniProt Accession Number
1	25	7.0	Bad	81.56	5.69	Bad	Glutathione S-transferase Mu7-like protein	A0A061IN16
2	25	7.5	Ugly	102.7	6.02	Bad	Actin, cytoplasmic 1	A0A069C7Y3
3	30	7.6	Ugly	38.03	6.08	Bad	Purine nucleoside phosphorylase-like protein	A0A061ILE8
4	50	9.4	Bad	72.13	7.23	Ugly	Pyruvate kinase	A0A098KXF7
5	25	6.3	Bad	38.03	6.08	Bad	Purine nucleoside phosphorylase-like protein	A0A061ILE8

[1] Theoretical values according to the unmodified full length protein according to UniProt; [2] Theoretical values calculated using the ExPASy computation tool (http://web.expasy.org/compute_pi/).

3. Materials and Methods

Chinese hamster ovary cells (CHO DG44) were used for the production of a monoclonal antibody. The culture conditions were 37 °C, 5% carbon dioxide, and 130 rpm. The cultivations were carried out in shake flasks in a serum-free medium.

The ATP system applied consisted of 44.5% broth, 15.5% PEG400 (Merck KGaA, Darmstadt, Germany), and 40% of a 40 wt% phosphate buffer. All the components were weighed. The extraction was carried out at pH 6.0 in 50-mL beakers at room temperature. The system was mixed for 15 min at 140 rpm in an incubator shaker. Phase separation took place within 30 min in a separatory funnel.

The broth was diafiltrated using a SARTOFLOW® Slice 200 Benchtop system from Sartorius Stedim (Germany). A 10 kDa Hydrosart® (Sartorius Stedim, Göttingen, Germany) was utilized as a membrane module.

The iCCC (integrated counter-current chromatography) is run by using Fractogel® EMD SO_3^-(s) and Fractogel® EMD Phenyl(s) (Merck KGaA, Darmstadt, Germany). The buffers consisted of a 20 mM sodium phosphate buffer (Na_2HPO_4, NaH_2PO_4) as well as a 20 mM sodium phosphate buffer with 1 M Na_2SO_4.

The product was quantified by Protein A chromatography (PA ID Sensor Cartridge, Applied Biosystems, Bedford, MA, USA). Dulbecco's PBS buffer (Sigma-Aldrich, St. Louis, MO, USA) was used as a loading buffer at pH 7.4 and as an elution buffer at pH 2.6. The absorbance was monitored at 280 nm.

The size exclusion chromatography was done by using a Yarra™ 3 μm SEC-3000 column (Phenomenex Ltd., Aschaffenburg, Germany) with 0.1 M Na_2SO_4, 0.1 M Na_2HPO_4, and 0.1 M NaH_2PO_4 (Merck KGaA, Germany) as a buffer system.

Isoelectric focusing was carried out using IPG strips (ReadyStripTM IPG Strips, linear, pH 3–10, BIO-RAD, Hercules, CA, USA) and an isoelectric focusing unit of Hoefer (Hoefer Inc., Holliston, MA, USA). A subsequent SDS PAGE was carried out using gels (Criterion TGX Precast Gel, 4–15% Bis-Tris, BIO-RAD), buffers, and an electrophoresis chamber from BIO-RAD. The resulting gels were colored by Coomassie Brilliant Blue G-250 (VWR International, Radnor, PA, USA).

For the identification of proteins, selected 2D GE spots were cut out and reduced into 1-mm² pieces. After reduction of the disulfide bonds with 10 mM DL-dithiothreitol (Sigma-Aldrich) and alkylation with 50 mM iodoacetamide (Sigma-Aldrich), an in-gel proteolytic digestion was performed with 8 ng/μL trypsin (Promega, Madison, WI, USA) at 37 °C overnight. The peptides were extracted from the gel with 65% acetonitrile and 5% acetic acid in water and the solvent was evaporated to complete dryness. The peptides were re-suspended in 20 μL 0.1% formic acid (Fluka) and subjected to LC-MS/MS analysis with a nano-flow ultra-performance liquid chromatography (nano-UPLC) system (nanoACQUITY, Waters, Manchester, UK) coupled via an electrospray-ionization (ESI) source to a tandem mass spectrometer (MS/MS) consisting of a quadrupole and a orbitrap mass analyzer (Orbitrap QExcactive, Thermo Scientific, Bremen, Germany). Four microliters of each sample were loaded onto a reversed-phase (RP) trapping column (Symetry C18 Trap Column; 100 Å, 5 μm, 180 μm × 20 mm) and washed with 1% buffer B for 5 min. The peptides were eluted onto a RP capillary column (nanoAcquity Peptide BEH analytical column; 130 Å, 1.7 μm, 75 μm × 200 mm) and separated by a gradient from 3 to 35% buffer B in 35 min (250 nL/min). Eluting peptides were ionized and desorbed by ESI in the positive mode using a fused-silica emitter (I.D. 10 μm, New Objective, Woburn, MA, USA) at a capillary voltage of 1800 V. Data-dependent acquisition mode was used with the following parameters: MS level over a m/z range from 400 to 1500, with a resolution of 70,000 FWHM at m/z 200. Maximum injection time was set to 120 ms for an AGC target of 1E6. For MS/MS analysis the top 12 signals were isolated in a 2 m/z window and fragmented with a normalized

HCD collision energy of 25. Fragment spectra were recorded with a resolution of 17,500 FWHM at m/z 200. Maximum injection time was set to 60 ms for an AGC target 5E5.

LC–MS raw data were processed with MaxQuant (Max Planck Institute of Biochemistry, Planegg, Germany) algorithms (version 1.5.8.3). Protein identification was carried out with Andromeda against a hamster (*Cricetulus griseus*) (www.uniprot.org, downloaded on 31 January 2017) and a contaminant database. The searches were performed using a precursor mass tolerance set to 10 ppm and fragment mass tolerance set to 20 ppm. For peptide identification, two missed cleavages were allowed, a carbamidomethylation on the cysteine as a fixed modification and oxidation of the methionine as a variable modification. A maximum of five modifications per peptide were allowed.

4. Conclusions

The presented approach of integrating USP and DSP is based on the classification and characterization of impurities generated during USP. This will lead to a deeper quantitative process understanding and identification of issues in the DSP early on. Here, the HCPs were categorized into "The Good, the Bad, and the Ugly" by evaluating their physicochemical properties compared to the monoclonal antibody. In this approach "Good" impurities possess a MW lower than 15 kDa and a pI lower than 4.75. "Ugly" impurities on the other hand exhibit a pI of 7.3–9.3, whereas "Bad" impurities feature a pI between 4.75 and 7.3 as well as between 9.3 and 10.0. In order to evaluate the classification system for the generated HCPs, orthogonal analytical methods are of utmost importance. IEX and SEC analysis were conducted for the identification of impurities. Theoretical pI and MW calculated based on the amino acid sequence differ from the experimental values obtained in 2D gel electrophoresis. This is due to not considering posttranslational modifications, as well as in vivo and ex vivo proteolytic processing.

Nevertheless, it is possible to characterize HCP based on pI and MW properties. In order to fully categorize the separation efficiency of each unit operation in the DSP as well as of their combinations, the HCP profile has to be determined with the aforementioned analytical methods in future approaches. This portfolio can of course be extended by adding supplementary methods like NMR technologies, preferably online [49].

Considering the significant amount of work in terms of characterization, monitoring, and removal of impurities and contaminations created by the USP step, as well as the time and cost associated with their removal, it may be worthwhile to reflect in more detail how these impurities and product variations are generated in the first place. Work to this end already started some time ago. Initial results and corresponding concepts for a more balanced integrated process design will be presented in the near future.

Acknowledgments: The authors would especially like to acknowledge Petra Gronemeyer (now Boehringer/ Biberach) for her outstanding contribution to this topic during her PhD studies, for which she has been highly esteemed at conferences.

Author Contributions: Martin Kornecki conceived and designed the experiment as well as wrote the paper. Martin Kornecki performed the SDS-PAGE experiments. Fabian Mestmäcker performed the chromatographic (iCCC, IEX, HIC) experiments. Laura Heikaus de Figueiredo performed the LC-MS/MS experiments and analyzed the data. All mentioned authors interpreted the data. Hartmut Schlüter as well as Jochen Strube substantively revised the work and contributed the materials and analysis tools. Jochen Strube is responsible for conception and supervision.

Appendix A

Table A1. Peptides and their corresponding proteins identified via LC-MS/MS in spots of 2D gel of the broth. Molecular weight (MW) and isoelectric point (pI) of the unmodified full length protein according to UniProt.

#	Gel MW	Gel pI	MW (UniProt)	pI (UniProt)	Primary Accession Number (UniProt)	Number of Unique Peptides	Protein
1	25	7.2	25.76	6.45	A0A061HUZ2	9	Platelet-activating factor
			81.56	5.69	A0A06IIN16	11	Glutathione S-transferase Mu 7-like protein
			25.88	6.43	A0A061HYZ1	9	Peroxiredoxin-6-like protein
2	25	7.9	30.28	7.22	A0A06IIFC9	4	Carbonic anhydrase
			89.52	6.23	A0A061IJC4	4	Glutathione S-transferase Mu 1-like protein
			81.56	5.69	A0A06IIN16	4	Glutathione S-transferase Mu 7-like protein
3	30	7.6	72.13	7.23	A0A098KXF7	8	Pyruvate kinase
			38.03	6.08	A0A061ILE8	6	Purine nucleoside phosphorylase-like protein
			32.23	9.11	A0A061IAK4	5	L-lactate dehydrogenase A chain
4	50	9.6	45.28	8.48	A0A061IB69	7	Fructose-bisphosphate aldolase
			72.13	7.23	A0A098KXF7	15	Pyruvate kinase
			102.7	6.02	A0A069C7Y3	5	Actin, cytoplasmic 1
5	25	6.6	27.39	6.34	A0A06I2E1	8	Proteasome subunit
			89.52	6.23	A0A06IIJC4	8	Glutathione S-transferase Mu 1-like protein
			81.56	5.69	A0A06IIN16	8	Glutathione S-transferase Mu 7-like protein
6	45	6.7	50.57	5.93	G3GR73	11	Rab GDP diss. inhib.
			52.79	6	A0A098KXB1	10	Cytosol aminopeptidase-like protein
			44.67	7.54	A0A061IJI8	9	Alpha-enolase
7	50	6.1	52.79	6	A0A098KXB1	20	Aminopeptidase
			72.13	7.23	A0A098KXF7	29	Pyruvate kinase
			145.1	8.37	A0A061HU29	15	Glucose-6-phosphate 1-dehydrogenase
8	57	6	73.86	5.56	A0A061I5D1	22	Heat shock protein
			74.72	5.29	A0A061HWC7	9	Plastin-3
			69.64	5.57	A0A061I5U1	9	Heat shock-related protein 2
9	80	6.1	72.13	7.23	A0A098KXF7	11	Pyruvate kinase
			117.7	5.42	G3IBG3	8	Ubiquitin activating enzyme E1
			73.86	5.56	A0A06I5D1	7	Heat shock protein
10	70	5.6	73.86	5.56	A0A061I5D1	9	Heat shock protein
			68.43	5.55	A0A06II1Q2	5	Vitamin K-dependent protein S
			85.71	5.2	A0A061IAX6	5	Dipeptidyl peptidase 3
11	25	6	25.88	6.43	A0A061HYZ1	9	Peroxiredoxin
			89.52	6.23	A0A06IIJC4	19	Glutathione S-transferase Mu 1-like protein
			81.56	5.69	A0A06IIN16	14	Glutathione S-transferase Mu 7-like protein
12	55	7.8	72.13	7.23	A0A098KXF7	37	Pyruvate kinase
			52.79	6	A0A098KXB1	10	Cytosol aminopeptidase-like protein
			73.86	5.56	A0A061I5D1	4	Heat shock protein
13	50	8.6	52.79	6	A0A098KXB1	4	Cytosol aminopeptidase-like protein
			72.13	7.23	A0A098KXF7	19	Pyruvate kinase
			145.1	8.37	A0A061HU29	2	Glucose-6-phosphate 1-dehydrogenase
14	50	9.2	72.13	7.23	A0A098KXF7	20	Pyruvate kinase
			44.67	7.54	A0A061IJI8	3	Alpha-enolase
			42.69	8.78	A0A061HV36	3	Eukaryotic translation initiation factor 2 subunit 3-like protein

Table A2. Peptides and their corresponding proteins identified via LC-MS/MS in spots of 2D gel of the diafiltrated broth. Molecular weight (MW) and isoelectric point (pI) of the unmodified full length protein according to UniProt.

#	Gel MW	Gel pI	MW (UniProt)	pI (UniProt)	Primary accession number (UniProt)	Number of Unique Peptides	Protein
1	25	7	26.96	5.38	A0A061I6A0	5	Glutathione S-transferase A4-like protein
			81.56	5.69	A0A061IN16	8	Glutathione S-transferase Mu 7-like protein
2	25	7.5	38.03	6.08	A0A061ILE8	8	Purine nucleoside phosphorylase-like protein
			38.03	6.08	A0A061ILE8	6	Purine nucleoside phosphorylase
			102.7	6.02	A0A069C7Y3	2	Actin, cytoplasmic 1
3	30	7.4	43.35	6.48	A0A061IJG8	2	Prostaglandin reductase 1-like protein
			45.28	8.48	A0A061IB69	1	Fructose-bisphosphate aldolase
4	50	9.4	89.52	6.23	A0A061IJC4	2	Glutathione S-transferase
5	25	6.6	38.03	6.08	A0A061ILE8	7	Purine nucleoside phosphorylase
			89.52	6.23	A0A061IJC4	5	Glutathione S-transferase
6	37	9.4	45.28	8.48	A0A061IB69	4	Fructose-bisphosphate aldolase
			43.35	6.48	A0A061IJG8	2	Prostaglandin reductase 1-like protein
			361.89	4.81	A0A061IH02	2	Desmoglein-4-like protein
7	30	7	38.03	6.08	A0A061ILE8	4	Purine nucleoside phosphorylase
			128.68	6.78	A0A061IK77	3	Exosome component 10 isoform 1
			11.37	11.36	G3H2T6	2	Histone H4
8	30	6.8	27.79	4.7	A0A061IGS6	4	Protein sigma
			102.7	6.02	A0A069C7Y3	5	Actin, cytoplasmic 1
			361.89	4.81	A0A061IH02	4	Desmoglein-4-like protein
9	17	6.6	11.37	11.36	G3H2T6	4	Histone H4
			14.99	10.2	A0A061IP52	2	Histone H2B
10	30	5.6	52.25	5.35	A0A061IML2	13	Annexin
			268.7	5.69	A0A061IP39	10	Filamin-B isoform 4
			50.99	6.94	A0A061I8I4	4	Cathepsin F
11	30	4.5	52.25	5.35	A0A061IML2	2	Annexin
			14.73	9.87	A0A061IQB8	3	Ubiquitin-60S
12	30	2.8	38.03	6.08	A0A061ILE8	8	Purine nucleoside phosphorylase
			89.52	6.23	A0A061IJC4	8	Glutathione S-transferase
			101.51	5.12	A0A061IRD9	5	AP complex subunit beta
13	15	6.7	38.03	6.08	A0A061ILE8	4	Purine nucleoside phosphorylase
			89.52	6.23	A0A061IJC4	4	Glutathione S-transferase
14	15	6.1	38.31	5.33	A0A061IEW1	3	Nuclear migration protein nudC-like protein
			38.31	5.33	A0A061IEW1	5	Nuclear migration protein nudC-like protein
			89.52	6.23	A0A061IJC4	4	Glutathione S-transferase
			54.11	5.01	A0A061IDB2	3	Prelamin-A/C-like isoform 1
15	12	5.6	17.16	7.8	A0A061I0I3	4	SH3 binding protein
			17.19	5.94	G3HBD4	3	Nucleoside diphosphate kinase
			23.42	5.1	G3GXB0	3	Rho GDP
16	17	6.6	89.52	6.23	A0A061IJC4	8	Glutathione S-transferase
			102.7	6.02	A0A069C7Y3	2	Actin, cytoplasmic 1
			14.73	9.87	A0A061IQB8	3	Ubiquitin-60S
17	16	9.2	102.7	6.02	A0A069C7Y3	3	Actin, cytoplasmic 1
			23.42	5.1	G3GXB0	3	Rho GDP

Table A3. Peptides and their corresponding proteins identified via LC-MS/MS in spots of 2D gel of the HIC fraction. Molecular weight (MW) and isoelectric point (pI) of the unmodified full length protein according to UniProt.

#	Gel MW	Gel pI	MW (UniProt)	pI (UniProt)	Primary Accession Number (UniProt)	Number of Unique Peptides	Protein
1	25	6.9	-	-	-	-	-
2	25	7.6	11.37	11.36	G3H2T6	2	Histone H4
			102.7	6.02	A0A069C7Y3	2	Actin, cytoplasmic 1
3	30	7.6	38.03	6.08	A0A061LE8	2	Purine nucleoside
			102.7	6.02	A0A069C7Y3	1	Actin, cytoplasmic 1
4	50	8.4	44.67	7.54	A0A061JJ8	8	Alpha-enolase
			72.13	7.23	A0A098KXF7	8	Pyruvate kinase
			38.03	6.08	A0A061LE8	2	Purine nucleoside
5	25	6.3	38.03	6.08	A0A061LE8	6	Purine nucleoside
6	25	8.4	38.03	6.08	A0A061LE8	4	Purine nucleoside
7	50	8	44.67	7.54	A0A061JJ8	1	Alpha-enolase
8	47	7.6	44.67	7.54	A0A061JJ8	5	Alpha-enolase
			102.7	6.02	A0A069C7Y3	3	Actin, cytoplasmic 1
			72.13	7.23	A0A098KXF7	2	Pyruvate kinase
9	50	7.2	59.76	9.22	A0A061CE4	4	ATP synthase subunit
			14.73	9.87	A0A061IQB8	2	Ubiquitin-60S ribosomal protein L40-like isoform 2
			102.7	6.02	A0A069C7Y3	2	Actin, cytoplasmic 1
10	25	5.1	-	-	-	-	-
11	50	4.8	211.66	5.42	A0A061I4N6	1	CAP-Gly domain-containing linker protein 1
12	52	4	-	-	-	-	-

(-) Spots, which were not able to be identified.

References

1.   EvaluatePharma. *World Preview 2016, Outlook to 2022*; EvaluatePharma: London, UK, 2016; pp. 1–39.
2.   EvaluatePharma. *World Preview 2015, Outlook to 2020*; EvaluatePharma: London, UK, 2015; pp. 1–39.
3.   Li, F.; Vijayasankaran, N.; Shen, A.; Kiss, R.; Amanullah, A. Cell culture processes for monoclonal antibody production. *mAbs* **2010**, *2*, 466–479. [CrossRef] [PubMed]
4.   Gronemeyer, P.; Ditz, R.; Strube, J. Trends in Upstream and Downstream Process Development for Antibody Manufacturing. *Bioengineering* **2014**, *1*, 188–212. [CrossRef]
5.   Sommerfeld, S.; Strube, J. Challenges in biotechnology production—Generic processes and process optimization for monoclonal antibodies. *Chem. Eng. Process. Process Intensif.* **2005**, *44*, 1123–1137. [CrossRef]
6.   Birch, J.R.; Racher, A.J. Antibody production. *Adv. Drug Deliv. Rev.* **2006**, *58*, 671–685. [CrossRef] [PubMed]
7.   Liu, H.F.; Ma, J.; Winter, C.; Bayer, R. Recovery and purification process development for monoclonal antibody production. *mAbs* **2010**, *2*, 480–499. [CrossRef] [PubMed]
8.   Shukla, A.A.; Thömmes, J. Recent advances in large-scale production of monoclonal antibodies and related proteins. *Trends Biotechnol.* **2010**, *28*, 253–261. [CrossRef] [PubMed]
9.   Jain, E.; Kumar, A. Upstream processes in antibody production: Evaluation of critical parameters. *Biotechnol. Adv.* **2008**, *26*, 46–72. [CrossRef] [PubMed]
10. Strube, J.; Grote, F.; Josch, J.P.; Ditz, R. Process development and design of downstream processes. *Chemie-Ingenieur-Technik* **2011**, *83*, 1044–1065. [CrossRef]
11. Gagnon, P. Technology trends in antibody purification. *J. Chromatogr. A* **2012**, *1221*, 57–70. [CrossRef] [PubMed]
12. Kelley, B. Industrialization of mAb production technology: The bioprocessing industry at a crossroads. *mAbs* **2009**, *1*, 440–449. [CrossRef]
13. Chon, J.H.; Zarbis-Papastoitsis, G. Advances in the production and downstream processing of antibodies. *New Biotechnol.* **2011**, *28*, 458–463. [CrossRef] [PubMed]
14. Park, J.H.; Jin, J.H.; Lim, M.S.; An, H.J.; Kim, J.W.; Lee, G.M. Proteomic Analysis of Host Cell Protein Dynamics in the Culture Supernatants of Antibody-Producing CHO Cells. *Sci. Rep.* **2017**, *7*, 44246. [CrossRef] [PubMed]
15. Reinhart, D.; Damjanovic, L.; Kaisermayer, C.; Kunert, R. Benchmarking of commercially available CHO cell culture media for antibody production. *Appl. Microbiol. Biotechnol.* **2015**, 4645–4657. [CrossRef] [PubMed]
16. Strube, J.; Sommerfeld, S.; Lohrmann, M. Process Development and Optimization for Biotechnology Production—Monoclonal Antibodies. In *Bioseparation and Bioprocessing*, 2nd ed.; Subramanian, G., Ed.; Wiley-VCH: Weinheim, Germany, 2007.
17. Strube, J.; Grote, F.; Ditz, R. Bioprocess Design and Production Technology for the Future. In *Biopharmaceutical Production Technology*; Subramanian, G., Ed.; Wiley-VCH: Weinheim, Germany, 2012.
18. GE Healthcare. *Strategies for Protein Purification. Handbook*; GE Healthcare: Little Chalfont, UK, 2010.
19. Levy, N.E.; Valente, K.N.; Choe, L.H.; Lee, K.H.; Lenhoff, A.M. Identification and Characterization of Host Cell Protein Product-Associated Impurities in Monoclonal Antibody Bioprocessing. *Biotechnol. Bioeng.* **2014**, *111*, 904–912. [CrossRef] [PubMed]
20. Del Val, I.J.; Kontoravdi, C.; Nagy, J.M. Towards the implementation of quality by design to the production of therapeutic monoclonal antibodies with desired glycosylation patterns. *Biotechnol. Prog.* **2010**, *26*, 1505–1527. [CrossRef] [PubMed]
21. Hinz, D.C. Process analytical technologies in the pharmaceutical industry: The FDA's PAT initiative. *Anal. Bioanal. Chem.* **2006**, *384*, 1036–1042. [CrossRef] [PubMed]
22. Mercier, S.M.; Rouel, P.M.; Lebrun, P.; Diepenbroek, B.; Wijffels, R.H.; Streefland, M. Process analytical technology tools for perfusion cell culture. *Eng. Life Sci.* **2016**, *16*, 25–35. [CrossRef]
23. Hakemeyer, C.; McNight, N.; St. John, R.; Meier, S.; Trexler-Schmidt, M.; Kelley, B.; Zettl, F.; Puskeiler, R.; Kleinjans, A.; Lim, F.; et al. Process characterization and Design Space definition. *Biologicals* **2016**, *44*, 306–318. [CrossRef] [PubMed]
24. Frenzel, A.; Hust, M.; Schirrmann, T. Expression of recombinant antibodies. *Front. Immunol.* **2013**, *4*, 1–20. [CrossRef] [PubMed]

25. Shields, R.L.; Lai, J.; Keck, R.; O'Connell, L.Y.; Hong, K.; Gloria Meng, Y.; Weikert, S.H.A.; Presta, L.G. Lack of fucose on human IgG1 N-linked oligosaccharide improves binding to human Fc\gammaRIII and antibody-dependent cellular toxicity. *J. Biol. Chem.* **2002**, *277*, 26733–26740. [CrossRef] [PubMed]

26. Richter, V.; Kwiatkowski, M.; Omidi, M.; Omidi, A.; Robertson, W.D.; Schlüter, H. Mass spectrometric analysis of protein species of biologics. *Pharm. Bioprocess.* **2013**, *1*, 381–404. [CrossRef]

27. Hakemeyer, C.; Pech, M.; Lipok, G.; Herrmann, A. Characterization of the influence of cultivation parameters on extracellular modifications of antibodies during fermentation. *BMC Proc.* **2013**, *7*, P85. [CrossRef]

28. Kunert, R.; Reinhart, D. Advances in recombinant antibody manufacturing. *Appl. Microbiol. Biotechnol.* **2016**, *100*, 3451–3461. [CrossRef] [PubMed]

29. Jefferis, R. Glycosylation as a strategy to improve antibody-based therapeutics. Nature reviews. *Drug Discovery* **2009**, *8*, 226–234. [CrossRef] [PubMed]

30. Alt, N.; Zhang, T.Y.; Motchnik, P.; Taticek, R.; Quarmby, V.; Schlothauer, T.; Beck, H.; Emrich, T.; Harris, R.J. Determination of critical quality attributes for monoclonal antibodies using quality by design principles. *Biologicals* **2016**, *44*, 1–15. [CrossRef] [PubMed]

31. Brunner, M.; Fricke, J.; Kroll, P.; Herwig, C. Investigation of the interactions of critical scale-up parameters (pH, pO_2 and pCO_2) on CHO batch performance and critical quality attributes. *Bioprocess Biosyst. Eng.* **2016**, 1–13. [CrossRef] [PubMed]

32. Chee Furng Wong, D.; Tin Kam Wong, K.; Tang Goh, L.; Kiat Heng, C.; Gek Sim Yap, M. Impact of dynamic online fed-batch strategies on metabolism, productivity and N-glycosylation quality in CHO cell cultures. *Biotechnol. Bioeng.* **2005**, *89*, 164–177. [CrossRef] [PubMed]

33. Gao, S.X.; Zhang, Y.; Stansberry-Perkins, K.; Buko, A.; Bai, S.; Nguyen, V.; Brader, M.L. Fragmentation of a highly purified monoclonal antibody attributed to residual CHO cell protease activity. *Biotechnol. Bioeng.* **2011**, *108*, 977–982. [CrossRef] [PubMed]

34. Gramer, M.J.; Goochee, C.F. Glycosidase activities of the 293 and NS0 cell lines, and of an antibody-producing hybridoma cell line. *Biotechnol. Bioeng.* **1994**, *43*, 423–428. [CrossRef] [PubMed]

35. Robert, F.; Bierau, H.; Rossi, M.; Agugiaro, D.; Soranzo, T.; Broly, H.; Mitchell-Logean, C. Degradation of an Fc-fusion recombinant protein by host cell proteases: Identification of a CHO cathepsin D protease. *Biotechnol. Bioeng.* **2009**, *104*, 1132–1141. [CrossRef] [PubMed]

36. Tait, A.S.; Hogwood, C.E.M.; Smales, C.M.; Bracewell, D.G. Host cell protein dynamics in the supernatant of a mAb producing CHO cell line. *Biotechnol. Bioeng.* **2012**, *109*, 971–982. [CrossRef] [PubMed]

37. Hogwood, C.E.M.; Tait, A.S.; Koloteva-Levine, N.; Bracewell, D.G.; Smales, C.M. The dynamics of the CHO host cell protein profile during clarification and protein A capture in a platform antibody purification process. *Biotechnol. Bioeng.* **2013**, *110*, 240–251. [CrossRef] [PubMed]

38. Singh, N.; Arunkumar, A.; Chollangi, S.; Tan, Z.G.; Borys, M.; Li, Z.J. Clarification technologies for monoclonal antibody manufacturing processes: Current state and future perspectives. *Biotechnol. Bioeng.* **2016**, *113*, 698–716. [CrossRef] [PubMed]

39. Valente, K.N.; Lenhoff, A.M.; Lee, K.H. Expression of difficult-to-remove host cell protein impurities during extended Chinese hamster ovary cell culture and their impact on continuous bioprocessing. *Biotechnol. Bioeng.* **2015**, *112*, 1232–1242. [CrossRef] [PubMed]

40. Wang, X.; Hunter, A.K.; Mozier, N.M. Host cell proteins in biologics development: Identification, quantitation and risk assessment. *Biotechnol. Bioeng.* **2009**, *103*, 446–458. [CrossRef] [PubMed]

41. Eggersgluess, J.K.; Richter, M.; Dieterle, M.; Strube, J. Multi-stage aqueous two-phase extraction for the purification of monoclonal antibodies. *Chem. Eng. Technol.* **2014**, *37*, 675–682. [CrossRef]

42. Gronemeyer, P.; Ditz, R.; Strube, J. Implementation of aqueous two-phase extraction combined with precipitation in a monoclonal antibody manufacturing process. *Chimica Oggi/Chem. Today* **2016**, *34*, 66–70.

43. Eggersgluess, J.A.N.K.; Both, S.; Strube, J. Process Development for the Extraction of Biomolecules. *Chimica Oggi/Chem. Today* **2012**, *30*, 4.

44. Asenjo, J.A.; Andrews, B.A. Aqueous two-phase systems for protein separation: A perspective. *J. Chromatogr. A* **2011**, *1218*, 8826–8835. [CrossRef] [PubMed]

45. Azevedo, A.M.; Gomes, A.G.; Rosa, P.A.J.; Ferreira, I.F.; Pisco, A.M.M.O.; Aires-Barros, M.R. Partitioning of human antibodies in polyethylene glycol-sodium citrate aqueous two-phase systems. *Sep. Purif. Technol.* **2009**, *65*, 14–21. [CrossRef]

46.   Zobel, S.; Helling, C.; Ditz, R.; Strube, J. Design and operation of continuous countercurrent chromatography in biotechnological production. *Ind. Eng. Chem. Res.* **2014**, *53*, 9169–9185. [CrossRef]

47.   Gronemeyer, P.; Ditz, R.; Strube, J. DoE based integration approach of upstream and downstream processing regarding HCP and ATPE as harvest operation. *Biochem. Eng. J.* **2016**, *113*, 158–166. [CrossRef]

48.   Ahmed, U.; Saunders, G. The Effect of NaCl Concentration on Protein Size Exclusion Chromatography. Application Note. Available online: http://cn.agilent.com/cs/library/applications/SI-02416.pdf (accessed on 17 July 2017).

49.   Roch, P.; Mandenius, C.-F. On-line monitoring of downstream bioprocesses. *Curr. Opin. Chem. Eng.* **2016**, *14*, 112–120. [CrossRef]

13

Antibody-Drug Conjugates: The New Frontier of Chemotherapy

Sara Ponziani [1,†], Giulia Di Vittorio [2,†], Giuseppina Pitari [1], Anna Maria Cimini [1],
Matteo Ardini [1], Roberta Gentile [2], Stefano Iacobelli [2], Gianluca Sala [2,3], Emily Capone [3],
David J. Flavell [4], Rodolfo Ippoliti [1] and Francesco Giansanti [1,*]

[1] Department of Life, Health and Environmental Sciences, University of L'Aquila, I-67100 L'Aquila, Italy;
     sara.ponziani@guest.univaq.it (S.P.); giuseppina.pitari@univaq.it (G.P.);
     annamaria.cimini@univaq.it (A.M.C.); matteo.ardini@univaq.it (M.A.); rodolfo.ippoliti@univaq.it (R.I.)
[2] MediaPharma SrL, I-66013 Chieti, Italy; g.divittorio@mediapharma.it (G.D.V.);
     r.gentile@mediapharma.it (R.G.); s.iacobelli@mediapharma.it (S.I.); g.sala@unich.it (G.S.)
[3] Department of Medical, Oral and Biotechnological Sciences, University of Chieti-Pescara,
     I-66100 Chieti, Italy; caponemily@gmail.com
[4] The Simon Flavell Leukaemia Research Laboratory, Southampton General Hospital,
     Southampton SO16 6YD, UK; davidf@leukaemiabusters.org.uk
*   Correspondence: francesco.giansanti@cc.univaq.it
†   These authors contributed equally to this work.

Abstract: In recent years, antibody-drug conjugates (ADCs) have become promising antitumor agents to be used as one of the tools in personalized cancer medicine. ADCs are comprised of a drug with cytotoxic activity cross-linked to a monoclonal antibody, targeting antigens expressed at higher levels on tumor cells than on normal cells. By providing a selective targeting mechanism for cytotoxic drugs, ADCs improve the therapeutic index in clinical practice. In this review, the chemistry of ADC linker conjugation together with strategies adopted to improve antibody tolerability (by reducing antigenicity) are examined, with particular attention to ADCs approved by the regulatory agencies (the U.S. Food and Drug Administration (FDA) and the European Medicines Agency (EMA)) for treating cancer patients. Recent developments in engineering Immunoglobulin (Ig) genes and antibody humanization have greatly reduced some of the problems of the first generation of ADCs, beset by problems, such as random coupling of the payload and immunogenicity of the antibody. ADC development and clinical use is a fast, evolving area, and will likely prove an important modality for the treatment of cancer in the near future.

Keywords: Mabs; Antibody-Drug Conjugate; cancer therapy; drug targeting; payload; cross-linking

1. Introduction

The twentieth century has been characterized by basic and applied research leading to the discovery and use of an increasing number of cytotoxic chemotherapeutic compounds with the ability to rapidly kill dividing cancer cells in preference to non-dividing healthy cells. The well-known drawback of chemotherapy is due to the fact that these drugs, in addition to damaging cancer cells, also damage healthy tissues; thus, causing side effects, sometimes with serious consequences.

The challenge is, therefore, to search for drug delivery systems that achieve high cytotoxic efficacy against cancer cells, but with limited systemic toxicity. Antibody-drug conjugates (ADCs) offer the promise of achieving this objective and increase the therapeutic index significantly.

The approach to targeted chemotherapy comes from Paul Ehrlich's concept of the "magic bullet" formulated at the beginning of the twentieth century [1]. The principle of this concept, to avoid side effects, drugs must be guided and released into the tumor sites through association with ligands that are overexpressed or selectively expressed in the tumor. Ehrlich's proposal has been translated into practical applications for therapy due to the development of monoclonal antibodies in the mid-70s, combining the selectivity of recognition to the power of chemotherapeutic drugs [2]. To become a pharmacologically active drug, monoclonal antibodies can be linked to either a radioisotope (giving rise to Antibody radioimmunoconjugates, RAC), to a highly potent cytotoxic drug (antibody-drug conjugates, ADCs) or protein toxins (producing immunotoxins) [3,4].

The production of ADCs face several vital issues, such as the target cell selection, the nature of antigen, structure and stability of the antibody, the linker chemistry, and finally the cytotoxic payload.

One of the first problems encountered in the use of antibodies was the fact that murine antibodies are foreign proteins recognized as non-self by the human immune system that responds by producing human anti-mouse antibodies (HAMA). HAMAs can have toxic effects due to immune-complex formation in the patient and, thus, prevent further administration. With the technology of recombinant DNA, Phage display, and transgenic mice, it is now possible to create of completely human antibodies that are not immunogenic and greatly ameliorate such toxicities.

Chemotherapeutic drugs include antimetabolites (methotrexate, 6-mercaptopurine, 5-fluorouracile, cytarabine, gemcitabine, etc.), molecules interfering with microtubule polymerization (vinca alkaloids, taxanes), and molecules inducing damages on DNA (anthracyclines, nitrogen mustards). The most recent generation of chemotherapeutic molecules include both DNA damaging/alkylating agents (i.e., duocarmycin from Medarex/Bristol Mayer Squibb, Syntarge, calicheamicin from Wyeth/Pfizer, indolino-benzodiazepine from Immunogen), and molecules interfering with microtubule structure (i.e., maytansinoids, from immunogen, auristatin derivatives from Seattle Genetics). These compounds can kill cells with extremely high potency so that severe side effects greatly limit the administrable dose as a free drug. These compounds are therefore considered as ideal payload components of ADCs with high therapeutic index [5].

The conjugation strategy and chemistry chosen to represent a key factor for the success of ADCs, the homogeneity of ADC molecules being one of the main challenges in ADC design [2]. In deciding in which chemical conjugation process to use, it is necessary to develop a strategy that allows the reaction of those residues placed on the surface of the antibody through a chemical reactive group present on the linker. These strategies, depending on the type of residue (mainly amino groups of lysines or sulfhydryl groups of cysteines) that can lead to the production of mixed species whose Drug-Antibody Ratio (DARs) is variable. When the DAR is poorly controlled, this phenomenon can reduce the efficacy of the ADCs and furthermore increase aggregation possibility, the overall rate of clearance and release of the payload systemically at an early stage [6], although higher DAR values are beneficial for the overall potency. To improve the technology, focusing on obtaining homogeneous ADCs with a high therapeutic index, site-specific conjugation technologies have now been developed [7].

2. Basic Characteristics of the Conjugate

An ADC is composed of three different components (Figure 1): a monoclonal antibody, the payload, and the linker that joins the first two components. Different types of conjugation chemistry exist: as in the most common, linkage is obtained through lysine (ε-amine-group, $-NH_2$ in the deprotonated form) or cysteine (sulfhydryl-group, $-SH$). However, other conjugation strategies may also be pursued (see below). Whatever the conjugation strategy, it is vital that this does not affect the integrity and functionality of the antibody.

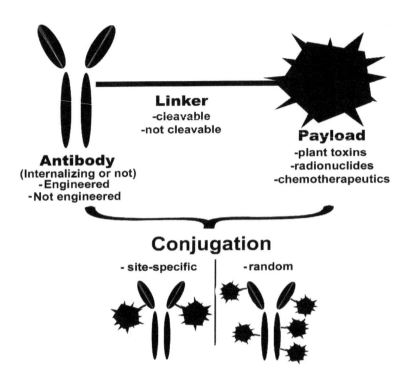

Figure 1. Schematic representation of various types of antibody-drug conjugates (ADCs) and their components.

2.1. Monoclonal Antibody

In the development of ADCs for cancer treatment, the choice of the antigen and, consequently, selection of the appropriate antibody plays a key role.

The antibody is chosen based on the molecular target recognition, with the highest affinity and selectivity for the target. Ideally, it should recognize an overexpressed target only at the tumor site to avoid delivering the pharmacological load inappropriately to non-target sites. For example, the (human epidermal growth factor receptor 2) (HER2) receptor is more than 100 times overexpressed in tumor tissues in comparison to the equivalent normal non-cancerous tissue [8].

The antigen against which the antibody is directed on the cancer cell should be present in high copy number ($>10^5$/cell.) [9]. So far, several antigens have been reported overexpressed in cancer tissues that can be exploited as targets for ADCs [10]. The antigen must be recognized and bound by the antibody with a reasonable affinty (Kd $\leq$ 10 nM) to ensure rapid uptake in the target cell [11].

In the first generation of ADCs, in many cases murine antibodies being recognized as foreign proteins generated a strong immune response with the production of anti-human antibodies that potentially reduced their therapeutic efficacy. This problem has been partially solved through the use of genetic engineering in second-generation ADCs, utilizing a mouse-human chimeric antibody format. The "humanized" chimeric antibody contains the mouse light and heavy chain variable regions that are linked to human constant regions. The chimeric ADCs showed promising results in cancer treatment but sometimes the problem of decreased efficiency and human anti-chimeric response were still present.

To overcome this problem, many efforts have been made to design a humanized monoclonal antibody, which contain only murine complementary determining regions (CDRs) regions combined with the human variable region [8] or fully human antibodies [12].

Usually, the antibodies used to construct ADCs are of the IgG1 class (Immunoglobulin G Subclass 1) (~150 kDa), but since antibodies in ADCs exploit the Fab region to recognize the antigen present at the end of light chains, only this region is essential to the antibody to carry out its function as a specific carrier. Therefore, in some cases, smaller antibody formats (i.e., antibody fragments that maintain the binding affinity for the receptor) have been used to create ADCs. These fragments can be obtained by IgG cleavage following papain digestion or recombinant production to produce Fabs and scFvs [13].

Selected antibodies and their derived ADCs can be directed against antigens that may or may not induce internalization through receptor-mediated endocytosis (RME), and by this criterion, ADCs can be classified as internalizing or non-internalizing.

2.1.1. Internalizing ADCs

Internalizing ADCs exploit RME to be internalized by target cells. In this case, the antibody performs a fundamental role as it favors the internalization of the target antigen receptor, which represents a crucial step for most ADCs to be effective. Although, as in the case of the anti-HER3 antibody EV20, the binding to the receptor and the internalization of receptor/antibody complex can alone induce cell death and inhibition of tumor growth [14–16].

Following internalization, the ADC can follow different endocytic routes that crucially may have profound effects on their cytotoxic efficacy. Clathrin-mediated and caveolae-mediated endocytosis (CME) in which the receptor mediates endocytosis and, alternatively, clathrin-caveolin-independent endocytosis, where the receptor does not mediate endocytosis [17]. The most common route to reach the cell cytoplasm, adopted by various ADCs, is CME, which is target antigen dependent. Molecules, such as epsin, dynamin, adaptor protein 2 (AP2), and phosphatidylinositol (4,5) bis-phosphate (PIP2) may increase accumulation of ADCs on the surface of cellular membrane [18] and assist the internalization of the ADC into the endo-lysosomal vesicle compartment.

Early endosomes form just below the membrane surface and usually endo-lysosomal vesicles containing ADCs progress to form late endosomes, whose lumens are acidic and may lead to the dissociation of antibodies from their receptors thus playing a vital role in recycling of antigen back to the membrane surface and subsequently lead to fusion of the late endosomal vesicle with lysosomes. The resulting pH decrease may also result in degradation of the ADC due to the numerous proteolytic enzymes present in the acidic lysosomal compartment with subsequent release of the drug payload. [19] (Figure 2).

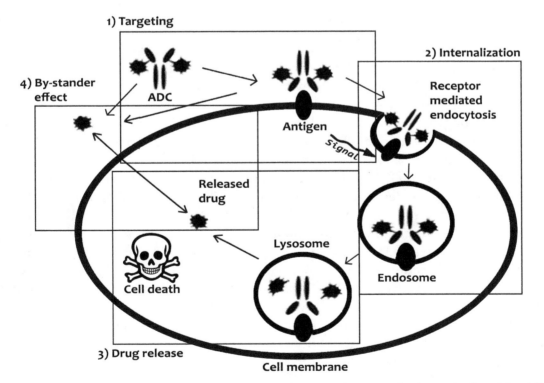

Figure 2. Schematic illustration of the mechanism of drug delivery and release mediated by ADCs.

Release of the drug within endolysosomal vesicles then results in the passive transport of drug payload into the cytosol where it can exert its pharmacological effect, killing the cancer cells via a molecule specific mechanism [20,21].

2.1.2. Non-Internalizing ADCs

The main pharmacological action of ADCs constructed with non-internalizing antibodies, relies on the cytotoxic payload exerting a bystander effect upon reaching the target tumor site. In this instance, once the ADC reaches the tumor site, proteolytic enzymes, or the reducing conditions in the tumor extracellular environment, act to liberate the drug payload, which facilitate the entry of drugs into the cells, by diffusion, pinocytosis, or other mechanisms. Once the released drugs start kill cancer cells, they release additional reducing agents or proteases, which in turn catalyze further release of drugs (Figure 2). This type of conjugates may also allow a by-stander effect on non-target cancer cells that are near the main target tumor mass, due to diffusion of the released drug into neighboring tumor cells of the drug [22].

It has been reported that an ADC directed against the alternatively spliced extracellular domain A of fibronectin induces a potent anticancer effect following the release of its payload after tumor cell death in the extracellular milieu. This allows the diffusion of the cytotoxic drug also into neighboring cells, and amplification of the process determined by a further release of reducing agents (e.g., cysteine, glutathione) [23].

2.2. Linkers

The linker component of the ADC, through which the covalent chemical bond between the drug and the antibody is created, should be chosen rationally, based on the mechanism of action of the antibody (whether internalizing or not) and limit potential chemical modifications to the drug in order to avoid loss of cytotoxicity. One of the main aims for the effective systemic delivery of an ADC is that the drug is released only at the target site; the linker, thus, must be stable enough in a biological environment (i.e., blood circulation) to avoid unwanted release of the pharmacological molecule.

There are two types of linkers available: cleavable and non-cleavable (Figure 3). The former can be used either in the design of either an internalizing or not internalizing ADC, because the release of the payload is required to take place in either the extracellular tumor environment, or within the lysosome or cytosol. This is possible because the extracellular environment of the tumor is highly reducing due to the presence of glutathione, which allows the release of payloads linked to the antibody via thiolic bonds. It also allows payload release via the degradation of peptide bonds in the presence of proteases such as Cathepsin B, whose overexpression in cancer drives its normal lysosomal localization towards extracellular secretion [24]. A cleavable linker, therefore, exploits differential conditions of reducing power or enzymatic degradation that can be present either outside or inside the target cell. Due to the chemical reactions needed to release the payload, the site of conjugation on the antibody is crucial to induce both stability in the plasma and availability to reduction or degradation on/into the target cell [25,26]. Non-cleavable linker-based ADC must, however, be internalizing, because to release their cytotoxic payload, the antibody component needs to be degraded by lysosomal or cytoplasmic proteases [27]. Furthermore, drugs linked to such linkers usually cannot exert a by-stander effect because upon degradation of the antibody by cellular proteases, they are released as fragments of antibody peptides that have a poor ability to permeate the cells. This type of non-cleavable linker has a higher efficiency for the treatment of tumors that express an antigen at high levels (to achieve a good clinical response and tumor regression, 99% of targeted cancer cells must be eliminated) or for hematological tumors [28,29].

A Disulfide linkers

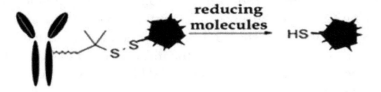

B Cathepsin B-responsive linker (Val-Cit)

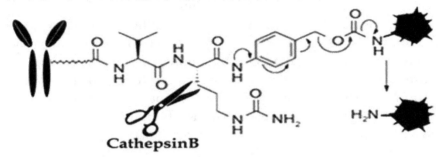

C Glycosidase-sensitive linker

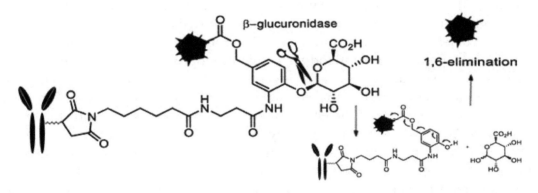

D Hydrazone linker

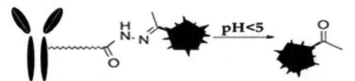

Figure 3. Available cleavable linkers in ADC (**A**) Disulfide linker, cleaved by reducing agents; (**B**) cathepsin B responsive linker, cleaved by Cathepsin B; (**C**) glycosidase-sensitive linker, cleaved by gluconidase; (**D**) hydrazone linker, cleaved by acidic environment.

2.2.1. Cleavable Linkers

Figure 3 above summarizes the most commonly used cleavable linkers that are described in detail in the sections that follow.

Disulfide Linkers

This type of linker is glutathione-sensitive. The disulfides are stable at physiological pH, in the systemic blood stream, but they are vulnerable to nucleophilic attack by thiols. Human serum albumin (HSA) represents the main thiol in plasma, being its concentration as high as >400 mM. Notwithstanding this high concentration, HSA fails to break the disulfide bond of ADC because its residue containing free thiol (Cys34) is found near a cleft in the molecule that is not significantly exposed to the solvent [30]. Conversely, disulfide-linked drugs resist reductive cleavage in the circulation because the glutathione (GSH) concentration in the blood (5 μmol/L) is lower than in the cytoplasm (1–10 mmol/L) allowing GSH thiol groups to be very effective in the cell cytoplasm also due to its well exposed position and its small size [31]. This difference in reductive potential between plasma and cytosol allows for the selective release of the intracellular payload of the ADCs. In addition, cancer cells cause oxidative stress that generates high GSH levels. Low glutathione levels in healthy tissues therefore discriminate release of the payload, also allowing the selective release of payload in close proximity to the tumor. ADCs with disulfide linkers are often associated with maytansinoid payloads, which were originally developed by Immunogen in 1992 [32]. To increase the stability of the bond, methyl groups may be added to surround disulfides in the linker structure [33], such as in the case of N-succinimidyl-4-(2-pyridyldithio)pentanoate (SPP) containing a single methyl, or N-succinimidyl-4-(2-pyridyldithio)butanoate (SPDB) containing two methyl groups.

Some ADC designs use a direct disulfide bond between the drug and the antibody. In this variety of ADC, the release of the drug is completely dependent on a strongly reducing tumor microenvironment [34]. Recently, ADCs with a direct disulfide bond between engineered cysteine residues and the thiols of maytansinoids payloads have been investigated [30]. By protecting disulfides reduction through antibody hindrance, these ADCs have good in vivo stability in mouse plasma. The results demonstrate that the DM3 payload is more stable than the DM1, given that only 10% of disulfide bonds are cleaved in plasma, a property that confers increased in vivo therapeutic activity in a murine model [35]. The structure of the whole antibody thus represents a protective environment significantly reducing the reductive release of the payload in the blood stream, but this in turn may limit the efficiency of release once at the tumor site. Other studies have shown that by creating an ADC using a small immunoprotein (SIP) antibody (small immunoprotein, comprised of an IgG, including variable regions from heavy and light chains linked through peptide plus additional C3 or C4 heavy chain proteins; see also below) and comparing the results with an analogous ADC constructed with intact IgG, the release of the drug by the ADC-SIP occurs faster. This is probably due to a more stable interchain disulfide bond in the SIP. However, by analyzing the stability of ADCs in mouse plasma, a half-life greater than 48 h with IgG and less than 3 h with SIP was determined. An analysis of the in vivo efficacy of the above compounds showed that the ADC-SIP experienced an accumulation and therefore a greater release than the IgG-ADC, despite there being a global accumulation of ADC-IgG after 24 h that was greater in the tumor than that observed for the ADC-SIP [23].

Cathepsin B-Sensitive Linker

The cysteine protease Cathepsin B is normally found inside late endosomes and lysosomal compartments in mammals. It is also implicated in tumor progression, being overexpressed by many cancers [36]. The carboxydipeptidase activity of Cathepsin B allows the splitting of a dipeptide linker that can bind a payload to the terminal C. This enzyme has various substrate target peptide sequences with Phe-Arg being the most common [36]. In addition, it also preferentially recognizes sequences such as valine-citrulline (Val-Cit) and phenylalanine-lysine (Phe-Lys) where the protease breaks a peptide bond on the C-terminal side of Val-Cit, Val-Ala, or Phe-Lys. Some studies have shown that a high pH basic environment increases the cleavage capacity [3] and that the hydrophobic residues Phe, Val, and Ala allow cleavage with cathepsin B that has the effect of increasing the stability in plasma. Sometimes, however, the payload can be too bulky in which case the use of a spacer that is stable and that does not alter the drugs chemistry, and functionality is necessary. One of the most used conjugation reagents is para-aminobenzyl carbamate (PABC) (Figure 4), that possesses a self-cleavage ability allowing it to release the unmodified payload [35]. For example, linkers containing Phe-Lys-PABC and Val-Cit-PABC, used for ADC with monomethyl-auristatin E (MMAE) payload, have a half-life in plasma for Phe-Lys-PABC of 12 h compared to 80 h for Val-Cit-PABC 80 h. This shorter half-life indicates that the linker with Phe-Lys-PABC is probably non-specific with the danger that it may exert off-target toxicity [37].

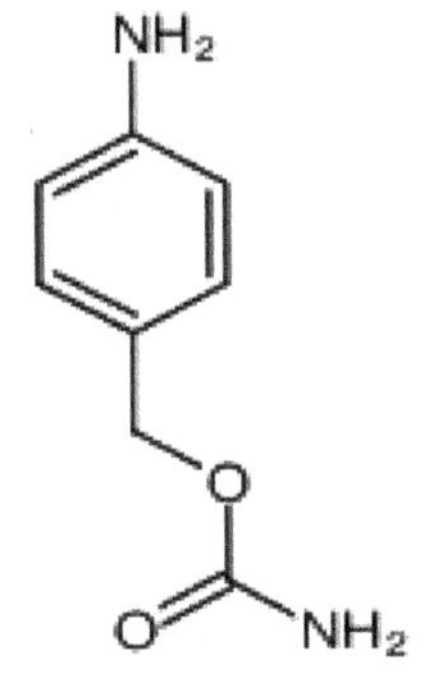

Figure 4. PABC, p-aminobenzyl carbamate, CAS#:918132-66-8.

To summarize, it has been shown that if these types of linker are coupled with paminobenzyloxycarbonyl (PABC) they work more efficiently as cleavable linkers (i.e., Val-Ala-PABC) for ADCs [38]. The PABC group acts as a spacer separating the toxic payload from Val-Cit sequence so that the active site of cathepsin B can gain better access to the cleavage sequence, thus, more effectively exploiting its protease activity, particularly if a large molecular sized payload is used. PABC is furthermore a self-immolate linker that, upon Cathepsin B cleavage, can undergo hydrolysis releasing the free drug to which it is attached (i.e., monomethyl-auristatin E (MMAE)) [39,40].

Hydrazone Linker

Hydrazone linkers or other similar molecules that are pH-dependent, have quite a stable structure at neutral pH (i.e., in the bloodstream at pH 7.4) and are hydrolyzed when they reach an acidic cellular compartment such as the lysosome (pH < 5) or late endosomes (pH 5.5–6.2). However, the degradation of this linker is not confined to the lysosome, but may, on occasion, also occur extracellularly. ADCs with a hydrazone linker hydrolyze only slowly under physiological conditions, with the slow release of the toxic payload [41]. A study with an antibody directed against mucin, conjugated via an acid-labile linker, showed good therapeutic effects in a preclinical pancreatic cancer model [42] where the tumor microenvironment is significantly more acidic than in normal tissues, due to the enhanced glycolysis taking place in the tumor with the consequent production of lactate to a level sufficient to induce extracellular cleavage of the linker. In mouse models, the slow release of the circulatory payload has produced promising results, but only in the presence of payloads with moderate cytotoxic activity. Payloads with higher cytotoxic activity, now widely used for the production of ADCs, demand the use linkers with higher stability to avoid the undesired release of the payload and resultant non-specific systemic toxicity [37].

Glycosidase-Sensitive Linkers

Glycosidases comprise hydrolytic lysosomal enzymes, such as β-glucuronidases that degrade β-glucuronic acid residues into polysaccharides. They are found in lysosomes and work under hydrophilic environments. β-glucuronidases, like cathepsin B, are also secreted in the necrotic areas of some tumors. They are also enzymatically active in the extracellular environment [43]. ADCs that contain β-glucuronic acid can reach a DAR = 8 without causing aggregation and without reducing the hydrophobicity of the ADC. Indeed, this type of linker greatly reduce plasma clearance of ADCs, thus increasing their efficacy in vivo [44]. It is also established that the use of Poly (Ethylene Glycol) PEG linkers increases the hydrophilicity of β-glucuronic acid and, thereby, increases the activity and efficiency of the ADC [30].

Another type of hydrolytic lysosomal enzyme, the β-galactosidases that degrade β-galactoside, are also overexpressed in some types of cancer [45]. An ADC based on trastuzumab linked to MMAE using a β-galactoside linker was shown to be more potent than an equivalent ADC based on a Val-Cit-PABC linker. This formulation of ADC-β-galactoside-DM1 has also been shown to be more efficient in vivo for the treatment of HER2+ breast tumors than the approved trastuzumab emtansine (T-DM1) [35].

2.2.2. Non-Cleavable Linkers

The most used non-cleavable linkers are alkylic and polymeric. For example, the MCC amine-to-sulfhydryl bifunctional cross-linker contains a cyclohexane ring structure that through steric hindrance protects the resulting thioether bond from hydrolysis [46]. The greatest advantage of non-cleavable versus cleavable linkers is their improved plasma stability; that results in reduced off-target toxicity in comparison to conjugates with cleavable linkers and thus provides greater stability and tolerability [47,48]. It is noteworthy that non-cleavable ADCs often have less activity against tumors due to the heterogeneity of target antigen expression where a bystander effect is an important contributor to therapeutic efficacy [49]. As described earlier, non-cleavable linkers require mAb degradation within the lysosome after ADC internalization to release the drug to the site of pharmacological activity in the cytosol. If the payload is linked to a charged amino acid such as lysine) with a Pi < 9.5, this will prevent escape of the drug by diffusion through the cell membrane and result in higher levels of drug-accumulation in the tumor cell which as a consequence should overcome the limitations of any bystander effect. In summary the major advantage of non-cleavable linkers is that they minimize drug release into the circulation thus limiting non-specific toxicity whilst maintaining, good in vivo stability [50].

Usually, non-cleavable linkers contain a thioether or maleimidocaproyl group. Examples of non-cleavable linker-based ADCs containing monomethyl auristatin F (MMAF), an anti-mitotic drug, where it was demonstrated that the drug is more potent if linked via a simple alkyl chain to the antibody. Conjugation effected with a non-reducible thioether linker demonstrated very good activity in both *in vitro* and in vivo [51].

2.3. Payloads

Currently, most ADCs are constructed with two main families of highly toxic compounds, acting either on microtubule or DNA structure. Among the first group, auristatins and maytansines payloads both act as tubulin inhibitors and have been widely used for construction of ADCs. Both molecules are potently cytotoxic against rapidly dividing cancer cells and have reduced toxicity to normal cells. Alternatively, calicheamicins and PBDs are DNA-damaging agents, inducing cell death by apoptotic mechanisms in all cells including cancer stem cells (CSCs), and for this reason, they do exert severe side effects. There is also a third category of drug that targets specific enzymes essential for cell survival. In general, the payloads suitable for an ADC must have: (a) good solubility in aqueous solutions allowing an easier conjugation to the antibody and ensuring enough solubility to ADC under physiological conditions; (b) a significantly higher cytotoxic activity (half maximal inhibitory concentration (IC_{50}) ranging from 0.01 to 0.1 nM) in comparison to clinically standard chemotherapeutic agents; (c) induce cancer cell death by apoptotic mechanisms; and (d) possess an appropriate functional group to facilitate conjugation to the antibody.

The most widely used commercialized drugs for ADC formulation comprise microtubule-targeting agents. The choice of tubulin inhibitors as payloads is appropriate since rapid cellular proliferation is one of the major discriminating features between cancerous and normal cells and antimitotic agents are in principle less toxic to the normal cells [52]. Vinca alkaloid, laulimalide, taxane, maytansine, and colchicine have all defined binding sites on microtubules. These molecules (Figure 5) can be grouped in two main categories depending on their mechanism of action: tubulin polymerization promoters (microtubule stabilizers) and tubulin polymerization inhibitors (microtubule destabilizers) [53]. In particular, microtubule stabilizers inhibit the formation of microtubules acting on the β-subunit of α-β tubulin dimers determining unregulated microtubule growth, as in case of Auristatin. In contrast, the mechanism of action of microtubule destabilizers is to block the polymerization of tubulin dimers by inhibiting the formation of mature microtubules, as is the case for maytansinoids (Figure 6).

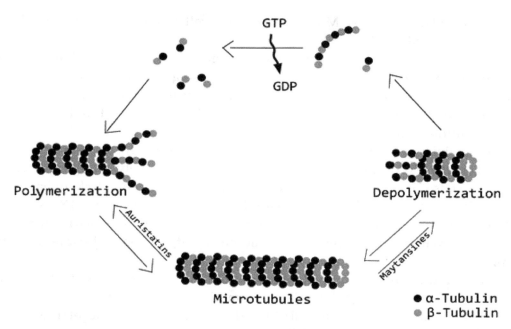

Figure 5. Mechanism of action of tubulin inhibitors payloads: polymerization promoters (microtubule stabilizers) and tubulin polymerization inhibitors (microtubule destabilizers). In the figure are two exemplifying drugs acting on microtubule formation: auristatins alters the formation of microtubules by binding on the β-subunit of α-β tubulin dimers; thus, producing uncontrolled growth of microtubules. Maytansines, on the contrary, stop tubulin dimers formation impairing the production of mature microtubules.

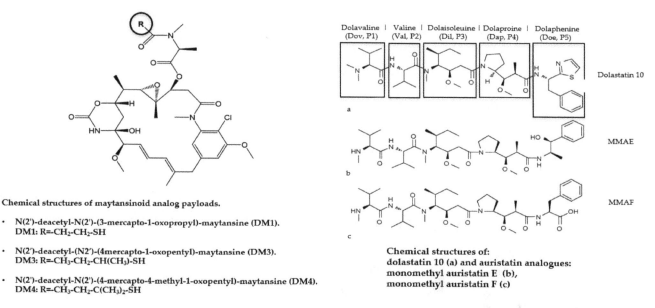

Chemical structures of maytansinoid analog payloads.

- N(2')-deacetyl-N(2')-(3-mercapto-1-oxopropyl)-maytansine (DM1).
  DM1: R=-CH₂-CH₂-SH

- N(2')-deacetyl-(N2')-(4mercapto-1-oxopentyl)-maytansine (DM3).
  DM3: R=-CH₃-CH₂-CH(CH₃)-SH

- N(2')-deacetyl-N(2')-(4-mercapto-4-methyl-1-oxopentyl)-maytansine (DM4).
  DM4: R=-CH₃-CH₂-C(CH₃)₂-SH

Chemical structures of:
dolastatin 10 (a) and auristatin analogues:
monomethyl auristatin E (b),
monomethyl auristatin F (c)

Figure 6. Classical microtubule-targeting agents: maytansinoids (**left**) and auristatin families (**right**).

Auristatin is a dolastatin synthetic analog. The original drug was isolated from *Dolabella auricularia* (sea hare) as dolastatin peptides, which successfully improved its water solubility to give auristatin [54]. Auristatins block tubulin assembly and induce cell cycle arrest in G2/M phase, causing cells to undergo apoptosis.

To prevent lysosomal payload degradation and to enhance drug efficacy two innovative auristatin derivatives (monomethyl auristatin E (MMAE) and monomethyl auristatin F (MMAF)) have been developed by Seattle Genetics. These two compounds are synthetic drugs derived by design from structure-activity relationship (SAR) analysis. These two new molecules are different due to a phenylalanine present at the C-terminus of MMAF that allows this latter compound to be more membrane impermeable. In contrast, MMAE can exit the cell and thus diffuse to nearby cells killing them through bystander effects [53].

Maytansinoids are derivatives of natural cytotoxic agents named maytansines, a family of toxins originally isolated from the cortex of *Maytenus serrata* possessing macrolide structure. Maytansine and maytansinoids alter microtubule polymerization thus inhibit the maturation of microtubules by binding to or in close proximity to the vinblastine-binding site on the β-subunit of tubulin. This consequently induces cell death through mitotic arrest [54].

ADCs that containing maytansinoid, are unfortunately substrates for multidrug resistance protein 1 (MDR1), a critical protein of the cell membrane that acts by actively pumping a wide variety of xenobiotics out of cells. To prevent this problem a series of hydrophilic linkers have been used in ADC chemistry. These linkers allow for an increased drug content (DAR) in ADCs s and subsequent increases in the amount of drug delivered to each target cell. The increased polarity introduced by such linkers allows the formation of maytansinoid metabolites that are poor substrates for efflux pumps thus overcoming MDR [55].

Maytansines are difficult to conjugate because they do not have reactive chemical groups. To overcome this problem, a series of derivatives containing SH groups have been created examples of which are, DM1 and DM4 that are substituted by methyl disulfide at the maytansine C3 *N*-acyl-*N*-methyl-L-alanyl ester side chain [56].

A third type of antimitotic payload includes tubulysins characterized by higher affinity of binding to the vinca domain of tubulin if compared with vinblastine. These agents exert a rapid disruption of the cytoskeleton and subsequent disassembly of the mitotic apparatus in proliferating cancer cells. This results in a block at G2/M of the cell cycle and subsequent apoptotic cell death [57] (Figure 7).

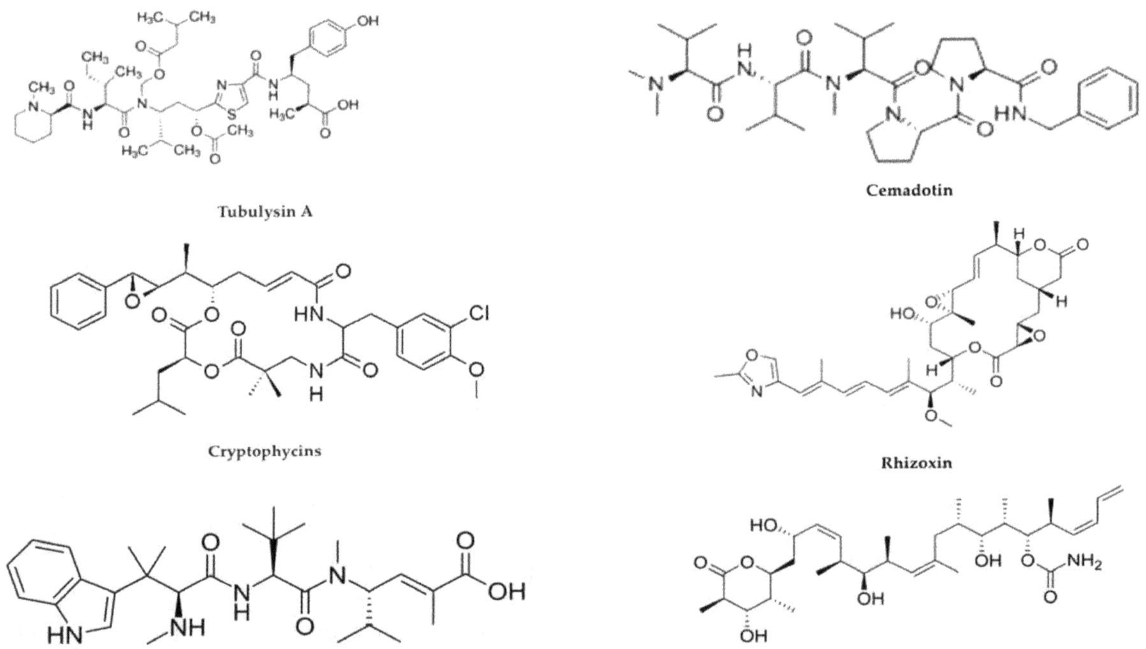

Figure 7. Other microtubule-targeting agents.

Tubulysins possess high degree of selective cytotoxicity against human cancer cells due to their rapid rate of division. Furthermore, they may also be effective against cancer cells overexpressing the P-glycoprotein or which possess mutations in tubulin gene. Tubulysins are comprised of a family with 14 different isoforms characterized by conserved core structure made of an L-isoleucine (Ile), a tubuvaline (Tuv), and an *N*-methylD-pipecolic acid (Mep) unit.

The first targeted drug (EC0305) based on tubulysin has been recently obtained by linking Tubulysin B to folic acid conjugate. Now several tubulysin D-based ADCs are under study [53].

To complete the family of drugs that bind to microtubules the following compounds are also worth mentioning:

Cryptophycins, a class of cytotoxins more potent than MMAE and DM1, isolated from *Nostoc cyanobacteria* induce tubulin depolymerization binding to microtubules. Cryptophycin-1 is the main component, acting on many solid tumors and additionally MDR cancer cells.

Hemiasterlin from marine sponges are naturally occurring tripeptides acting as potent inhibitors of cell growth. They bind to the tubulin vinca-site thus disrupting normal microtubule dynamics and consequently inhibiting tubulin polymerization. Taltobulin (HTI-286) is a fully synthetic analog of hemiasterlin and has been shown to be to be active against a variety of MDR cancer cell lines [53].

Cemadotin (LU103793) is a more hydrophilic synthetic pentapeptide analogous of dolastatin 15, possessing strong antiproliferative activity through inhibition of microtubule assembly and tubulin polymerization by binding at a novel site on tubulin. Cemadotin has been shown to be an effective payload for ADC construction [53].

Rhizoxin, a compound isolated from Rhizopus microspores (a fungus able to be infectious for humans causing mycosis) that binds to tubulin and causes inhibition of microtubule assembly [58].

Discodermolide is so far the most efficient natural promoter of tubulin assembly considered to be a very promising candidate for future ADC development [53].

There are furthermore other tubulin inhibitors that have been investigated for their possible use in ADC construction, such as taccalonolide A or B, taccalonolide AF or AJ, colchicine, epothilone A and B, taccalonolide AI-epoxide, CA-4, laulimalide, paclitaxel, and docetaxel, together with their synthetic analogous [53,59].

The second category of payload used for ADC construction is comprised of DNA-damaging drugs. This class of payload may be more effective than microtubule inhibitors with IC_{50} values in the picomolar, as opposed to the nanomolar range for microtubule inhibitors. This would make ADCs constructed with DNA damaging drug payloads more potent and therefore better suited for targeting antigens that are expressed at low levels on tumors. Furthermore, DNA-damaging drugs are fully capable of apoptotically killing non-dividing cells including cancer stem cells when used in combination with drugs that inhibit DNA repair and furthermore are capable of killing target cells at any point in the cell cycle [60].

There are at least four mechanisms of action exerted by DNA-damaging agents, which are as follows: (a) DNA double-strand breakage, (b) DNA alkylation, (c) DNA intercalation, and (d) DNA cross-linking. The most used DNA-damaging payloads are pyrrolobenzodiazepine, duocarmycins, doxorubicin, and calicheamicins [61] (Figure 8).

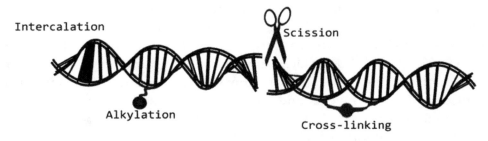

Figure 8. The four main mechanisms of action of DNA-damaging agents: DNA double-strand breakers, DNA alkylators, DNA intercalators, and DNA cross-linkers. DNA-damaging agents. These drugs can act at any phase of tumor cell life cycle.

Pyrrolobenzodiazepines (PBDs) were originally isolated from *Streptomyces* sp. and are natural products, possessing antibiotic and antitumor properties. PBD molecules bind in the minor groove of double- stranded DNAs to the C2-amino groups of guanine residues.

PBDs forms an adduct PBD/DNA in the minor groove of DNA, leading to decreased DNA repair and interfering with transcription factors binding to DNA, as well as to some enzyme functions including RNA polymerase and endonucleases.

Currently, additional to natural isolated monomeric forms of PBDs, synthetic PBD dimers are available, which in addition to forming monoadducts are also capable of forming intrastrand or interstrand DNA cross-links [62] (Figure 9).

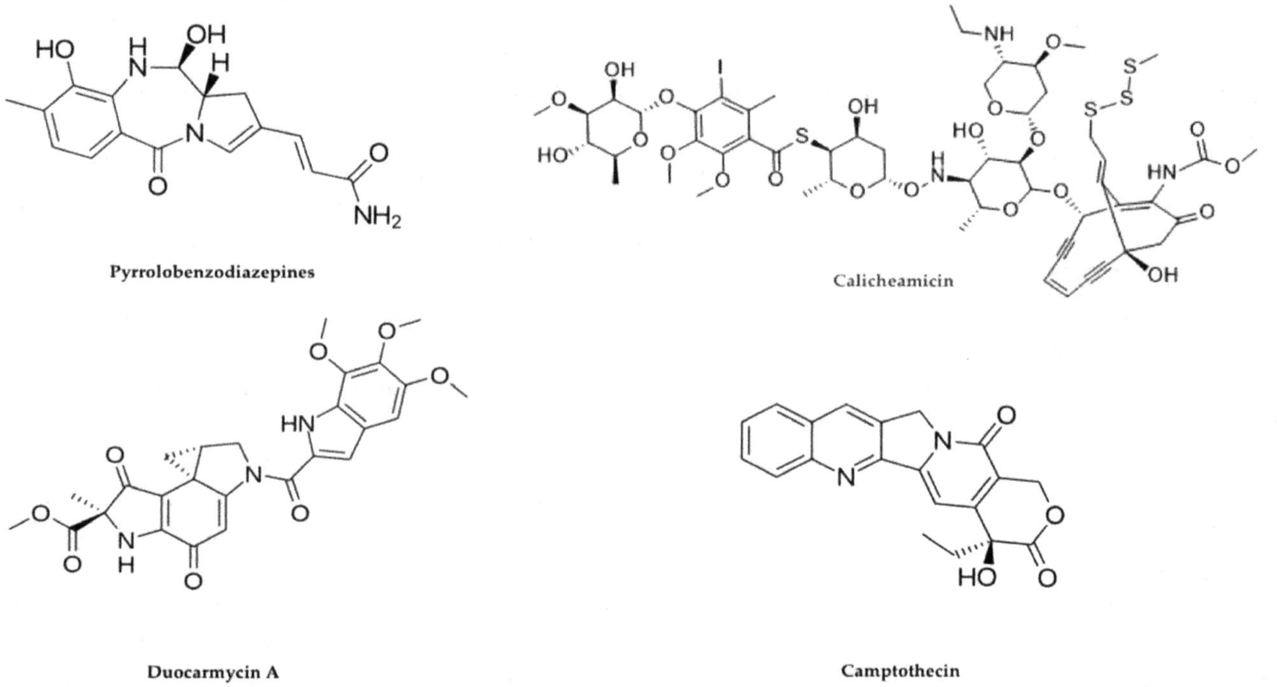

Figure 9. Examples of DNA-damaging drug payloads.

Duocarmycins, metabolites originally isolated from *Streptomyces* sp. are powerful cytotoxic substances because their mechanism of action involves alkylation of the DNA minor groove to form a stable adduct. Duocarmycins specifically bind to a sequence of five-base-pair rich in AT-rich where the central pyrroloindole may be easily accommodated. This results in irreversible DNA modification compromising its architecture that finally leads to DNA cleavage and apoptotic cell death. There are also synthetic analogs of duocarmycins available, such as adozelesin, bizelesin, and carzelesin.

Duocarmycins have impressively high cell cycle-independent cytotoxicity against a variety of proliferating cancer cells *in vitro* with IC$_{50}$ values in the pM range [63].

The duocarmycin analogous DUBA (duocarmycin-hydroxybenzamide-azaindole), representing the duocarmycin final active drug metabolite, has been used to produce different new-generation ADCs that have been tested *in vitro* and in vivo to verify their therapeutic efficacy. An example is represented by SYD983, an anti-HER2 ADC, exerting clear anti-tumor activity in a mouse xenograft model (BT-474) and showing enough stability in human and macaque primate plasma [64].

The high toxicity of duocarmycins and their analogous makes them desirable candidates to maximize ADC cell-killing activity and also suggests that they may be effective agents to overcome multi drug resistant (MDR) tumor cells [65].

Calicheamicins (LL-E33288) are a class of antibiotics that were discovered in Texas following a search for novel fermentation-derived antitumor antibiotics that led to *Micromonospora echinospora*. These compounds are a class of enediyne-containing DNA-cleaving antitumor agent with a potency 4000–10,000 times greater than DNA intercalating drugs, such as Adriamycin and other similar.

The mechanism of action of calicheamicins after cell entry and nuclear diffusion is due to drug targeting and binding to the minor groove of DNA, causing double-strand breaks that induce apoptotic cell death [66].

Calicheamicins are extremely powerful drugs acting at sub-pM concentrations but also unfortunately exert significant non-specific toxicity, damaging the DNA of all cells. Their high toxicity means that they cannot be used directly as a single therapeutic agent in cancer treatment. Their inherent characteristics (i.e., high cytotoxicity, relatively small molecular size, mechanism of action) have however made calicheamicins useful payloads for the construction of ADCs [54].

Camptothecin (CPT) is a natural compound isolated from *Camptotheca acuminata* and is an inhibitor of the nuclear enzyme topoisomerase I. CPT molecules inhibit both DNA and RNA synthesis in mammalian cells, and have demonstrated to be strongly cytotoxic against a wide range of experimental tumors. Unfortunately, several clinical trials have shown considerable toxicity problems in patients due to their low solubility and resultant adverse side effects. To circumvent these limitations, camptothecin analogs topotecan (TPT) and irinotecan (camptothecin-11, CPT-11) that show improved water solubility have been approved by the FDA. These molecules were tested in clinical practice, and demonstrated significant antitumor activity and reduced toxicity [67].

SN-38 and DX-8951f are two additional CPT-analogs that have been used as ADC payloads. SN-38, an active CPT-11 metabolite that exploits inhibition of DNA topoisomerase to exert its anticancer activity [68].

In addition to all of the above-mentioned payloads, other molecules available also act as DNA-damaging agents for incorporation into newly emerging ADCs. Among these compounds, particular mention should be given to iSGD-1882 (DNA minor groove cross-linker derived from PBD dimers), centanamycin (binds to DNA and alkylates or intercalates into DNA), PNU-159682 (an anthracycline metabolite) [69], and uncialamycin (an enediyne natural product isolated from Streptomyces uncialis) [70], all active on different cancer cell lines, and finally indolinobenzodiazepine dimers (IGNs) bind to the DNA minor groove leading to DNA cross-linking [71].

Alternative Payloads

In addition to all the payloads discussed above, other molecules are available whose cytotoxicity is based on different mechanisms of action that include the direct induction of apoptosis, spliceosome, and RNA polymerase inhibition.

Bcl-2 family members, including Bcl-xL, are overexpressed in cancer and the BH3- binding domain on Bcl-xL has been targeted. Examples of such targeting agents comprise two anti-EGFR-Bcl-xL ADCs both of which possessed reasonable anti-tumor activity [72].

The spliceosome is an attractive target in cancer therapy, and thailanstatins have been shown to inhibit RNA splicing by the binding to different spliceosome subunits [61]. Thailanstatin A in fact was demonstrated to bind to the SF3b subunit of the spliceosome blocking RNA splicing and was used in the generation of an ADC (anti-Her2-thailanstatin). The Spliceostatins are potent spliceosome inhibitors of natural origin with interesting and potentially useful anticancer activities [61].

The final class of promising payloads are the transcription inhibitors targeting RNA polymerase II. Example of these compounds are the amatoxins, macrocyclic peptides produced by mushrooms of the genus Amanita, that are powerful and selective inhibitors of RNA polymerase II, thus resulting in the inhibition of protein synthesis [73].

β-amanitin has been covalently coupled to a MUC1-targeting mAb and this ADC has proven to be specifically cytotoxic against the human breast carcinoma cell lineT47D [74].

α-amanitin was efficiently targeted to cancer cells through an anti-HER2 mAb, with an IC_{50} value in the pM range. Moreover, α-amanitin has also been covalently linked to an EpCAM-targeting mAb, showing effective antiproliferative activity both *in vitro* and in vivo. An anti-PSMA-α-amanitin ADC has been recently observed to have in vivo antitumor activity when coupled using a stable and cleavable linker [56].

Amatoxins are highly water soluble, a property that facilitates the conjugation process and reduces ADC aggregation. Their low molecular weight, after release, allows for rapid kidney excretion in the urine. Amatoxins are also highly active against MDR cancer cells because they represent poor substrates for MDR mechanistic processes [71].

It should also be mentioned that payloads for conjugation to antibody can also include proteinaceous enzymes from plants (e.g., saporin, ricin A chain) [4,20] or bacterial toxins (PE, Pseudomonas exotoxin, DT, Diphtheria toxin) which induce cell death by irreversibly inhibiting protein synthesis catalytically [75,76]. Although this latter class of toxin molecule when conjugated to an antibody is commonly known as an immunotoxin, it is not considered a small molecule drug. The enzymatic nature of proteinaceous toxins as a payload represents added value since a single molecule may be sufficient to fatally intoxicate an individual cell. A variety of different linkers and payloads has been investigated over the years and because these are totally protein constructs, fully recombinant toxins are possible making this a promising production strategy [4].

The Figure 10 below summarizes all the payload categories discussed above in Section 2.3.

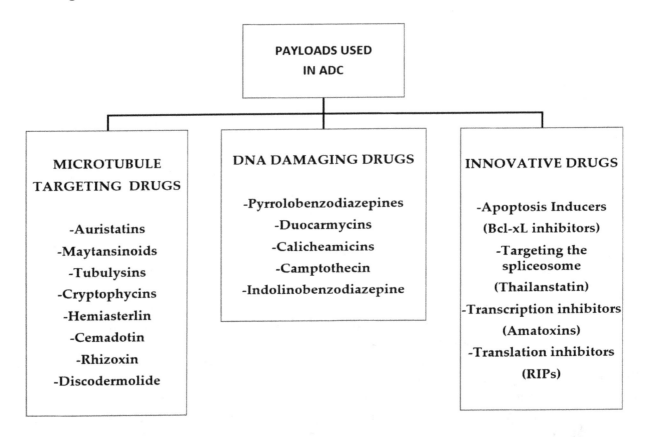

Figure 10. Summary diagram of the different classes of cytotoxic molecules used in ADC construction.

3. Conjugation Strategies

Most ADCs exploit the presence of lysine and cysteine residues within the polypeptide structure of the antibody as the point of conjugation. The average IgG_1 molecule for example, possesses approximately 90 lysine residues, but only 30 of these are accessible for conjugation, so theoretically the number of covalently coupled payloads could range from 1 to 30. Amide or amidine bond formation on the side chain of lysine is the most common reaction to effect covalent cross-linking of the antibody to the payload through exploitation of the reactive groups of linkers (i.e., N-hydroxysuccinimide esters, NHS; imidoesters) [77]. Figure 11 shows the main reactions used in the cross-linking procedures.

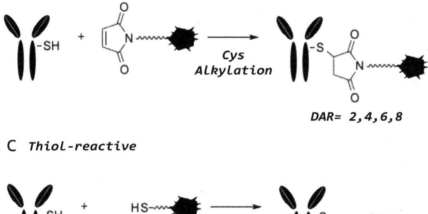

A *Lysine amide coupling*

DAR= 3,5-4

B *Maleimide alkylation*

Cys Alkylation

DAR= 2,4,6,8

C *Thiol-reactive*

DAR= 2-5

Figure 11. Main reactions used in the cross-linking procedures. (**A**) Lysine amide coupling, (**B**) Maleimide Alkylation, and (**C**) thiol-reactive conjugation.

The lysine-amide coupling conjugation is not site-specific and requires a pre-conjugation derivatization of the antibody and/or the payload in order for conjugation to proceed, very often using thiolic or citrulline-valine as linkers [77]. Alternatively, conjugation via cysteines requires that a partial reduction of the antibody is undertaken or a thiol-containing reagent (e.g., Trout's reagent) is used to introduce additional-SH groups available for the conjugation. This may cause destabilization of the whole IgG molecule and introduce structural heterogeneity into the final product. IgG_1 has four disulfide bridges, two that link the heavy to the light chains, and two in the hinge region, which bond together the two half-heavy chains of the whole antibody [78]. As one of the fundamental points of conjugation chemistry is the precise control of the drug Antibody Ratio (DAR), a recently used strategy is to achieve site-specific coupling of the payload by engineering the structure of the antibody. For example, the substitution of three cysteines in the hinge region with three serines yields an IgG molecule that fully retains its interactions between heavy and light chains [79]. Thus, through such modification of the cysteine residues, this leaves only two reactive cysteines, one on each chain, to yield an ADC product containing up to two molecules of drug per antibody. By refining the conjugation conditions, it is possible to obtain an extremely homogeneous product with the presence of the only conjugate with exactly two molecules of drug per antibody molecule (DAR 2) [23,34,79].

4. Site-Specific Enzymatic Conjugation

It is possible to use enzymatic methods to perform a site-specific controlled conjugation. This requires enzymes that react with the antibody and can induce a site- or amino acid sequence-specific modification. The most used enzymes are: sortase, transglutaminase, galactosyltransferase, and syaliltransferase. Sortase A from *Staphylococcus aureus* binds the LPXTG sequence and breaks the bond between glycine and threonine linking an oligoglycine (oligo-G) that can be used to bind the desired payload. A transglutaminase derived from *Streptomyces mobaraensis* catalyzes transpeptidation and recognizes an LLQG motif that has been inserted into a genetically engineered antibody, giving rise to a convenient site-specific ADC conjugation site. An application of a transglutaminase conjugation method gave rise to improvements in DAR for ADCs constructed with a branched linker that allowed for the loading of multiple payload molecules. Anami and coworkers developed an innovative conjugation method utilizing a branched linker on an anti-HER2 monoclonal antibody with MTGase, without a reduction in antibody binding affinity leading to the production of a homogeneous ADC molecular population with a remarkable increased DAR (up to 8) using monomethyl auristatin F as the payload [80].

The linkers used contain a lysine scaffold to generate a branch point and PEG spacers to increase ADC mobility. For MTGase-mediated antibody-linker conjugation, the presence of a primary amine is necessary as well as the presence of two reactive azide groups to link with the payloads [46]. Using MTGase this azide-linker can be bound to the glutamine residue Q295 in the IgG heavy chain. To generate an ADCs with DAR 2 the chosen payloads can be bound through azide-alkyne cyclization using a linear or branched linker to generate a DAR 4 ADC. This improved ADC showed increased *in vitro* cytotoxicity against HER2-expressing breast cancer cell lines compared to ADCs produced by more traditional methods [46].

An *N*-Glycan engineering strategy takes advantage of conserved Asn297 (N297) within the Fc domain in all IgG classes. In order to create a reactive aldehyde group on the *N*-glycan terminus it is possible to employ either β-1,4-galactosyltransferase (GalT) or α-2,6-sialyltransferase (SialT) enzymes to achieve this. The aldehyde groups enzymatically created are then used to conjugate amino-oxy-functionalized payloads [80]. Recently Bruins and coworkers used a mushroom tyrosinase to oxidize the exposed tyrosine residues on antibody to generate a 1,2-quinone, which can then be subjected to a nucleophilic reaction with thiols or amines from the side chains of amino acids such as cysteine, lysine, histidine, or any thus modified payload [81]. A further new recent strategy to improve ADC stability is site-specific conjugations using antibody engineered to incorporate non-natural amino acids (nnAA). The introduction of nnAA with orthogonal reactive functional groups (aldehyde, ketone, azido, or alkynyl tag) increases the homogeneity of ADCs and enables novel bioorthogonal chemistry that utilizes reactive groups that are different from the classical thiol or amine reactions. The most used nnAA or strategies are: seleno-cysteine, p-azidomethyl-L-phenylalanine (pAMF) p-acetyl phenylalanine (p-AcPhe), FGE (formylglycine generating enzyme) azide or alkynyl nnAA or glycan. To improve ADC stability, Transtuzumab was engineered to introduce p-AcPhe that could react through the carbonyl group (ketone) with a drug containing an alkoxy-amine to produce an oxime [82]. To achieve this, engineered new cell lines or cell free protein expression systems (OCFS: Open Cell Free Synthesis) were generated that possess the transcriptional machinery capable of inserting the a nnAA exactly where desired. In this system, the most important element needed for nnAA incorporation is a aminoacyl tRNA synthetase (aaRS) that charges a specific tRNA with the nnAA [83,84].

5. Approved ADCs and Future Perspectives

The ADC gemtuzumab ozogamicin, also known with the commercial name of Mylotarg® produced by Pfizer Inc., was the first ADC approved twenty years ago by the U.S. Food and Drug Administration (FDA). Mylotarg® was used to target the CD33 (Cluster of differentiation 33, sialic acid binding Ig-like lectin 3 (Siglec3)).

myeloid associated leukocyte differentiation antigen expressed by myeloid leukemia cells (CD33[+] AML). Currently, Mylotarg® is indicated for the treatment of patients diagnosed since at least two years with recurrent or refractory CD33[+] AML [85].

The Mylotarg® ADC was produced using a random conjugation technique with an amide bond interposed between the cleavable linker, hydrazone acetyl butyrate with the antibody attached to the calicheamicin payload via a lysine sidechain on the antibody [86]. The history of its approval has been complicated due to unexpected toxicities, in particular veno occlusive disease (VOD) in the liver in a significant proportion of patients. Myelotarg was initially approved by the FDA in the USA in 2000 but then voluntarily withdrawn from the market in 2011 following toxicity-related deaths and a lack of good clinical evidence showing its therapeutic benefits. Subsequently however, lower dose studies have demonstrated its safety and have clearly shown it to be of clinical benefit in a subset of AML patients [87].

In 2017, Myelotarg was once again approved by the FDA [88] and immediately following this approval another calicheamicin-based ADC using the same linker technology (linker-antibody bond and cytotoxin, bystander effect) inotuzumab ozogamicin (also known as Besponsa®) directed against the B-cell restricted differentiation antigen CD22 [89]. Besponsa®, was approved for use in the EU for the treatment of acute lymphoblastic leukemia currently under orphan drug status [90,91].

The second US, EU, and Japan approved ADC was brentuximab vedotin (Seattle Genetics, Inc. and Takeda Pharmaceutical Company Ltd.). The commercial name for this ADC is ADCETRIS® (Seattle Genetics Inc., n.d.) and is indicated for the treatment of Hodgkin's lymphoma targeting the Reed-Sternberg cell-associated antigen, CD30. This ADC was constructed using a protease-cleavable mc-VC-PABC linker and Monomethyl auristatin E (MMAE) as the cytotoxic drug payload [92]. The chemistry of linking method to provide a bystander effect is achieved through a dithiol bond via to a cysteine residue on the antibody. Adcetris® (brentuximab vedotin) has been approved by FDA in 2011 [93].

The final and most recent approved ADC at the time of writing is trastuzumab-emtansine (Roche Registration GmbH) sold under the commercial name Kadcyla®. The Trastuzumab (commercial name Herceptin) is a monoclonal antibody used as a naked antibody to treat HER2[+] breast cancer by targeting the antigen HER-2 (Human Epidermal growth factor Receptor) and triggering host-mediated antibody dependent cellular cytotoxicity (ADCC) while simultaneously downregulating EGFR-mediated growth signaling thereby inhibiting tumor growth [94]. The ADC Kadcyla® uses a maytansinoid derivative as the anti-neoplastic drug payload (DM-1) and a non-cleavable SMCC (amide antibody-linker) as linker. This ADC shows reduced bystander effect, strongest activity compared to Herceptin in certain conditions [86] and has been approved in the US, EU and Japan since 2013 [95–97].

Over the past two years, the FDA approved two new ADCs: Polivy® (Polatuzumab vedotin) and Lumoxiti® (Moxetumomab pasudotox). The Polivy® is a humanized monoclonal antibody, directed against CD79B (an antigen expressed by Large B-Cell lymphoma). Polivy is the first commercial therapeutic ADC produced using a site-specific covalent bond conjugated to the synthetic monomethyl auristatin E (MMAE) via engineered cysteines (THIOMABs) and using a protease-cleavable peptide linker to increase the plasma stability [98].

The Lumoxiti® is the first approved recombinant ADC. It is an innovative linkerless ADC is produced by genetic fusion between the Fv fragment of an anti-CD22 monoclonal with the 38 kDa fragment (PE38) of Pseudomonas exotoxin A [99].

We can underline that all the above-described approved ADCs (except the unique recombinant linkerless ADC Lumoxiti®) were developed using conventional random conjugation methods [100]. Table 1 reports shows all the approved and marketed ADCs.

Table 1. ADCs currently approved for clinical use.

Name	Antigen Target	Type of Cancer Target	Linker Type	Status
Mylotarg® (*Gemtuzumab ozogamicin*)	CD33	Myeloid leukemia B-cell lymphoma	Cleavable linker (hydrazone acetyl butyrate)	marketed
Besponsa® (*Inotuzumab ozogamicin*)	CD22	Lymphoblastic B leukemia	Cleavable linker (hydrazone acetyl butyrate)	marketed
Adcetris® (*Brentuximab vedotin*)	CD-30	Hodgkin's lymphoma	Protease-cleavable mc-VC PABC	marketed
Kadcyla® (*Trastuzumab emtansine*)	HER-2	HER2+ Breast cancer	Non cleavable thioether linker	marketed
Polivy® (*Polatuzumab vedotin*)	CD79B	Large B Cell lymphoma	Protease-cleavable	marketed
Lumoxiti® (*Moxetumomab pasudotox*)	CD22	Refractory hairy cell leukemia	Recombinant covalently fused (linkerless)	marketed

6. Future Perspectives

The approved ADCs are mostly indicated for the treatment of hematological malignancies and, with a few exceptions, their clinical activity has largely failed for solid tumors. The reasons for these failures may be attributed to the large molecular size of the ADC molecule that shows poor penetration into the tumor mass, thus resulting in poor in vivo efficacy [11]. For this reason, other forms of reduced sized antibodies such as single chain fragments of variable regions (scFv), i.e., v regions joined by a linker peptide, have been investigated, Also in the form of heterodimers of IgG and IgE, a small divalent immunoprotein (SIP, 75 kDa) or "minibody", a homodimer stabilized by a disulfide bond to its C-terminal [13]. The most explored antibody derivative variants are the dsFv and scFv. They are made of V_h and V_L domains linked through an interchain disulfide bond (dsFv) genetically engineered and linked covalently with a hydrophilic linker to form an scFv. Due to their modular nature, they can undergo multimerization into homo and hetero oligomers (diabody, triabody, tetrabody) strengthening antigen binding affinity and diversifying the different functionalities. The sdAbs (single domain antibodies) are smaller than scFvs, comprising 15-KDa V_h, V_l, or V_{hh} domains, also termed nanobodies, and containing the antigen domain in the terminal region of the hinge. Similarly, to scFv, these nanobodies can form homodimers increasing the binding affinity for the target antigen or formed into heterodimers with bispecific properties. Bispecific antibodies can interact simultaneously with two antigens on the same target cell, a property that potentially allows for an increase in the therapeutic window while decreasing the non-specific effects on non-target cells [101]. SIP antibodies have high affinity to their antigen and their turnover occurs in the liver. The technology for producing SIP antibodies was developed by Neri et al. [79] against fibronectin and other vascular antigens. These antigens, common in tumors, are stable and accessible. In addition, SIP have two C-terminal cysteines that allows a disulfide bridge with various payloads [102]. All these small fragments of antibodies as Fab, diabody and scFv, penetrate more rapidly into solid tumors but have a reduced serum half-life and undergo rapid renal elimination. This means that they are often eliminated before adequate absorption takes place at the tumor site.

Depending on the tumor under treatment, it is necessary to adequately choose and modify the Fc portion on the antibody to have the best possible response, especially to take advantage of the effect of the ADCC combined with other mechanisms of cell killing exerted via direct antibody-mediated cell signaling [2].

In addition to the above-mentioned ADCs, there are also other constructs and strategies to attack cancer cells that involve the conjugation of toxins or chemotherapeutic drugs to ligands or proteins that are overexpressed on the target cell. The most used ligands as carriers can be proteins or peptides. Another strategy is to use peptide-drug-conjugates that are made up of small, synthetic peptides [103–108]. These molecules appear to have an even faster penetration and elimination than the small antibody fragments we have described [102].

Nanomedicine is one of the formulation-based technologies to increase bioavailability of drugs. Nanotechnology can provide new treatment options for tumors due to the great potential for selective targeting and controlled drug release. Increasingly more attention is being paid to antibodies and their fragments as targeting ligands able to bind specific receptors that are overexpressed on tumor cells [109] for the delivery of nanoparticles.

Non-targeted nanoparticles such as liposomal-based preparations [110] polymeric [111] and metallic nanoparticles [112,113] are readily available for the conjugation with antibodies and drugs, potentially opening the possibility to develop theragnostic (therapeutics and diagnostics) agents. These formulations can reduce the toxicity profiles of the payloads and improve the therapeutic widow. One example is Doxil1, which has been on the market for 20 years as a liposomal preparation of doxorubicin, and is now being improved by PEGylation [114].

Antibody conjugate nanoparticles (ACNPs) are formed from a combination of ADC and nanotechnologies. ACNPs similarly to ADCs use antibodies to specifically target cancer cells for the delivery of encapsulated drugs.

Many ACNPs have been tested in clinical trials, but to date none has yet reached phase III trials [115].

In recent years, great progress has been made in developing effective nanoparticle-based drug targeting using conjugated antibodies. In addition, the use of antibody fragments combined with advances in molecular design are overcoming some of the problems associated with the large molecular size of unmodified antibodies [109].

With the adoption of strategies that improve the ability of ACNP to reach the tumor site to facilitate active targeting together with additional studies that are still needed to define and refine conjugation technology, size, shape and surface charge of nanoparticles will likely lead in the future to useful outcomes for these targeting reagents.

7. Conclusions

More than 80 ADCs are currently under investigation and are in various stages of clinical development for cancer treatment [116]. Current evidence indicates that the field of ADCs is a very promising one, even though in past years they have faced a number of clinical failures. Recent advances in technology now provide all of the necessary elements required for the facile production of humanized monoclonal antibodies, site-specific conjugation protocols, various potent cytotoxic payloads with different mechanisms of action, adaptable linker technologies, together with advanced analytic techniques [117]. With the availability of the new technologies and biomarker selection strategies, ADCs are set to represent an important contribution to the future of immuno-oncology.

Author Contributions: Conceptualization, F.G. and R.I.; Methodology, G.S. and S.I.; Software, S.P.; Validation, F.G., R.I.; Resources, S.P., R.G. and G.D.V.; Data Curation, S.P., G.P., E.C., M.A., R.G.; Writing-Original Draft Preparation, S.P., G.D.V., F.G., D.J.F. and R.I.; Writing-Review & Editing, A.M.C., G.S., S.I., D.J.F. and R.I.; Supervision, F.G., D.J.F. and R.I.; Project Administration, R.I., and S.I.; Funding Acquisition, R.I., G.S. and S.I. All authors have read and agreed to the published version of the manuscript.

References

1. Strebhardt, K.; Ullrich, A. Paul Ehrlich's magic bullet concept: 100 years of progress. *Nat. Rev. Cancer* **2008**, *8*, 473–480. [CrossRef] [PubMed]
2. Hoffmann, R.M.; Coumbe, B.G.T.; Josephs, D.H.; Mele, S.; Ilieva, K.M.; Cheung, A.; Tutt, A.N.; Spicer, J.F.; Thurston, D.E.; Crescioli, S.; et al. Antibody structure and engineering considerations for the design and function of Antibody Drug Conjugates (ADCs). *OncoImmunology* **2018**, *7*, e1395127. [CrossRef] [PubMed]
3. Sochaj, A.M.; Świderska, K.W.; Otlewski, J. Current methods for the synthesis of homogeneous antibody-drug conjugates. *Biotechnol. Adv.* **2015**, *33*, 775–784. [CrossRef] [PubMed]
4. Giansanti, F.; Flavell, D.J.; Angelucci, F.; Fabbrini, M.S.; Ippoliti, R. Strategies to Improve the Clinical Utility of Saporin-Based Targeted Toxins. *Toxins (Basel)* **2018**, *10*, 82. [CrossRef] [PubMed]
5. Panowski, S.; Bhakta, S.; Raab, H.; Polakis, P.; Junutula, J.R. Site-specific antibody drug conjugates for cancer therphy. *mAbs* **2014**, *6*, 34–45. [CrossRef] [PubMed]
6. Singh, S.K.; Luisi, D.L.; Pak, R.H. Antibody-Drug Conjugates: Design, Formulation and Physicochemical Stability. *Pharm. Res.* **2015**, *32*, 3541–3571. [CrossRef]
7. Zhou, Q. Site-specific conjugation for ADC and beyond. *Biomedicines* **2017**, *5*, 64. [CrossRef]
8. Khongorzul, P.; Ling, C.J.; Khan, F.U.; Ihsan, A.U.; Zhang, J. Antibody-Drug Conjugates: A Comprehensive Review. *Mol. Cancer Res.* **2020**, *18*, 3–19. [CrossRef]
9. Chari, R.V.J.; Miller, M.L.; Widdison, W.C. Antibody-drug conjugates: An emerging concept in cancer therapy. *Angew. Chem. Int. Ed. Engl.* **2014**, *53*, 3796–3827. [CrossRef]
10. Weidle, U.H.; Maisel, D.; Klostermann, S.; Schiller, C.; Weiss, E.H. Intracellular proteins displayed on the surface of tumor cells as targets for therapeutic intervention with antibody-related agents. *Cancer Genom. Proteom.* **2011**, *8*, 49–63.
11. Gauzy-Lazo, L.; Sassoon, I.; Brun, M.P. Advances in Antibody-Drug Conjugate Design: Current Clinical Landscape and Future Innovations. *Slas Discov.* **2020**, *20*, 2472555220912955. [CrossRef] [PubMed]
12. Brüggemann, M.; Osborn, M.J.; Ma, B.; Hayre, J.; Avis, S.; Lundstrom, B.; Buelow, R. Human antibody production in transgenic animals. *Arch. Immunol. Exp. (Warsz)* **2015**, *63*, 101–108. [CrossRef] [PubMed]
13. Aguiar, S.; Dias, J.; Manuel, A.M.; Russo, R.; Gois, P.M.P.; da Silva, F.A.; Goncalves, J. Chimeric Small Antibody Fragments as Strategy to Deliver Therapeutic Payloads. *Adv. Protein Chem. Struct. Biol.* **2018**, 143–182. [CrossRef]
14. Sala, G.; Rapposelli, I.G.; Ghasemi, R.; Piccolo, E.; Traini, S.; Capone, E.; Rossi, C.; Pelliccia, A.; Di Risio, A.; D'Egidio, M.; et al. EV20, a NovelAnti-ErbB-3 Humanized Antibody, Promotes ErbB-3 Down-Regulation and Inhibits Tumor Growth In Vivo. *Transl. Oncol.* **2013**, *6*, 676–684. [CrossRef]
15. Prasetyanti, P.R.; Capone, E.; Barcaroli, D.; D'Agostino, D.; Volpe, S.; Benfante, A.; van Hooff, S.; Iacobelli, V.; Rossi, C.; Iacobelli, S.; et al. ErbB-3 activation by NRG-1β sustains growth and promotes vemurafenib resistance in BRAF-V600E colon cancer stem cells (CSCs). *Oncotarget* **2015**, *6*, 16902–16911. [CrossRef]
16. Ghasemi, R.; Rapposelli, I.G.; Capone, E.; Rossi, C.; Lattanzio, R.; Piantelli, M.; Sala, G.; Iacobelli, S. Dual targeting of ErbB-2/ErbB-3 results in enhanced antitumor activity in preclinical models of pancreatic cancer. *Oncogenesis* **2014**, *3*, e117. [CrossRef]
17. Conner, S.D.; Schmid, S.L. Regulated portals of entry into the cell. *Nature* **2003**, *422*, 37–44. [CrossRef]
18. Kalim, M.; Chen, J.; Wang, S.; Lin, C.; Ullah, S.; Liang, K.; Ding, Q.; Chen, S.; Zhan, J. Intracellular trafficking of new anticancer therapeutics: Antibody-drug conjugates. *Drug Des. Devel.* **2017**, *11*, 2265–2276. [CrossRef]
19. Rusten, T.E.; Vaccari, T.; Stenmark, H. Shaping development with ESCRTs. *Nat. Cell Biol.* **2011**, *14*, 38–45. [CrossRef]
20. Capone, E.; Giansanti, F.; Ponziani, S.; Lamolinara, A.; Iezzi, M.; Cimini, A.; Angelucci, F.; Sorda, R.; Laurenzi, V.; Natali, P.G.; et al. EV20-Sap, a novel anti-HER-3 antibody-drug conjugate, displays promising antitumor activity in melanoma. *Oncotarget* **2017**, *8*, 95412–95424. [CrossRef]
21. Capone, E.; Lamolinara, A.; D'Agostino, D.; Rossi, C.; De Laurenzi, V.; Iezzi, M.; Sala, G.; Iacobelli, S. EV20-mediated delivery of cytotoxic auristatin MMAF exhibits potent therapeutic efficacy in cutaneous melanoma. *J. Control Release* **2018**, *277*, 48–56. [CrossRef] [PubMed]
22. Staudacher, A.H.; Brown, M.P. Antibody drug conjugates and bystander killing: Isantigen-dependent internalisation required? *Br. J. Cancer* **2017**, *117*, 1736–1742. [CrossRef] [PubMed]

23. Dal Corso, A.; Gebleux, R.; Murer, P.; Soltermann, A.; Neri, V. A non-internalizing antibody-drug conjugate based on an anthracycline payload displays potent therapeutic activity in Vivo. *J. Control. Release* **2017**, *264*, 211–218. [CrossRef] [PubMed]

24. Mohamed, M.M.; Sloane, B.F. Cysteine cathepsins: Multifunctional enzymes in cancer. *Nat. Rev. Cancer* **2006**, *6*, 764–775. [CrossRef]

25. Lewis Phillips, G.D.; Li, G.; Dugger, D.L.; Crocker, L.M.; Parsons, K.L.; Mai, E.; Blättler, W.A.; Lambert, J.M.; Chari, R.V.; Lutz, R.J.; et al. Targeting HER2-positive breastcancer with trastuzumab-DM1, an antibody-cytotoxic drug conjugate. *Cancer Res.* **2008**, *68*, 9280–9290. [CrossRef]

26. Dorywalska, M.; Strop, P.; Melton-Witt, J.A.A.; Hasa-Moreno, A.; Farias, S.E.; Galindo Casas, M.; Delaria, K.; Lui, V.; Poulsen, K.; Loo, C.; et al. Effect of attachment site on stability of cleavable antibody drug conjugates. *Bioconjug. Chem.* **2015**, *26*, 650–659. [CrossRef]

27. Lu, J.; Jiang, F.; Lu, A.; Zhang, G. Linkers Having a Crucial Role in Antibody-Drug Conjugates. *Int. J. Mol. Sci.* **2016**, *17*, 561. [CrossRef]

28. Chari, R.V. Targeted cancer therapy: Conferring specificity to cytotoxic drugs. *Acc. Chem. Res.* **2008**, *41*, 98–107. [CrossRef]

29. Dorywalska, M.; Strop, P.; Melton-Witt, J.A.; Hasa-Moreno, A.; Farias, S.E.; Galindo Casas, M.; Delaria, K.; Lui, V.; Poulsen, K.; Sutton, J.; et al. Site-Dependent Degradation of a Non-Cleavable Auristatin-Based Linker-Payload in Rodent Plasma and Its Effect on ADC Efficacy. *PLoS ONE* **2015**, *10*, e0132282. [CrossRef]

30. Pillow, T.H.; Sadowsky, J.D.; Zhang, D.; Yu, S.F.; Del Rosario, G.; Xu, K.; He, J.; Bhakta, S.; Ohri, R.; Kozak, K.R.; et al. Decoupling stability and release in disulfide bonds with antibody-small molecule conjugates. *Chem. Sci.* **2017**, *8*, 366–370. [CrossRef]

31. Wu, B.; Zhang, G.; Shuang, S.; Choi, M.M. Biosensors for determination of glucose with glucose oxidase immobilized on an eggshell membrane. *Talanta* **2004**, *64*, 546–553. [CrossRef] [PubMed]

32. Chari, R.V.; Martell, B.A.; Gross, J.L.; Cook, S.B.; Shah, S.A.; Blättler, W.A.; McKenzie, S.J.; Goldmacher, V.S. Immunoconjugates containing novel maytansinoids: Promisinganticancer drugs. *Cancer Res.* **1992**, *52*, 127–131. [PubMed]

33. Saito, G.; Swanson, J.A.; Lee, K.D. Drug delivery strategy utilizing conjugation viareversible disulfide linkages: Role and site of cellular reducing activities. *Adv. Drug Deliv. Rev.* **2003**, *55*, 199–215. [CrossRef]

34. Giansanti, F.; Capone, E.; Ponziani, S.; Piccolo, E.; Gentile, R.; Lamolinara, A.; Di Campli, A.; Sallese, M.; Iacobelli, V.; Cimini, A.; et al. Secreted Gal-3BP is a novel promising target for non-internalizing Antibody-Drug Conjugates. *J. Control. Release* **2018**, *294*, 176–184. [CrossRef]

35. Bargh, J.; Isidro-Llobet, A.; Parker, J.; Spring, D. Cleavable linkers in antibody–drug conjugates. *Chem. Soc. Rev.* **2019**, *48*, 4361–4374. [CrossRef]

36. Dubowchik, G.M.; Mosure, K.; Knipe, J.O.; Firestone, R.A. Cathepsin B-sensitive dipeptide prodrugs. 2. Models of anticancer drugs paclitaxel (Taxol), mitomycin C and doxorubicin. *Bioorganic. Med. Chem. Lett.* **1998**, *8*, 3347–3352. [CrossRef]

37. Doronina, S.O.; Toki, B.E.; Torgov, M.Y.; Mendelsohn, B.A.; Cerveny, C.G.; Chace, D.F.; DeBlanc, R.L.; Gearing, R.P.; Bovee, T.D.; Siegall, C.B.; et al. Development of potent monoclonal antibody auristatin conjugates for cancer therapy. *Nat. Biotechnol.* **2003**, *21*, 778–784. [CrossRef]

38. Jain, N.; Smith, S.W.; Ghone, S.; Tomczuk, B. Current ADC Linker Chemistry. *Pharm. Res.* **2015**, *32*, 3526–3540. [CrossRef]

39. Dubowchik, G.M.; Firestone, R.A.; Padilla, L.; Willner, D.; Hofstead, S.J.; Mosure, K.; Knipe, J.O.; Lasch, S.J.; Trail, P.A. Cathepsin B-labile dipeptide linkers for lysosomal release of doxorubicin from internalizing immunoconjugates: Model studies of enzymatic drug release and antigen-specific in vitro anticancer activity. *Bioconjug. Chem.* **2002**, *13*, 855–869. [CrossRef]

40. Caculitan, N.G.; Dela, C.; Chuh, J.; Ma, Y.; Zhang, D.; Kozak, K.R.; Liu, Y.; Pillow, T.H.; Sadowsky, J.; Cheung, T.K.; et al. Cathepsin B Is Dispensable for Cellular Processing of Cathepsin B-Cleavable Antibody-Drug Conjugates. *Cancer Res.* **2017**, *77*, 7027–7037. [CrossRef]

41. Laguzza, B.C.; Nichols, C.L.; Briggs, S.L.; Cullinan, G.J.; Johnson, D.A.; Starling, J.J.; Baker, A.L.; Bumol, T.F.; Corvalan, J.R. New antitumor monoclonal antibody-vinca conjugates LY203725 and related compounds: Design, preparation, and representative in vivo activity. *J. Med. Chem.* **1989**, *32*, 548–555. [CrossRef] [PubMed]

42. Govindan, S.V.; Cardillo, T.M.; Sharkey, R.M.; Tat, F.; Gold, D.V.; Goldenberg, D.M. Milatuzumab-SN-38 conjugates for the treatment of CD74+ cancers. *Mol. Cancer* **2013**, *12*, 968–978. [CrossRef] [PubMed]

43. Tranoy-Opalinski, I.; Legigan, T.; Barat, R.; Clarhaut, J.; Thomas, M.; Renoux, B.; Papot, S. β-Glucuronidase-responsive prodrugs for selective cancer chemotherapy: An update. *Eur. J. Med. Chem.* **2014**, *74*, 302–313. [CrossRef] [PubMed]

44. Lyon, R.P.; Bovee, T.D.; Doronina, S.O.; Burke, P.J.; Hunter, J.H.; Neff-LaFord, H.D.; Jonas, M.; Anderson, M.E.; Setter, J.R.; Senter, P.D. Reducing hydrophobicity of homogeneous antibody-drug conjugates improves pharmacokinetics and therapeutic index. *Nat. Biotechnol.* **2015**, *33*, 733–735. [CrossRef]

45. Kolodych, S.; Michel, C.; Delacroix, S.; Koniev, O.; Ehkirch, A.; Eberova, J.; Cianférani, S.; Renoux, B.; Krezel, W.; Poinot, P.; et al. Development and evaluation of β-galactosidase-sensitive antibody-drug conjugates. *Eur. J. Med. Chem.* **2017**, *142*, 376–382. [CrossRef]

46. Lambert, J.M.; Chari, R.V. Ado-trastuzumab Emtansine (T-DM1): An antibody-drug conjugate (ADC) for HER2-positive breast cancer. *J. Med. Chem.* **2014**, *57*, 6949–6964. [CrossRef]

47. Kovtun, Y.V.; Audette, C.A.; Ye, Y.; Xie, H.; Ruberti, M.F.; Phinney, S.J.; Leece, B.A.; Chittenden, T.; Blättler, W.A.; Goldmacher, V.S. Antibody-drug conjugates designed toeradicate tumors with homogeneous and heterogeneous expression of the targetantigen. *Cancer Res.* **2006**, *66*, 3214–3221. [CrossRef]

48. Oflazoglu, E.; Stone, I.J.; Gordon, K.; Wood, C.G.; Repasky, E.A.; Grewal, I.S.; Law, C.L.; Gerber, H.P. Potent anticarcinoma activity of the humanized anti-CD70 antibody h1F6 conjugated to the tubulin inhibitor auristatin via an uncleavable linker. *Clin. Cancer Res.* **2008**, *14*, 6171–6180. [CrossRef]

49. Polson, A.G.; Calemine-Fenaux, J.; Chan, P.; Chang, W.; Christensen, E.; Clark, S.; de Sauvage, F.J.; Eaton, D.; Elkins, K.; Elliott, J.M.; et al. Antibody-drug conjugates for the treatment of non-Hodgkin's lymphoma: Target and linker-drug selection. *Cancer Res.* **2009**, *69*, 2358–2364. [CrossRef]

50. Sau, S.; Alsaab, H.O.; Kashaw, S.K.; Tatiparti, K.; Iyer, A.K. Advances in antibody-drugconjugates: A new era of targeted cancer therapy. *Drug Discov. Today* **2017**, *22*, 1547–1556. [CrossRef]

51. Doronina, S.O.; Mendelsohn, B.A.; Bovee, T.D.; Cerveny, C.G.; Alley, S.C.; Meyer, D.L.; Oflazoglu, E.; Toki, B.E.; Sanderson, R.J.; Zabinski, R.F.; et al. Enhanced activity of monomethylauristatin F through monoclonal antibody delivery: Effects of linker technology on efficacy and toxicity. *Bioconjug. Chem.* **2006**, *17*, 114–124. [CrossRef]

52. Lencer, W.I.; Blumberg, R.S. A passionate kiss, then run: Exocytosis and recycling of IgG by FcRn. *Trends Cell Biol.* **2005**, *15*, 5–9. [CrossRef]

53. Chen, H.; Lin, Z.; Arnst, K.E.; Miller, D.D.; Li, W. Tubulin inhibitor-based antibody-drug conjugates for cancer therapy. *Molecules* **2017**, *22*, 1281. [CrossRef]

54. Anderl, J.; Faulstich, H.; Hechler, T.; Kulke, M. Antibody–Drug Conjugate Payloads. *Methods Mol. Biol.* **2013**, *1045*, 51–70. [CrossRef]

55. Zakacs, G.; Paterson, J.K.; Ludwig, J.A.; Booth-Genthe, C.; Gottesman, M.M. Targeting multidrug resistance in cancer. *Nat. Rev. Drug Discov.* **2006**, *5*, 219–234. [CrossRef] [PubMed]

56. Leung, D.; Wurst, J.M.; Liu, T.; Martinez, R.M.; Datta-Mannan, A.; Feng, Y. Antibody Conjugates-Recent Advances and Future Innovations. *Antibodies (Basel)* **2020**, *9*, 2. [CrossRef] [PubMed]

57. Kaur, G.; Hollingshead, M.; Holbeck, S.; Schauer-Vukasinovic, V.; Camalier, R.F.; Domling, A.; Agarwal, S. Biological evaluation of tubulysin A: A potential anticancer and antiangiogenic natural product. *Biochem. J.* **2006**, *396*, 235–242. [CrossRef] [PubMed]

58. Prota, A.E.; Bargsten, K.; Diaz, J.F.; Marsh, M.; Cuevas, C.; Liniger, M.; Steinmetz, M.O. A new tubulin-binding site and pharmacophore for microtubule destabilizing anticancer drugs. *Proc. Natl. Acad. Sci. USA* **2014**, *111*, 13817–13821. [CrossRef] [PubMed]

59. Dumontet, C.; Jordan, M.A. Microtubule-binding agents: A dynamic field of cancer therapeutics. *Nat. Rev. Drug Discov.* **2010**, *99*, 790–803. [CrossRef]

60. Kastenhuber, E.R.; Lowe, S.W. Putting p53 in Context. *Cell* **2017**, *170*, 1062–1078. [CrossRef]

61. Yaghoubi, S.; Karimi, M.H.; Lotfinia, M.; Gharibi, T.; Mahi-Birjand, M.; Kavi, E.; Hosseini, F.; Sineh Sepehr, K.; Khatami, M.; Bagheri, N.; et al. Potential drugs used in the antibody-drug conjugate (ADC) architecture for cancer therapy. *J. Cell. Physiol.* **2020**, *235*, 31–64. [CrossRef]

62. Antonow, D.; Thurston, D.E. Synthesis of DNA-interactive pyrrolo[2,1-c][1,4]benzodiazepines (PBDs). *Chem. Rev.* **2011**, *111*, 2815–2864. [CrossRef]

63. Tietze, L.F.; Schmuck, K. Prodrugs for targeted tumor therapies: Recent developments in ADEPT, GDEPT and PMT. *Curr. Pharm. Des.* **2011**, *17*, 3527–3547. [CrossRef]

64. Dokter, W.; Ubink, R.; van der Lee, M.; van der Vleuten, M.; van Achterberg, T.; Jacobs, D.; Loosveld, E.; van den Dobbelsteen, D.; Egging, D.; Mattaar, E.; et al. Preclinical profile of theHER2-targeting ADC SYD983/SYD985: Introduction of a new duocarmycin-basedlinker-drug platform. *Mol. Cancer* **2014**, *13*, 2618–2629. [CrossRef]

65. Rinnerthaler, G.; Gampenrieder, S.P.; Greil, R. HER2 Directed Antibody-Drug-Conjugates beyond T-DM1 in Breast Cancer. *Int. J. Mol. Sci.* **2019**, *20*, 1115. [CrossRef]

66. Gebleux, R.; Casi, G. Antibody-drug conjugates: Current status and future perspectives. *Pharm. Ther.* **2016**, *167*, 48–59. [CrossRef]

67. Adams, D.J.; Dewhirst, M.W.; Flowers, J.L.; Gamcsik, M.P.; Colvin, O.M.; Manikumar, G.; Wani, M.C.; Wall, M.E. Camptothecin analogues with enhanced antitumor activity at acidic pH. *Cancer Chemother. Pharm.* **2000**, *46*, 263–271. [CrossRef]

68. Starodub, A.N.; Ocean, A.J.; Shah, M.A.; Guarino, M.J.; Picozzi, V.J.; Vahdat, L.T.; Thomas, S.S.; Govindan, S.V.; Maliakal, P.P.; Wegener, W.A. First-in-human trial of a novel anti-trop-2 antibody-SN-38 conjugate, sacituzumab govitecan, for the treatment of diverse metastatic solid tumors. *Clin. Cancer Res.* **2015**, *21*, 3870–3878. [CrossRef]

69. Yu, Q.; Ding, J. Precision cancer medicine: Where to target? *Acta Pharmacol. Sin.* **2015**, *36*, 1161–1162. [CrossRef]

70. Chowdari, N.S.; Pan, C.; Rao, C.; Langley, D.R.; Sivaprakasam, P.; Sufi, B.; Derwin, D.; Wang, Y.; Kwok, E.; Passmore, D.; et al. Uncialamycin as a novel payload for antibody drug conjugate (ADC) based targeted cancer therapy. *Bioorganic. Med. Chem. Lett.* **2019**, *29*, 466–470. [CrossRef]

71. Kim, E.G.; Kim, K.M. Strategies and advancement in antibody- drug conjugate optimization for targeted cancer therapeutics. *Biomol. Ther. (Seoul)* **2015**, *23*, 493–509. [CrossRef]

72. Hennessy, E.J. Selective inhibitors of Bcl-2 and Bcl-xL: Balancing antitumor activity with on-target toxicity. *Bioorganic. Med. Chem. Lett.* **2016**, *26*, 2105–2114. [CrossRef] [PubMed]

73. Hallen, H.E.; Luo, H.; Scott-Craig, J.S.; Walton, J.D. Gene family encoding the major toxins of lethal Amanita mushrooms. *Proc. Natl. Acad. Sci. USA* **2007**, *104*, 19097–19101. [CrossRef] [PubMed]

74. Danielczyk, A.; Stahn, R.; Faulstich, D.; Löffler, A.; Märten, A.; Karsten, U.; Goletz, S. PankoMab: A potent new generation anti-tumour MUC1 antibody. *Cancer Immunol. Immunother. CII* **2006**, *55*, 1337–1347. [CrossRef] [PubMed]

75. Kaplan, G.; Mazor, R.; Lee, F.; Jang, Y.; Leshem, Y.; Pastan, I. Improving the In Vivo Efficacy of an Anti-Tac (CD25) Immunotoxin by Pseudomonas Exotoxin A Domain II Engineering. *Mol. Cancer Ther.* **2018**, *17*, 1486–1493. [CrossRef]

76. Kaplan, G.; Lee, F.; Onda, M.; Kolyvas, E.; Bhardwaj, G.; Baker, D.; Pastan, I. Protection of the Furin Cleavage Site in Low-Toxicity Immunotoxins Based on Pseudomonas Exotoxin A. *Toxins* **2016**, *8*, 217. [CrossRef] [PubMed]

77. Tsuchikama, K.; An, Z. Antibody-drug conjugates: Recent advances in conjugation and linker chemistries. *Protein Cell* **2018**, *9*, 33–46. [CrossRef]

78. Liu, H.; May, K. Disulfide bond structures of IgG molecules: Structural variations, chemical modifications and possible impacts to stability and biological function. *mABs* **2012**, *4*, 17–23. [CrossRef]

79. Gébleux, R.; Wulhfard, S.; Casi, G.; Neri, D. Antibody Format and Drug Release RateDetermine the Therapeutic Activity of Noninternalizing Antibody-Drug Conjugates. *Mol. Cancer Ther.* **2015**, *14*, 2606–2612. [CrossRef]

80. Anami, Y.; Xiong, W.; Gui, X.; Deng, M.; Zhang, C.C.; Zhang, N.; An, Z.; Tsuchikama, K. Enzymatic conjugation using branched linkers for constructing homogeneous antibody-drug conjugates with high potency. *Org. Biomol. Chem.* **2017**, *15*, 5635–5642. [CrossRef]

81. Bruins, J.J.; Westphal, A.H.; Albada, B.; Wagner, K.; Bartels, L.; Spits, H.; van Berkel, W.J.H.; van Delft, F.L. Inducible, Site-Specific Protein Labeling by Tyrosine Oxidation-Strain-Promoted (4 + 2) Cycloaddition. *Bioconjug. Chem.* **2017**, *28*, 1189–1193. [CrossRef]

82. Axup, J.Y.; Bajjuri, K.M.; Ritland, M.; Hutchins, B.M.; Kim, C.H.; Kazane, S.A. Synthesis of site-specific antibody-drug conjugates using unnatural amino acids. *Proc. Natl. Acad. Sci. USA* **2012**, *109*, 16101–16106. [CrossRef] [PubMed]

83. Tian, F.; Lu, Y.; Manibusan, A.; Sellers, A.; Tran, H.; Sun, Y.; Phuong, T.; Barnett, R.; Hehli, B. A general approach to site-specific antibody drug conjugates. *Proc. Natl. Acad. Sci. USA* **2014**, *111*, 1766–1771. [CrossRef] [PubMed]

84. Zimmerman, E.S.; Heibeck, T.H.; Gill, A.; Li, X.; Murray, C.J.; Madlansacay, M.R.; Tran, C.; Uter, N.T.; Yin, G.; Rivers, P.J.; et al. Production of site-specific antibody-drug conjugates using optimized non-natural amino acids in a cell-free expression system. *Bioconjug. Chem.* **2014**, *25*, 351–361. [CrossRef]

85. Norsworthy, K.J.; Ko, C.W.; Lee, J.E.; Liu, J.; John, C.S.; Przepiorka, D.; Farrell, A.T.; Pazdur, R. FDA Approval Summary: Mylotarg for Treatment of Patients with Relapsed orRefractory CD33-Positive Acute Myeloid Leukemia. *Oncologist* **2018**, *23*, 1103–1108. [CrossRef] [PubMed]

86. Ricart, A.D. Antibody-drug conjugates of calicheamicin derivative: Gemtuzumab ozogamicin and inotuzumab ozogamicin. *Clin. Cancer Res.* **2011**, *17*, 6417–6427. [CrossRef] [PubMed]

87. Tanimoto, T.; Tsubokura, M.; Mori, J.; Pietrek, M.; Ono, S.; Kami, M. Differences in drugapproval processes of 3 regulatory agencies: A case study of gemtuzumabozogamicin. *Invest. New Drugs* **2013**, *31*, 473–478. [CrossRef]

88. FDA. FDA Approves Mylotarg for Treatment of Acute Myeloid leukemia [WWW]. 2017. Available online: https://www.fda.gov/newsevents/newsroom/pressannouncements/ucm574507.htm (accessed on 1 September 2017).

89. FDA. FDA Approves New Treatment for Adults with Relapsed or Refractory Acute Lymphoblastic Leukemia [WWW]. 2017. Available online: https://www.fda.gov/newsevents/newsroom/pressannouncements/ucm572131.htm (accessed on 17 August 2017).

90. EMA Besponsa. Inotuzumab ozogamicin [WWW]. 2017. Available online: http://www.ema.europa.eu/ema/index.jsp?curl=pages/medicines/human/medicines/004119/human_med_002109.jsp&mid=WC0b01ac058001d124 (accessed on 28 June 2017).

91. Lamb, Y.N. Inotuzumab Ozogamicin: First Global Approval. *Drugs* **2017**, *77*, 1603–1610. [CrossRef]

92. Moek, K.L.; de Groot, D.J.A.; de Vries, E.G.E.; Fehrmann, R.S.N. The antibody-drug conjugate target landscape across a broad range of tumour types. *Ann. Oncol.* **2017**, *28*, 3083–3091. [CrossRef]

93. Dan, N.; Setua, S.; Kashyap, V.K.; Khan, S.; Jaggi, M.; Yallapu, M.M.; Chauhan, S.C. Antibody-Drug Conjugates for Cancer Therapy: Chemistry to Clinical Implications. *Pharmaceuticals (Basel)* **2018**, *11*, 32. [CrossRef]

94. EMA Herceptin. Trastuzumab [WWW]. 2018. Available online: http://www.ema.europa.eu/ema/index.jsp?curl=pages/medicines/human/medicines/000278/human_med_000818.jsp&mid=WC0b01ac058001d124 (accessed on 14 May 2018).

95. EMA Kadcyla. Trastuzumab Emtansine [WWW]. 2018. Available online: http://www.ema.europa.eu/ema/index.jsp?curl=pages/medicines/human/medicines/002389/human_med_001712.jsp&mid=WC0b01ac058001d124 (accessed on 14 May 2018).

96. FDA Drug Approval Package. Kadcyla (Ado-Trastuzumab Emtansine) Injection [WWW]. 2013. Available online: https://www.accessdata.fda.gov/drugsatfda_docs/nda/2013/125427Orig1s000TOC.cfm (accessed on 18 May 2018).

97. PMDA Trastuzumab emtansine. Review Report [WWW]. 2013. Available online: http://www.pmda.go.jp/files/000153735.pdf (accessed on 14 May 2018).

98. Deeks, E.D. Polatuzumab Vedotin: First Global Approval. *Drugs* **2019**, *79*, 1467–1475. [CrossRef]

99. Dhillon, S. Moxetumomab Pasudotox: First Global Approval. *Drugs* **2018**, *78*, 1763–1767. [CrossRef] [PubMed]

100. Yoder, N.C.; Bai, C.; Tavares, D.; Widdison, W.C.; Whiteman, K.R.; Wilhelm, A.; Wilhelm, S.D.; McShea, M.A.; Maloney, E.K.; Ab, O.; et al. A Case Study Comparing Heterogeneous Lysine- and Site-Specific Cysteine-Conjugated Maytansinoid Antibody-Drug Conjugates (ADCs) Illustrates the Benefits of Lysine Conjugation. *Mol. Pharm.* **2019**, *16*, 3926–3937. [CrossRef] [PubMed]

101. Goulet, D.R.; Atkins, W.M. Considerations for the Design of Antibody-Based Therapeutics. *J. Pharm. Sci.* **2020**, *109*, 74–103. [CrossRef] [PubMed]

102. Deonarain, M.P. Miniaturised 'antibody'-drug conjugates for solid tumours? *Drug Discov. Today Technol.* **2018**, *30*, 47–53. [CrossRef]

103. Cimini, A.; Mei, S.; Benedetti, E.; Laurenti, G.; Koutris, I.; Cinque, B.; Cifone, M.G.; Galzio, R.; Pitari, G.; Di Leandro, L.; et al. Distinct cellular responses induced by saporin and a transferrin-saporinconjugate in two different human glioblastoma cell lines. *J. Cell Physiol.* **2012**, *227*, 939–951. [CrossRef]

104. Della Cristina, P.; Castagna, M.; Lombardi, A.; Barison, E.; Tagliabue, G.; Ceriotti, A.; Koutris, I.; Di Leandro, L.; Giansanti, F.; Vago, R.; et al. Systematic comparison of single-chain Fvantibody-fusion toxin constructs containing Pseudomonas Exotoxin A or saporinproduced in different microbial expression systems. *Microb. Cell Fact.* **2015**, *14*, 19. [CrossRef]

105. Giansanti, F.; Di Leandro, L.; Koutris, I.; Pitari, G.; Fabbrini, M.S.; Lombardi, A.; Flavell, D.J.; Flavell, S.U.; Gianni, S.; Ippoliti, R. Engineering a switchable toxin: Thepotential use of PDZ domains in the expression, targeting and activation ofmodified saporin variants. *Protein Eng. Des. Sel.* **2010**, *23*, 61–68. [CrossRef]

106. Giansanti, F.; Sabatini, D.; Pennacchio, M.R.; Scotti, S.; Angelucci, F.; Dhez, A.C.; Antonosante, A.; Cimini, A.; Giordano, A.; Ippoliti, R. PDZ Domain in the Engineeringand Production of a Saporin Chimeric Toxin as a Tool for targeting Cancer Cells. *J. Cell Biochem.* **2015**, *116*, 1256–1266. [CrossRef]

107. Provenzano, E.A.; Posteri, R.; Giansanti, F.; Angelucci, F.; Flavell, S.U.; Flavell, D.J.; Fabbrini, M.S.; Porro, D.; Ippoliti, R.; Ceriotti, A.; et al. Optimization of construct design and fermentation strategy for the production ofbioactive ATF-SAP, a saporin based anti-tumoral uPAR-targeted chimera. *Microbcell Fact.* **2016**, *15*, 194. [CrossRef]

108. Dhez, A.C.; Benedetti, E.; Antonosante, A.; Panella, G.; Ranieri, B.; Florio, T.M.; Cristiano, L.; Angelucci, F.; Giansanti, F.; Di Leandro, L.; et al. Targeted therapy of human glioblastoma via delivery of a toxinthrough a peptide directed to cell surface nucleolin. *J. Cell Physiol.* **2018**, *233*, 4091–4105. [CrossRef]

109. Marques, A.C.; Costa, P.J.; Velho, S.; Amaral, M.H. Functionalizing nanoparticles with cancer-targeting antibodies: A comparison of strategies. *J. Control. Release* **2020**, *320*, 180–200. [CrossRef] [PubMed]

110. El Maghraby, G.M.; Arafa, M.F. Liposomes for enhanced cellular uptake of anticancer agents. *Curr. Drug Deliv.* **2020**. [CrossRef] [PubMed]

111. Sun, H.; Erdman, W.; Yuan, Y.; Mohamed, M.A.; Xie, R.; Gong, S.; Cheng, C. Crosslinked polymer nanocapsules for therapeutic, diagnostic, and theranostic applications. *Wiley Interdiscip. Rev. Nanomed. Nanobiotechnol.* **2020**, e1653. [CrossRef] [PubMed]

112. Jindal, M.; Nagpal, M.; Singh, M.; Aggarwal, G.; Dhingra, G.A. Gold Nanoparticles- Boon in Cancer Theranostics. *Curr. Pharm. Des.* **2020**. [CrossRef]

113. Ardini, M.; Huang, J.; Sánchez, C.S.; Mousavi, M.Z.; Caprettini, V.; Maccaferri, N.; Melle, G.; Bruno, G.; Pasquale, L.; Garoli, D.; et al. Live Intracellular Biorthogonal Imaging by Surface Enhanced Raman Spectroscopy using Alkyne-Silver Nanoparticles Clusters. *Sci. Rep.* **2018**, *8*, 1265.

114. Wang, H.; Zheng, M.; Gao, J.; Wang, J.; Zhang, Q.; Fawcett, J.P.; He, Y.; Gu, J. Uptake and release profiles of PEGylated liposomal doxorubicin nanoparticles: A comprehensive picture based on separate determination of encapsulated and total drug concentrations in tissues of tumor-bearing mice. *Talanta* **2020**, *208*, 120358. [CrossRef]

115. Johnston, M.C.; Scott, C.J. Antibody conjugated nanoparticles as a novel form of antibody drug conjugate chemotherapy. *Drug Discov. Today Technol.* **2018**, *30*, 63–69. [CrossRef]

116. Coats, S.; Williams, M.; Kebble, B.; Dixit, R.; Tseng, L.; Yao, N.S.; Tice, D.A.; Soria, J.C. Antibody-Drug Conjugates: Future Directions in Clinical and Translational Strategies to Improve the Therapeutic Index. *Clin. Cancer Res.* **2019**, *12*. [CrossRef]

117. Drake, P.M.; Rabuka, D. Recent Developments in ADC Technology: Preclinical Studies Signal Future Clinical Trends. *Bio. Drugs* **2017**, *31*, 521–531. [CrossRef]

Permissions

All chapters in this book were first published by MDPI; hereby published with permission under the Creative Commons Attribution License or equivalent. Every chapter published in this book has been scrutinized by our experts. Their significance has been extensively debated. The topics covered herein carry significant findings which will fuel the growth of the discipline. They may even be implemented as practical applications or may be referred to as a beginning point for another development.

The contributors of this book come from diverse backgrounds, making this book a truly international effort. This book will bring forth new frontiers with its revolutionizing research information and detailed analysis of the nascent developments around the world.

We would like to thank all the contributing authors for lending their expertise to make the book truly unique. They have played a crucial role in the development of this book. Without their invaluable contributions this book wouldn't have been possible. They have made vital efforts to compile up to date information on the varied aspects of this subject to make this book a valuable addition to the collection of many professionals and students.

This book was conceptualized with the vision of imparting up-to-date information and advanced data in this field. To ensure the same, a matchless editorial board was set up. Every individual on the board went through rigorous rounds of assessment to prove their worth. After which they invested a large part of their time researching and compiling the most relevant data for our readers.

The editorial board has been involved in producing this book since its inception. They have spent rigorous hours researching and exploring the diverse topics which have resulted in the successful publishing of this book. They have passed on their knowledge of decades through this book. To expedite this challenging task, the publisher supported the team at every step. A small team of assistant editors was also appointed to further simplify the editing procedure and attain best results for the readers.

Apart from the editorial board, the designing team has also invested a significant amount of their time in understanding the subject and creating the most relevant covers. They scrutinized every image to scout for the most suitable representation of the subject and create an appropriate cover for the book.

The publishing team has been an ardent support to the editorial, designing and production team. Their endless efforts to recruit the best for this project, has resulted in the accomplishment of this book. They are a veteran in the field of academics and their pool of knowledge is as vast as their experience in printing. Their expertise and guidance has proved useful at every step. Their uncompromising quality standards have made this book an exceptional effort. Their encouragement from time to time has been an inspiration for everyone.

The publisher and the editorial board hope that this book will prove to be a valuable piece of knowledge for researchers, students, practitioners and scholars across the globe.

List of Contributors

Sonia Morè, Massimo Offidani and Attilio Olivieri
Clinica di Ematologia, Azienda Ospedaliero-UniversitariaOspedali Riuniti di Ancona, 60126 Ancona, Italy

Maria Teresa Petrucci and Francesca Fazio
Sezione di Ematologia, Dipartimento di Medicina Traslazionale e di Precisione, Azienda Ospedaliera Policlinico Umberto I, Università "Sapienza" di Roma, 00161 Roma, Italy

Laura Corvatta
UOC Medicina, Ospedale Profili Fabriano, 6004 Fabriano, Italy

Annina Lyly
Inflammation Centre, Skin and Allergy Hospital, Helsinki University Hospital, University of Helsinki, 00029 HUS Helsinki, Finland
Department of Otorhinolaryngology—Head and Neck Surgery, Helsinki University Hospital, University of Helsinki, 00029 HUS Helsinki, Finland

Anu Laulajainen-Hongisto
Department of Otorhinolaryngology—Head and Neck Surgery, Helsinki University Hospital, University of Helsinki, 00029 HUS Helsinki, Finland

Philippe Gevaert
Department of Otorhinolaryngology, Upper Airway Research Laboratory, Ghent University Hospital, 9000 Ghent, Belgium

Paula Kauppi
Heart and Lung Center, Pulmonary Department, University of Helsinki and Helsinki University Hospital, 00029 HUS Helsinki, Finland

Sanna Toppila-Salmi
Inflammation Centre, Skin and Allergy Hospital, Helsinki University Hospital, University of Helsinki, 00029 HUS Helsinki, Finland
Medicum, Haartman Institute, University of Helsinki, 00029 HUS Helsinki, Finland

Shun Xin Wang-Lin and Joseph P. Balthasar
Department of Pharmaceutical Sciences, University at Buffalo, State University of New York, Buffalo, NY 14214, USA

Donmienne Leung
Biotechnology Discovery Research, Lilly Research Laboratories, Lilly Biotechnology Center, Eli Lilly and Company, San Diego, CA 92121, USA

Jacqueline M. Wurst, Tao Liu and Ruben M. Martinez
Discovery Chemistry and Research Technology, Lilly Research Laboratories, Lilly Biotechnology Center, Eli Lilly and Company, San Diego, CA 92121, USA

Amita Datta-Mannan
Exploratory Medicine & Pharmacology, Lilly Research Laboratories, Lilly Corporate Center, Eli Lilly and Company, Indianapolis, IN 46225, USA

Yiqing Feng
Biotechnology Discovery Research, Lilly Research Laboratories, Lilly Technology Center North, Eli Lilly and Company, Indianapolis, IN 46221, USA

Steffen Zobel-Roos, Mourad Mouellef and Jochen Strube
Institute for Separation and Process Technology, Clausthal University of Technology, Leibnizstr. 15, 38678 Clausthal-Zellerfeld, Germany

Christian Siemers
Institute for Process Control, Clausthal University of Technology, Arnold-Sommerfeld-Straße 1, 38678 Clausthal-Zellerfeld, Germany

Ashley R. Sutherland and Madeline N. Owens
Department of Biochemistry, Microbiology and Immunology, University of Saskatchewan, Saskatoon, SK S7N 5E5, Canada

C. Ronald Geyer
Department of Pathology and LaboratoryMedicine, University of Saskatchewan, Saskatoon, SK S7N 5E5, Canada

Leticia Barboza Rocha, Bruna Alves Caetano, Thais Mitsunari, Juliana Moutinho Polatto, Daniela Luz and Roxane Maria Fontes Piazza
Laboratório de Bacteriologia, Instituto Butantan, São Paulo, 05503-900 SP, Brazil

Ricardo Palacios and Alexander Roberto Precioso
Divisão de Ensaios Clínicos e Farmacovigilância, Instituto Butantan, São Paulo, 05503-900 SP, Brazil

Luís Carlos de Souza Ferreira, Lennon Ramos Pereira, Jaime Henrique Amorim, Rubens Prince dos Santos Alves
Laboratório de Desenvolvimento de Vacinas, Instituto de Ciências Biomédicas, Universidade de São Paulo, São Paulo, 05508-000 SP, Brazil

Viviane Fongaro Botosso
Laboratório de Virologia, Instituto Butantan, São Paulo, 05503-900 SP, Brazil

Neuza Maria Frazatti Gallina
Divisão de Desenvolvimento Tecnológico e Produção; Instituto Butantan, São Paulo, 05503-900 SP, Brazil

Steffen Zobel-Roos and Jochen Strube
Institute for Separation and Process Technology, Clausthal University of Technology, Leibnizstr. 15, 38678 Clausthal-Zellerfeld, Germany

Celso Francisco Hernandes Granato
Departamento de Medicina, Disciplina de Doenças Infecciosas e Parasitárias, Universidade Federal de São Paulo, São Paulo, 04023-062 SP, Brazil

Danielle Bruna Leal Oliveira and Vanessa Barbosa da Silveira
Laboratório de Virologia Molecular e Clínica, Departamento de Microbiologia, Instituto de Ciências Biomédicas, Universidade de São Paulo, São Paulo, 05508-000 SP, Brazil

Vaneet K. Sharma, Sreenivas Avula and Antu K. Dey
IAVI, 125 Broad Street, New York, NY 10004, USA

Bijay Misra, Kaliappanadar Nellaiappan and Indu Javeri
CuriRx, Inc., 205 Lowell Street, Wilmington, MA 01887, USA

Kevin T. McManus and Michael S. Seaman
Center for Virology and Vaccine Research, Beth Israel Deaconess Medical Center, Boston, MA 02215, USA

Michel C. Nussenzweig
Laboratory of Molecular Immunology, The Rockefeller University, New York, NY 10065, USA
Howard Hughes Medical Institute, The Rockefeller University, New York, NY 10065, USA

Juliet Rashidian, Raul Copaciu, Qin Su, Brett Merritt, Claire Johnson, Aril Yahyabeik, Ella French and Kelsea Cummings
MilliporeSigma, 6600 Sierra College Blvd, Rocklin, CA 95677, USA

Roberta Gentile, Stefano Iacobelli and Giulia Di Vittorio
MediaPharma SrL, I-66013 Chieti, Italy

Souad Boune, Peisheng Hu, Alan L. Epstein and Leslie A. Khawli
Department of Pathology, Keck School of Medicine, University of Southern California, Los Angeles, CA 90089, USA

Marina Caskey and Jill Horowitz
Laboratory of Molecular Immunology, The Rockefeller University, New York, NY 10065, USA

André L. B. Bitencourt, Raquel M. Campos and Adriano Sebollela
Department of Biochemistry and Immunology, Ribeirao Preto Medical School, University of São Paulo, Ribeirão Preto, SP 14049-900, Brazil

Erika N. Cline and William L. Klein
Department of Neurobiology, Northwestern University, Evanston, IL 60208-3520, USA

Martin Kornecki and Fabian Mestmäcker
Institute for Separation and Process Technology, Clausthal University of Technology, Leibnizstr. 15, 38678 Clausthal-Zellerfeld, Germany

Laura Heikaus de Figueiredo and Hartmut Schlüter
Institute of Clinical Chemistry, Department for Mass Spectrometric Proteomics, University Medical Center Hamburg-Eppendorf, Martinistr. 52, 20246 Hamburg, Germany

Sara Ponziani, Giuseppina Pitari, Anna Maria Cimini, Matteo Ardini, Rodolfo Ippoliti and Francesco Giansanti
Department of Life, Health and Environmental Sciences, University of L'Aquila, I-67100 L'Aquila, Italy

Emily Capone
Department of Medical, Oral and Biotechnological Sciences, University of Chieti-Pescara, I-66100 Chieti, Italy

Gianluca Sala
MediaPharma SrL, I-66013 Chieti, Italy
Department of Medical, Oral and Biotechnological Sciences, University of Chieti-Pescara, I-66100 Chieti, Italy

David J. Flavell
The Simon Flavell Leukaemia Research Laboratory, Southampton General Hospital, Southampton SO16 6YD, UK

Index

Printed in the USA
CPSIA information can be obtained
at www.ICGtesting.com
JSHW051408091023
49903JS00006B/337

9 781639 277353